# Haemoglobinopathy Diagnosis

This book is dedicated to the past and present scientific staff of the Haematology Departments of the Princess Alexandra Hospital, Brisbane, Australia and St Mary's Hospital, Paddington, London, without whom it would not have been possible.

# Haemoglobinopathy Diagnosis

Barbara J. Bain MBBS FRACP FRCPath

*Professor of Diagnostic Haematology*
*St Mary's Hospital Campus of Imperial College*
*Faculty of Medicine, London*
*and Honorary Consultant Haematologist*
*St Mary's Hospital, London*

**Second Edition**

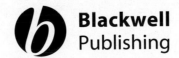

**Blackwell**
Publishing

© 2006 Barbara J. Bain
Published by Blackwell Publishing Ltd
Blackwell Publishing, Inc., 350 Main Street, Malden,
   Massachusetts 02148-5020, USA
Blackwell Publishing Ltd, 9600 Garsington Road, Oxford
   OX4 2DQ, UK
Blackwell Publishing Asia Pty Ltd, 550 Swanston Street,
   Carlton, Victoria 3053, Australia

First published 2001
Reprinted 2003
Second edition 2006

Library of Congress Cataloging-in-Publication Data

Bain, Barbara J.
   Haemoglobinopathy diagnosis / Barbara J. Bain.—2nd ed.
      p.   ;   cm.
   Includes bibliographical references and index.
   ISBN-10: 1-4051-3516-6
   ISBN-13: 978-1-4051-3516-0
   1. Hemoglobinopathy—Diagnosis.
   [DNLM:   1.  Hemoglobinopathies—diagnosis.   2.
Hematologic Tests—methods.   WH 190 B162h 2006]
I. Title.

   RC641.7.H35B73 2006
   616.1'51075

                              2005015281

ISBN-13: 9-7814-0513-516-0
ISBN-10: 1-4051-3516-6

A catalogue record for this title is available from the British
Library

Set in 9/12 Palatino by SNP Best-set Typesetter Ltd.,
   Hong Kong
Printed and bound in India by Replika Press Pvt., Ltd

Commissioning Editor: Maria Khan
Development Editor: Helen Harvey
Production Controller: Kate Charman

For further information on Blackwell Publishing, visit our
website:
http://www.blackwellpublishing.com

The publisher's policy is to use permanent paper from
mills that operate a sustainable forestry policy, and which
has been manufactured from pulp processed using acid-
free and elementary chlorine-free practices. Furthermore,
the publisher ensures that the text paper and cover board
used have met acceptable environmental accreditation
standards.

# Contents

# Preface to the first edition

It is now 6 years since colleagues at the Princess Alexandra Hospital, Brisbane, suggested that there was a need for a practical book on the laboratory diagnosis of haemoglobinopathies and that perhaps I might consider writing it. As the subject was one of considerable interest to me, I was happy to accept their suggestion. The book has been some time in the writing but here it is. I hope that it meets their expectations.

I am grateful to those with whom I have worked in this field of haematology. For over 25 years they have shared my pleasure in solving diagnostic problems and, at the same time, have joined in my efforts to provide an accurate, clinically relevant diagnostic service. It is to them that the book is dedicated.

I should like to thank particularly Ms Lorraine Phelan and Dr David Rees who have read the entire manuscript and have made many helpful suggestions. I am also grateful to the many colleagues who have contributed invaluable illustrations. They are individually acknowledged in the figure legends.

Barbara J. Bain
*London, 2000*

# Abbreviations and glossary

α the Greek letter, alpha

**α chain** the α globin chain which is required for the synthesis of haemoglobins A, F and A$_2$ and also the embryonic haemoglobin, Gower 2

**α gene** one of a pair of genes on chromosome 16 that encode α globin

**α thalassaemia** a group of thalassaemias characterized by absent or reduced α globin chain transcription, usually resulting from the deletion of one or more of the α globin genes; less often it results from the altered structure of an α gene or the mutation of locus control genes or genes encoding *trans*-acting factors

**α$^0$ thalassaemia** a thalassaemic condition in which there is no α globin chain translation from one or both copies of chromosome 16

**α$^+$ thalassaemia** a thalassaemic condition in which there is reduced translation of α chain from one or both copies of chromosome 16

β the Greek letter, beta

**β chain** the β globin chain which forms part of haemoglobin A and haemoglobin Portland 2 and is the only globin chain in the abnormal haemoglobin, haemoglobin H

**β gene** the gene on chromosome 11 that encodes β globin

**β thalassaemia** a thalassaemia characterized by reduced β globin synthesis, usually caused by the mutation of a β globin gene; less often it results from gene deletion or from deletion or mutation of the locus control region

γ the Greek letter, gamma

**γ chain** the γ globin chain which forms part of fetal haemoglobin (haemoglobin F) and the embryonic haemoglobin, haemoglobin Portland 1, and is the only globin chain in the abnormal variant, haemoglobin Bart's

**γ gene** one of a pair of very similar genes on chromosome 11 encoding γ globin chain

**γ thalassaemia** a thalassaemic condition resulting from reduced synthesis of γ globin chain

δ the Greek letter, delta

**δ chain** a β-like globin chain, which forms part of haemoglobin A$_2$

**δ gene** a gene of the β cluster on chromosome 11 that encodes δ globin

**δ thalassaemia** a thalassaemic condition resulting from reduced synthesis of δ globin chain and therefore of haemoglobin A$_2$

ε the Greek letter, epsilon

**ε chain** the ε globin chain which is synthesized during early embryonic life and forms part of haemoglobins Gower 1 and Gower 2

**ε gene** a gene of the α globin cluster on chromosome 16 that encodes ε globin chain

ζ the Greek letter, zeta

**ζ chain** the ζ globin chain which is synthesized in intrauterine life and forms part of haemoglobins Gower 1, Portland 1 and Portland 2

**ζ gene** a gene of the α globin gene cluster on chromosome 16 that encodes ζ globin chain

**ψ** the Greek letter, psi, used to indicate a pseudogene

**2,3-DPG** 2,3-diphosphoglycerate; a small molecule that interacts with haemoglobin, decreasing its oxygen affinity

**3′** the end of a gene where transcription ceases

**5′** the end of a gene where transcription starts

**acquired** a condition that is not present at birth or is not inherited

**affinity** the avidity of haemoglobin for oxygen

**ala** δ-aminolaevulinic acid; the first compound formed during the process of haem synthesis

**AML** acute myeloid leukaemia

**ARMS** amplification refractory mutation system; a PCR technique used, for example, for the detection of mutations causing β thalassaemia; it employs two primer sets, one amplifying normal sequences and one abnormal sequences

**balanced polymorphism** the stable persistence of two or more alleles of a gene in a significant proportion of a population; a potentially deleterious allele may show balanced polymorphism if the heterozygous state conveys an advantage

**base** a ring-shaped organic molecule containing nitrogen which is a constituent of DNA and RNA; DNA contains four bases — adenine, guanine, cytosine and thymine; RNA contains four bases — adenine, guanine, cytosine and uracil

**Bohr effect** the effect of pH on oxygen affinity; the alkaline Bohr effect is the reduction of oxygen affinity of haemoglobin as the pH falls from above to below the physiological pH; there is also an acid Bohr effect which is a rise of oxygen affinity as the pH falls further, to a pH level that is incompatible with life

**bp** base pair; the pairing of specific bases, e.g. adenine with thymine, in the complementary strands of the DNA double helix

**CAP** 7-methylguanosine cap

**carbonic anhydrase** a red cell enzyme that is the second most abundant red cell protein after haemoglobin; it may be apparent on haemoglobin electrophoretic strips if a protein rather than a haem stain is used

**carboxyhaemoglobin** haemoglobin that has been chemically altered by combination with carbon monoxide

**CE-HPLC** cation-exchange high performance liquid chromatography

**chromatography** a method of separating proteins from each other by means of physical characteristics, such as molecular weight, charge or hydrophobicity, or by means of differing affinity for lectins, antibodies or other proteins; in column chromatography, the proteins move through an absorbent column and emerge after different periods of time

*cis* on the same chromosome (see also *trans*)

*cis*-acting a DNA sequence that affects the expression of a gene on the same chromosome but not on the homologous chromosome (see also *trans-acting*)

**CO** carbon monoxide, the molecule composed of one carbon atom and one oxygen atom, formed by combustion of hydrocarbons

**$CO_2$** carbon dioxide, the molecule composed of one atom of carbon combined with two of oxygen

**codon** a triplet of nucleotides that encodes a specific amino acid or serves as a termination signal; there are 61 codons encoding 20 amino acids and three codons that act as termination or stop codons

**congenital** present at birth, often but not necessarily inherited

**cooperativity** the interaction between the four globin monomers that makes possible the Bohr effect and the sigmoid shape of the oxygen dissociation curve

**CT** computed tomography

**CV** coefficient of variation

**DCIP** 2,6-dichlorophenolindophenol

**deletion** loss of part of a chromosome, which may include all or part of a globin gene

**deoxyhaemoglobin** haemoglobin that is not combined with $O_2$

**DGGE** denaturing gradient gel electrophoresis; a molecular genetic technique for locating a mutation prior to precise analysis

**DNA** deoxyribonucleic acid; the major constituent of the nucleus of a cell; a polynucleotide strand that is able to replicate and that codes for the majority of proteins synthesized by the cell; the DNA molecule is a double helix of two complementary intertwined polynucleotides

**EDTA** ethylene diamine tetra-acetic acid

**EKLF** erythroid Kruppel-like factor

**electrophoresis** separation of charged suspended particles, such as proteins, by application to a membrane followed by exposure to a charge gradient, e.g. haemoglobin electrophoresis

**ELISA** enzyme-linked immunosorbent assay

**elution** removal of an absorbed substance from a chromatography column

**enhancer** a DNA sequence that influences the promoter of a nearby gene to increase transcription; an enhancer acts on a gene in *cis* and may be sited upstream, downstream or within a gene

**exon** a part of a gene that is represented in mature mRNA; most genes are composed of exons and non-translated introns

**FAB classification** French–American–British classification

**FBC** full blood count

**Fe** iron

**$Fe^{2+}$** ferrous or bivalent iron

**$Fe^{3+}$** ferric or trivalent iron

**fetal haemoglobin** haemoglobin F, the major haemoglobin present during intrauterine life, having two α chains and two γ chains

**GAP-PCR** a PCR technique in which there is amplification across a 'gap' created by deletion

**GATA 1** an erythroid-specific transcription factor

**gene** the segment of DNA that is involved in producing a polypeptide chain; it includes regions preceding and following the coding region (5' and 3' untranslated regions) as well as intervening sequences (introns) between individual coding segments (exons); genes mediate inheritance; they are located on nuclear chromosomes or, rarely, in a mitochondrion

**genetic code** the relationship between a triplet of bases, called a codon, and the amino acid that it encodes

**genotype** the genetic constitution of an individual (cf. phenotype)

**globin** the protein part of the haemoglobin molecule, usually composed of two pairs of non-identical chains, e.g. two α chains and two β chains

**H⁺** a proton

**haem** a porphyrin structure that contains iron and that forms part of the haemoglobin molecule

**haemoglobin** a complex molecule composed of four globin chains, each one enclosing a haem group

**haemoglobin A** the major haemoglobin component present in most adults, having two α and two β chains

**haemoglobin A₁c** glycosylated haemoglobin A

**haemoglobin A₂** a minor haemoglobin component present in most adults, and as an even lower proportion of total haemoglobin in neonates and infants, having two α chains and two δ chains

**haemoglobin Bart's** an abnormal haemoglobin with four γ chains and no α chains, present as the major haemoglobin component in haemoglobin Bart's hydrops fetalis and as a minor component in neonates with haemoglobin H disease or α thalassaemia trait

**haemoglobin Bart's hydrops fetalis** a fatal condition of a fetus or neonate with no α genes and, consequently, no production of haemoglobins A, A₂ or F

**haemoglobin C** a variant haemoglobin with an amino acid substitution in the β chain, mainly found in those of African ancestry

**haemoglobin Constant Spring** a variant haemoglobin with a structurally abnormal α chain which is synthesized at a reduced rate, leading to α thalassaemia

**haemoglobin D** the designation of a group of haemoglobin variants, some α chain variants and some β chain variants, that have the same mobility as haemoglobin S on electrophoresis at alkaline pH

**haemoglobin dissociation curve** a plot of the percentage saturation of haemoglobin against the partial pressure of oxygen

**haemoglobin E** a variant haemoglobin with an amino acid substitution in the β chain, mainly found in South-East Asia and parts of the Indian subcontinent

**haemoglobin F** fetal haemoglobin, the major haemoglobin of the fetus and neonate, which is present as a very minor component in most adults and as a larger proportion in a minority

**haemoglobin G** the designation of a group of haemoglobin variants, some α chain variants and some β chain variants, that have the same mobility as haemoglobin S on electrophoresis at alkaline pH

**haemoglobin Gower 1** an embryonic haemoglobin, having two ε chains and two ζ chains

**haemoglobin Gower 2** an embryonic haemoglobin, having two α chains and two ε chains

**haemoglobin H** a variant haemoglobin with four β chains and no α chains, present in haemoglobin H disease and, in small quantities, in α thalassaemia trait

**haemoglobin H disease** a haemoglobinopathy caused by marked underproduction of α chains, often consequent on deletion of three of the four α genes

**haemoglobin I** a group of variant haemoglobins that move more rapidly than haemoglobin A on electrophoresis at alkaline pH

**haemoglobin J** a group of variant haemoglobins that move more rapidly than haemoglobin A, but more slowly than haemoglobin I, on electrophoresis at alkaline pH

**haemoglobin K** a group of variant haemoglobins moving between haemoglobins A and J on electrophoresis at alkaline pH

**haemoglobin Lepore** a number of variant haemoglobins resulting from the fusion of part of a δ globin gene with part of a β globin gene, giving a δβ fusion gene and fusion protein that combines with α globin to form haemoglobin Lepore

**haemoglobin M** a variant haemoglobin that oxidizes readily to methaemoglobin

**haemoglobin N** a group of variant haemoglobins moving between haemoglobins J and I on electrophoresis at alkaline pH

**haemoglobin O-Arab** a β chain variant haemoglobin moving near haemoglobin C at alkaline pH and near haemoglobin S at acid pH

**haemoglobinopathy** an inherited disorder resulting from the synthesis of a structurally abnormal haemoglobin; the term can also be used to encompass the thalassaemias in which there is a reduced rate of synthesis of one of the globin chains

**haemoglobin Portland 1** an embryonic haemoglobin, having two ζ chains and two γ chains

**haemoglobin Portland 2** an embryonic haemoglobin, having two ζ chains and two β chains

**haemoglobin S** sickle cell haemoglobin, a variant haemoglobin with a tendency to polymerize at low oxygen tension, causing erythrocytes to deform into the shape of a sickle

**Hct** haematocrit

**HDW** haemoglobin distribution width

**heteroduplex analysis** a molecular genetic technique for locating a mutation prior to precise analysis

**heterozygosity** the state of having two different alleles of a specified autosomal gene (or, in a female, two different alleles of an X chromosomal gene)

**heterozygous** having two different alleles of a specified autosomal or X chromosome gene

**HIV** human immunodeficiency virus

**homologous** being equivalent or similar to another

**homologue** an equivalent or similar structure; the α1 and α2 genes are homologues, as are the two copies of a chromosome

**homology** the presence of structural similarity, implying a common remote origin; the δ and β genes show partial homology

**homozygosity** the state of having two identical alleles of a specified autosomal gene

**homozygous** having two identical alleles of a specified autosomal gene (or, in a female, two identical alleles of an X chromosome gene)

**HPLC** high performance liquid chromatography; a method of separating proteins, such as haemoglobin variants, from each other on the basis of characteristics such as size, hydrophobicity and ionic strength; a solution of proteins is eluted from a specially designed column by exposure to various buffers, different proteins emerging after varying periods of time

**HS1, HS2, HS3, HS4** hypersensitive sites 1, 2, 3 and 4

**HS –40** an upstream enhancer of α globin gene transcription

**HVR** hypervariable region

**IEF** isoelectric focusing; the separation of proteins in an electric field as they move through a pH gradient to their isoelectric points

**inherited** a characteristic that is transmitted from a parent by means of genes that form part of nuclear or mitochondrial DNA

**initiation** (i) the process by which RNA transcription from a gene commences; (ii) the process by which protein translation from mRNA commences

**initiation codon** the three nucleotide codon (ATG) at the 5′ end of a gene which is essential to permit initiation of transcription of a gene, i.e. initiation of polypeptide synthesis

**insertion** the insertion of a DNA sequence, e.g. from one chromosome into another

**intron** a sequence of DNA in a gene which is not represented in processed mRNA or in the protein product

**inversion** the reversal of the normal position of a DNA sequence on a chromosome

**isoelectric point** the pH at which a protein has no net charge

**IVS** intervening sequence; an intron

**kb** kilobase; a unit for measuring the length of DNA; one kilobase is 1000 nucleotide base pairs

**kDa** kilodalton; a unit for measuring molecular weight; one kilodalton is 1000 daltons

**LCR** locus control region; a DNA sequence upstream of genes of the β globin cluster that enhances transcription of the genes of this cluster

**LDH** lactate dehydrogenase

**MCH** mean cell haemoglobin

**MCHC** mean cell haemoglobin concentration

**MCV** mean cell volume

**methaemoglobin** oxidized haemoglobin which does not function in oxygen transport

**mis-sense mutation** a mutation that leads to the encoding of a different amino acid

**mRNA** messenger ribonucleic acid; ribonucleic acid that is transcribed in the nucleus, on a DNA template, and moves to the cytoplasm, becoming attached to ribosomes and serving as a template for the synthesis of proteins

**NO** nitric oxide

**nonsense mutation** a mutation that leads to no amino acid being encoded and therefore functions as a stop or termination codon, leading to the synthesis of a truncated polypeptide chain

**NRBC** nucleated red blood cell

$O_2$ oxygen

**ORF** open reading frame

**oxyhaemoglobin** haemoglobin combined with $O_2$

$P_{50}$ $Po_2$ at which haemoglobin is 50% saturated

$Pao_2$ partial pressure of oxygen in arterial blood

**partial pressure of oxygen** that part of the total blood gas pressure exerted by oxygen

**PAS** periodic acid–Schiff

**PCR** polymerase chain reaction; a method of making multiple copies of a DNA sequence

**PCV** packed cell volume

**phenocopy** a condition that simulates an inherited condition; a phenocopy may be acquired or may be a genetic characteristic that simulates another

**phenotype** the characteristics of an individual, which may be determined by the genotype, or may be an acquired characteristic (cf. genotype)

$Po_2$ partial pressure of oxygen

**polymorphism** the occurrence of a variant form of a gene in a significant proportion of a population

**promoter** a sequence of DNA at the 5′ end of a gene which is essential for initiation of transcription

**pseudogene** a non-functioning homologue of a gene

**purine** one of the two types of nitrogenous base found in nucleic acids; purines have a double ring structure (see also **pyrimidine**)

**pyrimidine** one of the two types of nitrogenous base found in nucleic acids; pyrimidines have a single ring structure (see also **purine**)

**RBC** red blood cell count

**RDW** red cell distribution width

**restriction endonuclease** an enzyme that recognizes specific sequences in a DNA molecule and cleaves the molecule in or very near the recognition site

**restriction fragment** a fragment of DNA produced by cleavage by a restriction endonuclease

**RFLP** restriction fragment length polymorphism; variation between homologous chromosomes with regard to the length of DNA fragments produced by application of a specific restriction endonuclease; can be used for the demonstration of heterozygosity or for the demonstration of a specific gene that removes or creates a specific cleavage site

**ribosome** a cytoplasmic structure on which proteins are translated from mRNA; ribosomes may be free within the cytosol or form part of the rough endoplasmic reticulum

**RNA** ribonucleic acid; a polynucleotide in which the nitrogenous bases are adenine, guanine, cytosine and uracil and the sugar is ribose; RNA is produced in the nucleus and in mitochondria from DNA templates

**rRNA** ribosomal RNA; RNA that, together with protein, constitutes the ribosomes

**sickle cell** an erythrocyte that becomes sickle- or crescent-shaped as a result of polymerization of haemoglobin S

**sickle cell anaemia** the disease resulting from homozygosity for haemoglobin S

**sickle cell disease** a group of diseases including sickle cell anaemia and various compound heterozygous states in which clinicopathological effects occur as a result of sickle cell formation

**sickle cell trait** heterozygosity for the $\beta^s$ gene that encodes the β chain of haemoglobin S

**SOP** standard operating procedure

**splicing** the process by which RNA sequences, corresponding to introns in the gene, are removed during processing of RNA

**SSP** stage selector protein

**sulphaemoglobin** haemoglobin that has been irreversibly oxidized and chemically altered by drugs or chemicals with incorporation of a sulphur atom into the haemoglobin molecule

**thalassaemia** a disorder, usually inherited, in which one or more of the globin chains incorporated into a haemoglobin molecule or molecules is synthesized at a reduced rate

**thalassaemia intermedia** a thalassaemic condition that is moderately severe, but nevertheless does not require regular blood transfusions to sustain life

**thalassaemia major** thalassaemia that is incompatible with more than a short survival in the absence of blood transfusion

**thalassaemia minor** an asymptomatic thalassaemic condition

**trait** a term applied to heterozygosity for an inherited characteristic; in the case of disorders of globin genes, the term would not be used if heterozygosity were associated with a significant phenotypic abnormality; rather it is used when homozygosity or compound heterozygosity produces a clinically significant abnormality but simple heterozygosity does not

*trans* having an influence on a DNA sequence on another chromosome (see also *cis*)

*trans*-acting a DNA sequence that affects the expression of a gene on another chromosome (see also *cis*-acting)

**transcript** an RNA molecule, corresponding to one gene, transcribed from nuclear DNA

**transcription** the synthesis of RNA on a DNA template

**transcription factor** a protein capable of enhancing transcription of one or more genes

**translation** the synthesis of protein from an mRNA template

**tRNA** transfer RNA; RNA molecules that bind to specific amino acids and transport them to ribosomes; there they bind to specific mRNA sequences, leading to incorporation of amino acids into peptide chains in the sequence specified by the mRNA

**unstable** a term applied to a haemoglobin that is abnormally prone to post-translational structural alteration, which may include loss of the normal tertiary or quaternary structure

**UTR** untranslated region

**variant** a term applied to any haemoglobin other than haemoglobins A, $A_2$, F and the normal embryonal haemoglobins

**WBC** white blood cell count

**yolk sac** part of an embryo; the initial site of formation of blood cells

# 1 Haemoglobin and the genetics of haemoglobin synthesis

## Haemoglobins and their structure and function

The haemoglobin molecule contained within red blood cells is essential for human life, being the means by which oxygen is transported to the tissues. Other functions include the transport of carbon dioxide ($CO_2$) and a buffering action (reduction of the changes in pH that would otherwise be expected when an acid or an alkali enters or is generated in a red cell). A normal haemoglobin molecule is composed of two dissimilar pairs of polypeptide chains, each of which encloses an iron-containing porphyrin designated haem (Fig. 1.1). Haemoglobin has a molecular weight of 64–64.5 kDa. Haem is essential for oxygen transport while globin serves to protect haem from oxidation, renders the molecule soluble and permits variation in oxygen affinity. The structure of the haemoglobin molecule produces an internal environment of hydrophobic radicals which protects the iron of haem from water and thus from oxidation. External radicals are hydrophilic and thus render the haemoglobin molecule soluble. Both haem and globin are subject to modification. The iron of haemoglobin is normally in the ferrous form ($Fe^{2+}$). Haem is able to combine reversibly with oxygen so that haemoglobin can function as an oxygen-transporting protein. Oxidation of iron to the ferric form ($Fe^{3+}$) is a less reversible reaction, converting haem to haematin and haemoglobin to methaemoglobin, a form of haemoglobin that cannot transport oxygen.

The haemoglobin molecule can also combine with $CO_2$, being responsible for about 10% of the transport of $CO_2$ from the tissues to the lungs; transport is by reversible carbamation of the N-terminal groups of the α chains of haemoglobin. Carbamated haemoglobin has a lower oxygen affinity than the non-carbamated form, so that binding of the $CO_2$ produced by the metabolic processes in tissues facilitates oxygen delivery to tissues. In addition, non-oxygenated haemoglobin can carry more $CO_2$ than oxygenated haemoglobin, so that unloading of oxygen to the tissues facilities the uptake and transport of $CO_2$. Because of its buffering action (mopping up of protons, $H^+$), haemoglobin also contributes to keeping $CO_2$ in the soluble bicarbonate form and thus transportable. The reaction $CO_2 + H_2O \rightarrow HCO_3^- + H^+$ is facilitated.

The haemoglobin molecule has a role in nitric oxide (NO) transport and metabolism. Haemoglobin is both a scavenger and an active transporter of NO. NO is produced in endothelial cells and neutrophils by the action of nitric acid synthase [1–3]. NO has a very high affinity for oxyhaemoglobin, so that blood levels are a balance between production and removal by binding to oxyhaemoglobin. NO is a potent vasodilator, this effect being limited by its binding to haemoglobin. The iron atom of a haem group of oxyhaemoglobin (preferentially the haem enclosed in the haem pocket of an α chain) binds NO. A haemoglobin molecule with NO bound to two haem groups strikingly favours the deoxy conformation, so that oxygen is readily released. NO-haemoglobin is subsequently converted to methaemoglobin with release of NO and the production of nitrate ions, which are excreted. As deoxyhaemoglobin has a much lower affinity for NO, hypoxic conditions may leave more NO free and lead to vasodilation of potential physiological benefit.

NO also causes S-nitrosylation of a conserved cysteine residue ($Cys^{93}$, E15) of the β globin chain of oxyhaemoglobin to form S-nitrosohaemoglobin. This occurs in the lungs. In this circumstance, the bioactivity of NO may be retained, with NO being delivered to low molecular weight thiol-containing molecules to reach target cells, such as the smooth muscle of blood vessels. Oxygenation of haemoglobin favours S-nitrosylation. Conversely, deoxygenation favours

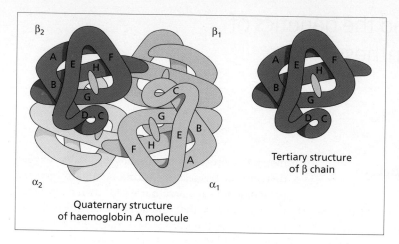

**Fig. 1.1** Diagrammatic representation of the tertiary structure of a haemoglobin monomer (a β globin chain containing a haem group) and the quaternary structure of haemoglobin; upper case letters indicate homologous α helixes.

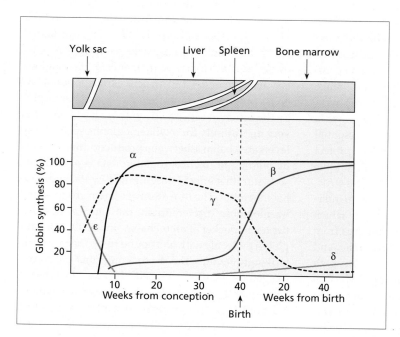

**Fig. 1.2** Diagrammatic representation of the sites and rates of synthesis of different globin chains *in utero* and during infancy.

the release of NO. This may be an important physiological process, with NO being released in peripheral tissues where it can facilitate arteriolar dilation. The oxy form of S-nitrosohaemoglobin is a vasoconstrictor, whereas the deoxy form is a vasodilator. Lack of oxygen could thus again favour vasodilation.

In normal circumstances, the ability of haemoglobin to scavenge or destroy NO is reduced by the barrier to NO diffusion provided by the red cell membrane; however, in chronic haemolytic anaemia, increased free plasma haemoglobin may lead to impaired vascular responses to NO [3]; inactivation of NO by haemoglobin in the plasma may contribute to the pulmonary hypertension that can be a feature of sickle cell anaemia, and also the hypertension that has been observed with some haemoglobin-based blood substitutes.

As a result of the synthesis of different globin chains at different stages of life (Fig. 1.2), there is a difference in the type of haemoglobin present in red

**Table 1.1** Haemoglobins normally present during adult, fetal and embryonic periods of life.

| Haemoglobin species | Globin chains | Period when normally present |
| --- | --- | --- |
| A | $\alpha_2\beta_2$* | Major haemoglobin in adult life |
| A$_2$ | $\alpha_2\delta_2$ | Minor haemoglobin in adult life; even more minor in fetal and neonatal life |
| F | $\alpha_2{}^G\gamma_2$ or $\alpha_2{}^A\gamma_2$ | Minor haemoglobin in adult life; major haemoglobin in fetal life with a declining percentage through the neonatal period |
| Gower 1 | $\zeta_2\varepsilon_2$ | Significant haemoglobin during early intrauterine life |
| Gower 2 | $\alpha_2\varepsilon_2$ | Significant haemoglobin during early intrauterine life |
| Portland or Portland 1† | $\zeta_2\gamma_2$ | Significant haemoglobin during early intrauterine life |

*Can also be designated $\alpha^A{}_2\beta^A{}_2$ to distinguish the globin chains of haemoglobin A from those of variant haemoglobins.
† Haemoglobin Portland 2 ($\zeta_2\beta_2$) has been observed in $\alpha$ thalassaemia syndromes, but is unlikely to occur in significant amounts during normal development.

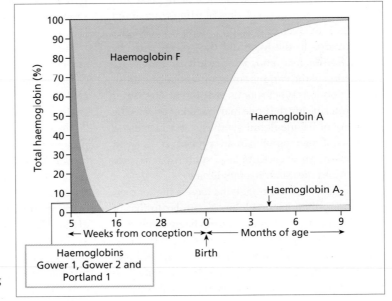

**Fig. 1.3** Diagrammatic representation of the average percentages of various haemoglobins present during the embryonic and fetal periods and during infancy.

cells between adult life and the fetal and neonatal periods (Table 1.1, Fig. 1.3). In adults, 96–98% of haemoglobin is haemoglobin A (A = adult), which has two alpha ($\alpha$) chains and two beta ($\beta$) chains. The name 'haemoglobin A' was given by Linus Pauling and colleagues in 1949 when they discovered that asymptomatic carriers of sickle cell disease had two different haemoglobins, which they designated haemoglobin A and haemoglobin S [4]. A minor haemoglobin, haemoglobin A$_2$, has two $\alpha$ chains and two delta ($\delta$)

chains. Its existence was first reported in 1955 by Kunkel and Wallenius [5]. A very minor haemoglobin in adults, but the major haemoglobin during fetal life and the early neonatal period, is haemoglobin F or fetal haemoglobin, which has two $\alpha$ chains and two gamma ($\gamma$) chains. There are two species of haemoglobin F, designated $^G\gamma$ and $^A\gamma$, with glycine and alanine, respectively, at position 136 of the $\gamma$ chain. In addition, the $^A\gamma$ chain shows polymorphism at position 75, which may be occupied by threonine rather than the more common isoleucine [6], a polymorphism that was previously referred to as haemoglobin F-Sardinia. In the early embryo, haemoglobin is synthesized in the yolk sac and specific embryonic haemoglobins are produced — Gower 1, Gower 2 and Portland (or Portland 1). They contain globin chains that are synthesized in significant amounts only during embryonic life, specifically zeta ($\zeta$) and epsilon ($\varepsilon$) chains (Table 1.1). Haemoglobins Gower 1 ($\zeta_2\varepsilon_2$) and Gower 2 ($\alpha_2\varepsilon_2$) were first described by Huehns and colleagues in 1961 [7], being named for Gower Street, in which University College Hospital is situated. Portland 1 ($\zeta_2\gamma_2$) was described in 1967 and was so named because it was first identified in the University of Oregon in Portland, Oregon [8]. By 5 weeks of gestation, $\zeta$ and $\varepsilon$ chains are already being synthesized in primitive erythroblasts in the yolk sac. From the sixth week onwards, these same cells start to synthesize $\alpha$, $\beta$ and $\gamma$ chains. Starting from about the 10th–12th week of gestation, there is haemoglobin synthesis in the liver and the spleen with the production of fetal and, later, adult haemoglobin. Production of the various embryonic, fetal and adult haemoglobins is synchronous in different sites. Later in intrauterine life the bone marrow takes over as the main site of haemoglobin synthesis and increasing amounts of haemoglobin A are produced. In adult life, bone marrow erythroblasts synthesize haemoglobin A and the minor haemoglobins.

The embryonic haemoglobins have a higher oxygen affinity than haemoglobin A, similar to that of haemoglobin F [9]. They differ from haemoglobins A and F in that they continue to bind oxygen strongly, even in acidotic conditions [9]. In the case of Gower 2, impaired binding to 2,3-diphosphoglycerate (2,3-DPG) is the basis of the increased oxygen affinity [10].

Haemoglobin can undergo post-translational modification (see also Chapter 6). Glycosylation occurs with the formation of haemoglobins $A_{1a-e}$, but principally haemoglobin $A_{1c}$. In normal individuals, haemoglobin $A_{1c}$ may constitute up to 4–6% of total haemoglobin, but in diabetics it can be much higher. In individuals with a shortened red cell life span it is lower. Another minor fraction, formed on ageing, is haemoglobin $A_{III}$, in which glutathione is bound to the cysteine at $\beta93$. Unmodified haemoglobin can be distinguished by use of the designation haemoglobin $A_0$. In the fetus, about 20% of haemo-

globin F shows acetylation of the $\gamma$ chain, but this is not a major feature of other normal human globin chains [6]. Exposure to carbon monoxide, the product of incomplete combustion of hydrocarbons, leads to the formation of carboxyhaemoglobin. In normal individuals, carboxyhaemoglobin comprises 0.2–0.8% of total haemoglobin, but, in heavy smokers, it may be as much as 10–15%. Small amounts of sulphaemoglobin and methaemoglobin are also formed in normal subjects. Methaemoglobin is usually less than 1% of total haemoglobin. Post-synthetic modification of a haemoglobin molecule can also occur as a consequence of a mutation in a globin gene; either the abnormal amino acid or an adjacent normal amino acid can undergo post-translational conversion to another amino acid (see below). In addition, some abnormal haemoglobins, in which there is a mutation of N-terminal amino acids, are particularly prone to acetylation, which occurs cotranslationally [11].

The structure of haemoglobin is highly complex and can be viewed at four levels.

**1** The primary structure is the sequence of the amino acids in the polypeptide which constitutes the globin chain.

**2** The secondary structure is the arrangement of the polypeptide globin chains into $\alpha$ helices separated by non-helical turns; in the case of the $\beta$ globin chain, there are eight $\alpha$ helices, designated A–H, whereas the $\alpha$ globin chain lacks the D helix residues; 70–80% of the amino acid residues of haemoglobin form part of the helices.

**3** The tertiary structure is the arrangement of the coiled globin chain into a three-dimensional structure which has a surface haem-containing pocket between the E and F helices; binding of haem between two specific histidine residues in the E and F helices, respectively (Fig. 1.4), is essential for maintaining the secondary and tertiary structure of haemoglobin.

**4** The quaternary structure is the relationship between the four globin chains, which is not fixed; the strong $\alpha_1\beta_1$ and $\alpha_2\beta_2$ bonds (dimeric bonds) hold the molecule together in a stable form, while the $\alpha_1\beta_2$ and $\alpha_2\beta_1$ bonds (tetrameric bonds) both contribute to stability, albeit to a lesser extent than the dimeric bonds, and permit the chains to slide on each other and rotate; alteration in the quaternary structure of haemoglobin is responsible for the sigmoid oxygen

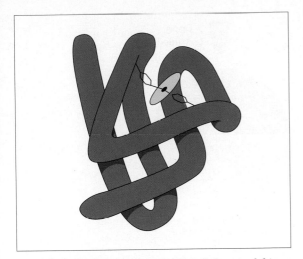

**Fig. 1.4** Diagrammatic representation of a haemoglobin molecule with a haem group within the haem pocket, showing the relationship of haem to two histidine residues of the globin chain (designated proximal and distal histidines).

dissociation curve, the Bohr effect and the variation of oxygen affinity consequent on interaction with 2,3-DPG (see below). Contacts between like chains, $\alpha_1\alpha_2$ and $\beta_1\beta_2$, are also of physiological significance.

The interaction between the four globin chains is such that oxygenation of one haem group alters the shape of the molecule in such a way that oxygenation of other haem groups becomes more likely. This is known as cooperativity and is reflected in the shape of the oxygen dissociation curve (Fig. 1.5). The cooperativity between the globin chains is shown diagrammatically in Fig. 1.6. It is consequent on the fact that, in the deoxygenated state, the $Fe^{2+}$ atom is out of the plane of the porphyrin ring of haem. Oxygenation of $Fe^{2+}$ causes it to move into the plane of the porphyrin ring and, because of the link between haem and the histidine residues of globin, there is an alteration in the tertiary structure of that haemoglobin monomer; this, in turn, causes the oxygenated monomer to alter its position in relation to other

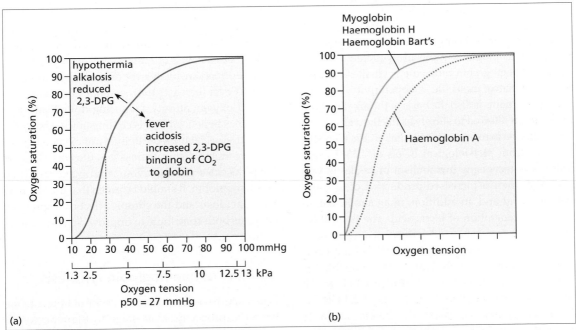

**Fig. 1.5** (a) Normal oxygen dissociation curve indicating the effects of alteration of pH, body temperature and 2,3-diphosphoglycerate (2,3-DPG) concentration on the oxygen affinity of haemoglobin. (b) Comparison of the hyperbolic oxygen dissociation curve characteristic of myoglobin and of abnormal haemoglobins that do not exhibit cooperativity, with the sigmoid dissociation curve characteristic of haemoglobin A; haemoglobins $A_2$ and F have dissociation curves similar to that of haemoglobin A but further to the right.

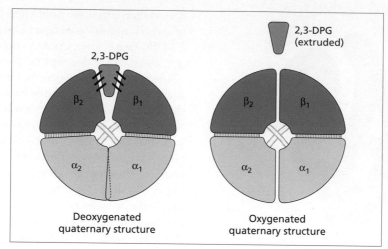

**Fig. 1.6** Diagrammatic representation of the effect of oxygenation and deoxygenation on the quaternary structure of haemoglobin. The haemoglobin dimers ($\alpha_1\beta_1$ and $\alpha_2\beta_2$) are stable, with the dimeric bonds between the $\alpha$ and $\beta$ chains having 34 contacts in both the deoxygenated and oxygenated forms. There are less strong $\alpha_2\beta_1$ and $\alpha_1\beta_2$ tetrameric bonds, with 17 contacts between the $\alpha$ and $\beta$ chains in the deoxy form and a different 17 contacts in the oxy form. There are also $\alpha_1\alpha_2$ bonds with four inter-chain contacts in the deoxy form only. 2,3-diphosphoglycerate (2,3-DPG) binds to the $\beta$ chains (three contacts with each chain) only in the deoxy form of the molecule. Oxygenation is associated with breaking and reforming of tetrameric ($\alpha_2\beta_1$ and $\alpha_1\beta_2$) contacts, breaking of $\alpha_1\alpha_2$ contacts, expulsion of 2,3-DPG and the assumption of a more compact form of the molecule. In the deoxygenated form, the $\alpha$ chains are closer together and there is a cleft between the $\beta$ chains, whereas, in the oxygenated form, the $\alpha$ chains are further apart and the $\beta$ cleft has disappeared.

haemoglobin monomers, i.e. the quaternary structure of the haemoglobin molecule is altered. The oxygenated haemoglobin molecule is smaller than the non-oxygenated molecule. Cooperativity between the globin chains is also the basis of the alkaline Bohr effect (often referred to simply as the Bohr effect), i.e. the reduction in oxygen affinity that occurs when the pH falls from physiological levels of 7.35–7.45 towards 6.0. Increasing metabolism in tissues lowers the pH as there is increased production of $CO_2$ and carbonic acid and, in addition, in anaerobic conditions, the generation of lactic acid. The Bohr effect therefore leads to enhanced delivery of oxygen to tissues, such as exercising muscle. Similarly, the quaternary structure of haemoglobin makes possible the interaction of haemoglobin with 2,3-DPG, which enhances oxygen delivery. Synthesis of 2,3-DPG is increased by hypoxia. Marked anaemia can cause respiratory alkalosis, which enhances 2,3-DPG synthesis, thus compensating to some extent for the anaemia. There is also increased 2,3-DPG synthesis in renal failure, again partly compensating for the anaemia.

Oxygen affinity is reduced not only by acidosis and increased levels of 2,3-DPG, but also by fever. All of these effects are likely to be of physiological significance. Fever increases the metabolic rate, so that decreased oxygen affinity, favouring downloading of oxygen, is beneficial in this circumstance. The lower pH in tissues favours the delivery of oxygen to sites of active metabolism, whereas the efflux of $CO_2$ in the lungs raises the pH and favours the uptake of oxygen by haemoglobin. It should be noted that the acute effect of acidosis and the chronic effect of respiratory alkalosis both contribute to improved oxygen delivery to tissues.

## Genetics of haemoglobin synthesis

Haem synthesis takes place in erythroid precursors, from the proerythroblast stage to the reticulocyte stage. Eight enzymes, under separate genetic control, are known to be necessary for haem synthesis [12]. Different stages of haem synthesis take place either in mitochondria or within the cytosol (Fig. 1.7). The first enzymatic reaction and the last three occur

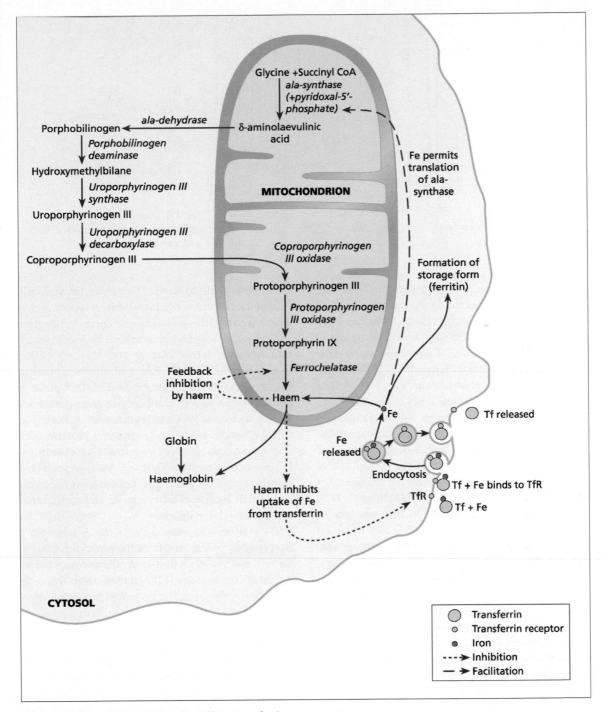

**Fig. 1.7** Diagrammatic representation of haem synthesis.

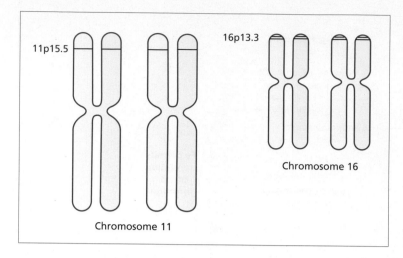

**Fig. 1.8** Diagram of chromosomes 11 and 16 showing the positions of the β and α globin gene clusters.

in the mitochondrion, whereas the four intermediate enzymatic reactions occur in the cytosol. The first rate-limiting step in haem synthesis is the formation of δ-aminolaevulinic acid (ala) by condensation of glycine and succinyl CoA. This reaction is under the control of ala-synthase with pyridoxal-5′-phosphate as cofactor. The rate of formation of ala is controlled by iron availability; iron deficiency causes iron regulatory proteins to bind to iron-responsive elements in the messenger RNA (mRNA) for ala-synthase with consequent repression of translation. Synthesis of ala is followed by its entry into the cytosol where two molecules combine, under the influence of ala-dehydrase, to form porphobilinogen. Four molecules of porphobilinogen in turn combine to form uroporphyrinogen III, which is then modified in two further steps to form coproporphyrinogen III. Coproporphyrinogen III enters the mitochondrion where it is converted to protoporphyrin IX. The final stage is the combination of ferrous ($Fe^{2+}$) iron with protoporphyrin IX to form haem, under the influence of ferrochelatase. Haem is also referred to as ferroprotoporphyrin.

The uptake of iron by erythroid cells is from transferrin (Fig. 1.7). A molecule of transferrin with its attached iron first binds to a membrane transferrin receptor. The whole complex is internalized, a process known as endocytosis. Iron is released from its carrier within the endocytotic vesicle and, following reduction to the ferrous form, is transferred to the mitochondrion for haem synthesis or is stored as fer-

ritin within the cytoplasm. The transferrin molecule then detaches from the transferrin receptor and is released from the cell surface. There is negative feedback control of haem synthesis by haem, which inhibits both ferrochelatase and the acquisition of iron from transferrin. Reduced cellular uptake of iron in turn inhibits the production of ala. Uptake of iron by erythroid cells is enhanced by iron deficiency and by increased levels of erythropoietin. Both lead to the combination of iron regulatory proteins with iron-responsive elements in the mRNA for the transferrin receptor protein. The mRNA is then protected from degradation, leading to increased expression of transferrin receptors on erythroid cell membranes and increased iron uptake.

The synthesis of α and β globin chains takes place in erythroid precursors, from the proerythroblast to the reticulocyte stage; δ chain synthesis ceases before the reticulocyte stage [13]. Synthesis is in the cytoplasm, on ribosomes. The genes for globin chain synthesis are located in two clusters, on chromosomes 11 and 16 (Figs 1.8 and 1.9). The α gene cluster is close to the telomere of chromosome 16, at 16p13.3. The distance from the telomere shows polymorphic variation, from 170 to 430 kilobases (kb), a kilobase being 1000 nucleotide bases. The β gene is at 11p15.5. In addition to the functional globin genes, these clusters contain 'pseudogenes', which are non-functional homologues of globin genes; they are transcribed but not translated. The α cluster of chromosome 16 extends over 28 kb and contains, in the following order,

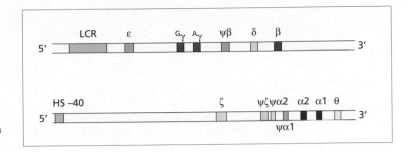

**Fig. 1.9** Diagrammatic representation of the α and β globin gene clusters.

**Table 1.2** Sequences showing CACCC, CCAAT and TATA homology in the promoters of globin genes; identical sequences in different genes are shown in bold red.

| Gene | CACCC homology box | CCAAT homology box | TATA homology box |
|---|---|---|---|
| ζ | | CCAAT | TATAAAC |
| α1 and α2 | | CCAAT | CATAAAC |
| ε | | CCAAT | AATAAAG |
| $^{G}$γ and $^{A}$γ | CACCC | CCAAT/CCAAT | AATAAAA |
| β | CACCC | CCAAT | CATAAAA |
| δ | | CCAAC | CATAAAA |

a ζ gene (also referred to as ζ2), a pseudo ζ gene (ψζ or ψζ1), two pseudo α genes, (ψα2 and ψα1) and two α genes, designated α2 and α1. The β cluster on chromosome 11 contains, in the following order, an ε gene, two γ genes, designated $^{G}$γ and $^{A}$γ, respectively, a pseudo β gene (ψβ), a δ gene and a β gene. There is wide variability of the α and β globin gene clusters between individuals and groups, with duplications and triplications of ζ, ψζ and α being quite common. The overall structure of the two clusters is remarkably conserved amongst vertebrates and this has led to the hypothesis that all the globin genes, as well as the gene for the unlinked but related protein, myoglobin, arose from a common ancestor by the processes of duplication, unequal crossing over and sequence divergence. Many primitive invertebrates have only a single globin gene, whereas fish and amphibians have α and β genes on the same chromosome. Birds have α and β genes on different chromosomes. All the human globin genes have three coding sequences (exons) and two intervening non-coding sequences (intervening sequences or introns) and are flanked by 5′ and 3′ non-coding se-

quences (referred to as untranslated regions, UTRs) (Fig. 1.10). The two α genes differ in structure in intron 2 and the 3′ UTR, but the coding sequences are identical. As for all genes, coding is by means of triplets of nucleotides, known as codons, which code for a specific amino acid. 5′ to each gene is the promoter, a sequence that binds RNA polymerase and transcription factors and is necessary for the initiation of transcription. Globin gene promoters share several conserved DNA sequences that bind crucial transcription factors [14,15]. These are summarized in Table 1.2.

The process by which globin chains are synthesized is shown diagrammatically in Fig. 1.10. Transcription is the process by which RNA is synthesized from a DNA template by the action of RNA polymerase. The entire globin gene, including the introns and the 5′ and 3′ UTRs, is transcribed. Transcription is controlled by interaction between the genes and transcription factors that bind to both promoters and upstream regulatory elements, referred to as the β-locus control region (β-LCR) for the β cluster and HS −40 for the α cluster. The β-LCR includes four

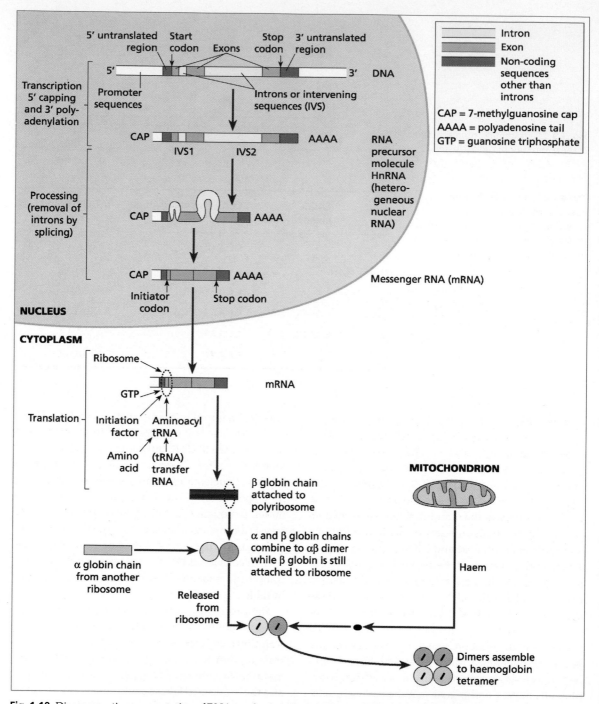

**Fig. 1.10** Diagrammatic representation of RNA synthesis and processing and β globin chain synthesis.

erythroid-specific DNase sites, designated HS1, HS2, HS3 and HS4, of which HS3 is probably the most important in opening the chromatin structure to permit access of transcription factors and HS2 is probably the most important in enhancing globin chain synthesis [16]. There are also enhancers within introns of genes and downstream of the β and $^A\gamma$ genes. *Trans*-acting factors, encoded by genes on chromosomes other than 11 and 16, are vital for the expression of globin genes. Relatively erythroid-specific *trans*-activating factors, including GATA1, NFE2, EKLF, SSP, Nrf-1, Nrf-2 and LCR-F1, contribute to the regulation of gene expression by interacting either with the LCRs or with the globin gene promoters to increase gene expression [17,18]. EKLF (erythroid Kruppel-like factor) is an enhancer of β chain synthesis and SSP (stage selector protein) is an enhancer of δ and γ chain synthesis [17]. In addition to transcription factors that are relatively specific to erythroid cells, globin gene expression is also influenced by general transcription factors, including AP-1, Sp1, YY1, USF and TAL-1/SCL [16–18]. Nascent RNA molecules resulting from transcription are large and unstable and are modified in the nucleus. Initially, the 5′ end acquires a 7-methylguanosine cap (CAP), which is probably added during transcription and has a role during translation; during this 'capping' process, methylation of adjacent ribose residues also occurs. Following this, the majority of transcripts acquire a 3′ polyadenosine tail with the addition of 75 to several hundred adenylate residues. There is an AAUAA sequence near the 3′ end (within the 3′ UTR) that serves as a signal for 3′ cleaving of the transcript and polyadenylation. Polyadenylation may have a role in transfer of the mRNA from the nucleus to the cytoplasm. The polyadenylate tail is also important for mRNA stability and enhances translation. Finally, the introns are excised to give a functional mRNA molecule which, in most cases, contains a single continuous open reading frame (ORF), encoding the sequence of the relevant protein, flanked by 5′ and 3′ UTRs.

Molecules of mRNA move from the nucleus to the cytoplasm where they bind to ribosomes and serve as templates for the assembly of the polypeptide sequences of the globin chain. Each nucleotide triplet serves as a template for a specific amino acid that is covalently bound to, and transported to, the ribosome by, transfer RNA (tRNA). tRNAs are specific for both a nucleotide triplet and an amino acid. Amino acids are thus assembled in the correct sequence, forming a polypeptide. This process is known as translation. An initiation codon, AUG, is essential for the initiation of translation; it is the first codon after the 5′ UTR and encodes methionine. Initiation requires the amino acid methionine, tRNA specific for methionine, guanosine triphosphate (GTP) and an initiation factor. When the nascent molecule reaches 20–30 amino acid residues, the methionine is removed through the action of methionine aminopeptidase. When the chain reaches 40–50 residues, cotranslational acetylation of the N-terminal residue can occur through the action of several acetyl transferases [19]. Whether this occurs to any great extent depends on the nature of the N-terminal residue. Thus the glycine of the γ chain is 10–15% acetylated, whereas the valine of normal α, β and δ chains is resistant to acetylation. There are 64 possible nucleotide triplets or codons, 61 of which encode amino acids (20 in all) and three of which do not; the latter serve as stop or termination codons, leading to termination of globin chain synthesis. Transcription thus continues until a termination codon, UAA, UAG or UGA, is encountered. The termination codon is followed by the 3′ UTR.

The rate-limiting step of globin chain translation is the commencement of elongation, i.e. the next step after initiation. Transcription from the two α genes is equal up to the eighth week of gestation, but thereafter the α2 gene becomes dominant and, in adult life, the ratio of α2 to α1 mRNA is 2.6–2.8:1 [20]. The translational efficiency differs somewhat so that the α2 gene directs the synthesis of about twice as much α chain as the α1 gene. There is more α than β mRNA, probably about 2.5 times as much, but β chain synthesis is more translationally efficient than α chain synthesis and α chains are therefore produced only slightly in excess of β chains [20]. The control of globin chain synthesis is probably mainly at the level of transcription, with translational control being less important. Translation is dependent on the presence of haem. In iron deficiency, the reduced availability of haem leads to inactivation of the initiation factor and thus reduced synthesis of globin chains. The α and β globin chains are synthesized on different polyribosomes. The combination of a free α

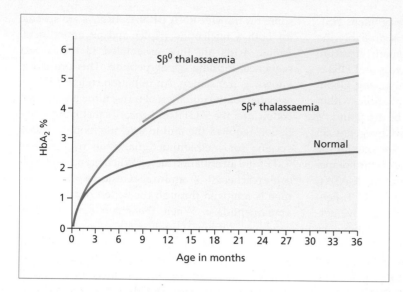

**Fig. 1.11** Diagram showing the rate of rise of haemoglobin $A_2$ in haematologically normal Jamaican babies and in babies with sickle cell/$\beta$ thalassaemia. (Modified from reference [21].)

chain with a $\beta$ chain that is still attached to the polyribosome, to form an $\alpha\beta$ dimer, may contribute to the release of the $\beta$ chain from the ribosome. Incorporation of haem probably occurs after release from the polyribosome.

Globin mRNA is unusually stable so that translation can continue for up to 3 days after cessation of transcription. Both the $\alpha$ and $\beta$ globin genes have structural determinants in their 3' UTRs that are important for mRNA stability [17].

## Normal haemoglobins

The normal haemoglobins beyond the neonatal period are haemoglobin A and two minor haemoglobins, haemoglobin $A_2$ and haemoglobin F.

### Haemoglobin $A_2$

In adults, haemoglobin $A_2$ comprises about 2–3.5% of total haemoglobin. The percentage is much lower at birth, about 0.2–0.3%, with a rise to adult levels during the first 2 years of life. The steepest rise occurs in the first year, but there is a continuing slow rise up to 3 years of age [21] (Fig. 1.11). In the normal adult population, the percentage of haemoglobin $A_2$ shows a Gaussian distribution. It has functional properties that are very similar to those of haemoglobin A [13] (similar cooperativity and interaction with

2,3-DPG), although, in comparison with haemoglobin A, it inhibits polymerization of haemoglobin S [22] and has a higher oxygen affinity [10]. It has a pancellular distribution.

The reduced rate of synthesis of haemoglobin $A_2$, in comparison with haemoglobin A, reflects the much slower rate of synthesis of the $\delta$ chain in comparison with the $\beta$ chain. This, in turn, appears to be consequent on a reduced rate of transcription of $\delta$ mRNA caused by a difference in the promoter region of these two genes; the $\delta$ gene has a CCAAC box rather than the CCAAT box of the $\beta$ gene [13] and, in addition, lacks the CACCC sequence that is present in the $\beta$ promoter (Table 1.2). The proportion of haemoglobin $A_2$ is reduced by absolute or functional iron deficiency (see Table 6.3) and by $\alpha$, $\delta$ and $\delta\beta$ thalassaemia trait (see Fig. 3.11). In $\gamma\delta\beta$ thalassaemia, the rate of synthesis, but not the proportion, of haemoglobin $A_2$ is reduced, as the synthesis of $\gamma$ and $\beta$ chains is reduced, as well as $\delta$ chain synthesis. The proportion of haemoglobin $A_2$ is increased in the great majority of patients with $\beta$ thalassaemia trait and in some patients with an unstable haemoglobin.

There are $\delta$ chain variants and $\delta$ thalassaemias. About 1% of individuals of African ancestry have the variant haemoglobin designated haemoglobin $A_2'$ ($A_2$ prime) or haemoglobin $B_2$ ($\delta^{16Gly\rightarrow Arg}$). It is readily detected by high performance liquid chromatography (Fig. 1.12) and isoelectric focusing. The $\delta$ thalas-

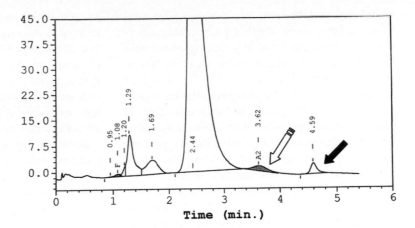

**Fig. 1.12** High performance liquid chromatography (HPLC) chromatogram showing a split haemoglobin $A_2$ resulting from heterozygosity for haemoglobin $A_2'$; the white arrow shows haemoglobin $A_2$ and the black arrow haemoglobin $A_2'$.

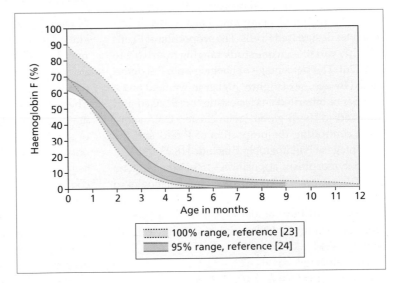

**Fig. 1.13** Rate of fall of the percentage of haemoglobin F postnatally in normal and premature babies; the pale blue represents premature babies while the deep blue represents normal babies. (Derived from references [23,24].)

saemias are also common in some ethnic groups, e.g. present in 1% of Sardinians [10]. The δ thalassaemias and δ chain variants are of no functional significance, although some variants are unstable or have increased oxygen affinity. However, their presence complicates the diagnosis of β thalassaemia trait (see p. 97).

## Haemoglobin F

Haemoglobin F is the major haemoglobin during intrauterine life. Its oxygen affinity is higher than that of haemoglobin A and this facilitates oxygen transfer from the mother to the fetus. However, it should be noted that fetal development appears to be normal in the offspring of mothers with very high levels of haemoglobin F. Its oxygen dissociation curve is sigmoid. The increased oxygen affinity, in comparison with haemoglobin A, is attributable to its weak affinity for 2,3-DPG [6]. In comparison with haemoglobin A, haemoglobin F is less efficient at transporting $CO_2$. A significant proportion of haemoglobin F is acetylated.

During the first year of life, the percentage of haemoglobin F falls progressively to values close to adult levels (Fig. 1.13) [23–25]. A slower fall to final adult levels may continue for several years, even up to puberty and beyond. The percentage of fetal haemoglobin present at birth is quite variable, usually being between 60% and 95%. During intrauterine life and at birth, haemoglobin F shows a $^G\gamma$ to $^A\gamma$ ratio of approximately 2:1 to 3:1. Within the first few months of birth, this changes to the adult ratio of approximately 2:3. In premature infants, there is initially a plateau phase in haemoglobin F concentration lasting 20–60 days, followed by a linear decrease similar to that in term babies [24]. At any given period after birth, the spread of values is greater than that in term babies. Initially, there are more high values but, after the first month of life, values both higher and lower than those of term infants are observed [24].

In normal adults, haemoglobin F is heterogeneously distributed, being found in a subset of erythrocytes designated F cells. The proportion of F cells is highly variable, in one study ranging from 0.6% to 22% [26]. The percentage of haemoglobin F is determined by age, sex (slightly higher in women) and a number of inherited characteristics both linked and unlinked to the β globin gene cluster. DNA sequences controlling the proportion of F cells and the percentage of haemoglobin F include [18,23–29]:

- a polymorphism at position −158 of the Gγ gene (C→T being associated with a higher haemoglobin F);
- variation of the number of repeats of a specific motif at −530 in the HS2 component of the β-LCR, namely $(AT)_x N_{12} GT(AT)_y$;
- a *trans*-acting locus at 6q22.3–23.2;
- a *trans*-acting locus at Xp22.2–22.3;
- a *trans*-acting locus on an autosome other than 6.

The percentage of haemoglobin F is also affected by any increase in the number of γ genes.

The mechanism by which the polymorphisms in the LCR at −530 base pairs (bp) to the Gγ gene influence γ chain synthesis appears to be that, in comparison with $(AT)_7 T_7$, the $(AT)_9 T_5$ sequence shows increased binding of BP-1, a negative *trans*-acting factor [30].

The distribution of the percentage of haemoglobin F in the population is skewed. In 85–90% of individuals, haemoglobin F is less than 0.6–0.7% and F cells are less than 4.5% [27,29]. The other 10–15% of the population have values above these levels. The upper limit of normal is rather arbitrarily taken as 1%. It would probably be more accurate to take 0.6% or 0.7% as the upper limit of normal, excluding the 11% of males and 21% of females who have a slight elevation of the percentage of F cells and the haemoglobin F percentage as an X-linked dominant characteristic [27]. However, as the measurement of a low percentage of haemoglobin F is very imprecise, 1% is a practical upper limit.

Haemoglobin F is more markedly increased in patients with various inherited abnormalities of β globin chain synthesis (see Table 3.12) and, less often, in various acquired conditions (see Table 6.2).

## Variant haemoglobins and abnormalities of globin gene synthesis

Nuclear DNA, including the DNA of globin genes, is subject to spontaneous mutation. This may be a point mutation (alteration of a single nucleotide) or a more extensive mutation, in which there is deletion, insertion or other alteration of more than one nucleotide. The types of mutation that may occur in globin genes are summarized in Table 1.3. In addition, expression of globin genes can be affected by DNA sequences outside the globin genes themselves, either enhancers acting in *cis* or genes on other chromosomes encoding *trans*-acting transcription factors (Tables 1.3 and 1.4).

Point mutations in globin genes sometimes have no effect on the amino acid sequence. This occurs because, as mentioned above, there is redundancy in the genetic code, with a number of nucleotide triplets coding for the same amino acid. When a 'same-sense' mutation occurs, the new codon resulting from the mutation codes for the same amino acid as the original codon and there is thus no effect on the final gene product. Similarly, mutation of a termination codon may be to a different termination codon. Many spontaneous mutations in globin genes are same-sense mutations. Point mutations may also result in a 'missense' mutation when the new codon codes for a different amino acid, leading to the production of a variant haemoglobin. The site of a mutation is critical, determining whether there is an effect on stability, oxygen affinity, solubility or other critical characteristics of the haemoglobin molecule. Because of the redundancy in the genetic code, different point mutations may give rise to the same variant

**Table 1.3** Types of mutation that can occur in globin genes and adjoining sequences.

| Type of mutation | Possible consequence | Example |
| --- | --- | --- |
| *Point mutations*<br>Within coding sequence, i.e. within an exon | **Same-sense or neutral mutation**, i.e. mutant codon codes for same amino acid as normal codon, so there are no consequences | Many mutations are of this type; more than one-third of theoretically possible point mutations would result in no alteration in the amino acid encoded |
| | **Mis-sense mutation**, i.e. mutant codon codes for a different amino acid from the normal codon; includes mis-sense mutations in which an abnormal amino acid interferes with the normal cleavage of the N-terminal methionine | Haemoglobin S, haemoglobin C, haemoglobin E<br>Haemoglobin Marseille and haemoglobin South Florida (altered amino acid near N-terminus plus persisting methionine residue at the N-terminus of the $\beta$ chain) |
| | **Nonsense mutation**, i.e. the mutant codon does not code for an amino acid and thus functions as a stop or termination codon, producing a shortened globin chain | Haemoglobin McKees Rocks (two amino acids shorter than normal); $\alpha2$ CD116 GAG$\rightarrow$TAG creating premature stop codon and causing $\alpha$ thalassaemia |
| | **New-sense mutation**, i.e. conversion of a stop codon to a coding sequence, producing an elongated globin chain | Haemoglobin Constant Spring, haemoglobin Icaria, haemoglobin Seal Rock, haemoglobin Koya Dora, haemoglobin Paksé |
| | Gene conversion* | Conversion of $^G\gamma$ gene to $^A\gamma$ gene, giving $^A\gamma^A\gamma$ genotype<br>Conversion of $^A\gamma$ gene to $^G\gamma$ gene, giving $^G\gamma^G\gamma$ genotype<br>Conversion of $\psi\zeta1$ to a gene that resembles $\zeta2$ but is still non-functional ($\zeta1$)<br>Conversion between the $\alpha2$ and $\alpha1$ genes so that the same mutation is present in both, e.g. $\alpha2^{Lys\rightarrow Glu}\alpha1^{Lys\rightarrow Glu}$, giving unusually high levels of haemoglobin I |
| | Gene conversion plus further point mutation* | Haemoglobin F-Port Royal, resulting from a further point mutation in a $^G\gamma^G\gamma$ gene complex |
| Within non-coding sequence, i.e. in an intron | Production of a new splice site leading to a structurally abnormal mRNA | Some $\beta$ thalassaemias |
| Mutation 5' or 3' to the gene (i.e. outside the gene) | Mutation of an enhancer | Some $\beta$ thalassaemias |
| | Reduced rate of synthesis of mRNA due to interference with 3'-end formation of mRNA | Some $\beta$ thalassaemias |

*Continued on p. 16.*

**Table 1.3** *Continued.*

| Type of mutation | Possible consequence | Example |
|---|---|---|
| *Deletion or duplication of one or more genes* | | |
| Deletion of one or more genes | Total loss of expression of relevant gene; occasionally, also loss of function of an adjacent structurally normal gene | Most α thalassaemias, some β thalassaemias, δβ thalassaemias and γδβ thalassaemias; deletion of $^{G}\gamma$ gene ($-^{A}\gamma$), homozygosity for which causes anaemia and a reduced haemoglobin F percentage in the neonate; deletion of ψζ1 |
| Deletion of genes with downstream enhancer being juxtaposed to remaining gene | Loss of β and δ gene function, but enhanced function of remaining $^{G}\gamma$ ($±^{A}\gamma$) gene | Deletional hereditary persistence of fetal haemoglobin |
| Duplication of α gene | Triple or quadruple α gene | ααα†/αα, ααα/ααα, αααα‡/αα or αααα/αααα |
| Triplication of entire α globin gene cluster | Six α genes on a single chromosome | αα:αα:αα/αα |
| Duplication of $^{G}\gamma$ gene | Double, triple or quadruple $^{G}\gamma$ gene so that there are three, four or five γ genes on a chromosome | $^{G}\gamma^{G}\gamma^{A}\gamma$, $^{G}\gamma^{G}\gamma^{G}\gamma^{A}\gamma$ (homozygotes have been described with a total of eight γ genes) or $^{G}\gamma^{G}\gamma^{G}\gamma^{G}\gamma^{A}\gamma$ |
| Duplication of the ζ or ψζ gene | Double, triple or quadruple ζ/ψζ gene | ζ2ψζ1ψζ1/ζ2ψζ1 or ζ2ψζ1ψζ1/ζ2ψζ1ψζ1 or four ζ-like genes per chromosome |
| *Abnormal cross-over during meiosis leading to gene fusion* | | |
| α2α1 fusion | Effective loss of one α gene but structurally normal α chain is encoded | $-\alpha^{3.7}$ thalassaemia |
| δβ fusion — simple cross-over | Reduced rate of synthesis of structurally abnormal globin chain | Haemoglobin Lepore, e.g. haemoglobin Lepore-Washington/Boston, haemoglobin Lepore-Baltimore and haemoglobin Lepore-Hollandia, or $\delta^{0}\beta^{+}$ thalassaemia [31] |
| δβδ fusion — double cross-over with δ sequences on either side of β sequences | Reduced rate of synthesis of structurally abnormal globin chain | Haemoglobin Parchman |
| βδ fusion (with preservation of intact δ and β genes on either side of fusion gene, with or without additional mutation) | | Anti-Lepore haemoglobins, e.g. haemoglobin Miyada, haemoglobin P-Nilotic, haemoglobin P-Congo, haemoglobin Lincoln Park |
| $^{A}\gamma\beta$ fusion | Synthesis of variant haemoglobin plus increased synthesis of haemoglobin F | Haemoglobin Kenya |
| $\beta^{A}\gamma$ fusion (with preservation of intact $^{G}\gamma$ and $^{A}\gamma$ genes and duplication of the δ gene) | | Haemoglobin anti-Kenya |
| $^{G}\gamma^{A}\gamma$ fusion (designated $-^{G}\gamma^{A}\gamma-$) | Reduced rate of synthesis of haemoglobin F | γ thalassaemia |

**Table 1.3** *Continued.*

| Type of mutation | Possible consequence | Example |
|---|---|---|
| *Deletion of DNA sequences but without a frame shift in coding sequence* | | |
| Deletion of part of a coding sequence, either three nucleotides or a multiple of three | One to five amino acids missing but sequence otherwise normal | Haemoglobin Gun Hill (an unstable haemoglobin with five amino acids missing) |
| *Deletion plus inversion* | | |
| Two deletions with inversion of intervening sequence | Deletion involving $^A\gamma$ and $\delta$ plus $\beta$ genes, respectively, but with preservation of an intervening region which is inverted | Indian type of deletional $^A\gamma\delta\beta^0$ thalassaemia |
| *Deletion plus insertion* | | |
| Deletion with insertion of extraneous DNA between breakpoints | Same functional effect as deletion | One type of $\alpha^0$ thalassaemia, _ _$_{MED}$ |
| *Insertion within a coding sequence but without a frame shift* | | |
| Insertion of nucleotides, either three or multiples of three, e.g. by tandem duplication | Up to five extra amino acids | Haemoglobin Koriyama (an unstable haemoglobin with insertion of five codons in $\beta$ gene, anti-Gun Hill); haemoglobin Grady (insertion of three codons in $\alpha$ gene) |
| *Frame shift mutations* | | |
| Alteration of the reading frame resulting from deletion, insertion, deletion plus insertion or deletion plus duplication | Abnormal amino acid sequence with an elongated globin chain (when a stop codon is out of phase and translation continues until another 'in-frame' stop codon is met); abnormal amino acid sequence with a truncated globin chain (when a premature stop codon is created) | Haemoglobin Wayne ($\alpha$ chain), haemoglobin Tak ($\beta$ chain), haemoglobin Cranston ($\beta$ chain), some $\beta$ thalassaemias, including some dominant $\beta$ thalassaemias, some $\alpha$ thalassaemias |
| *Chromosomal translocation* | | |
| Unbalanced translocation | Extra $\alpha$ genes on a chromosome other than chromosome 16 | Same significance as homozygous triplication of an $\alpha$ gene as there are a total of six $\alpha$ genes |
| | Loss of an $\alpha$ gene | $\alpha$ thalassaemia |
| *Deletion of a locus control region* | | |
| Locus control region deleted, with or without deletion of relevant genes | Deletion of the locus control region of the $\beta$ gene | $(\epsilon)\gamma\delta\beta^0$ thalassaemia |
| | Deletion of the $\alpha$ gene enhancer (HS –40) 40 kb upstream of the $\zeta 2$ gen | $\alpha^0$ thalassaemia |

*Gene conversion is non-reciprocal genetic exchange between allelic or non-allelic homologous sequences so that one gene comes to resemble another more closely or becomes identical to it; it is responsible for maintaining the similarity between pairs of identical or similar genes.

†Either $\alpha\alpha\alpha^{anti3.7}$ or $\alpha\alpha\alpha^{anti4.2}$.

‡Either $\alpha\alpha\alpha\alpha^{anti3.7}$ or $\alpha\alpha\alpha\alpha^{anti4.2}$.

**Table 1.4** Mutations occurring outside the globin gene clusters leading to abnormal globin gene synthesis.

| Mutation | Consequence |
| --- | --- |
| Mutation in $XH_2$ gene at Xq13.3, which encodes a *trans*-acting factor regulating α gene expression | Haemoglobin H disease plus dysmorphism and severe learning difficulties |
| Mutation in a putative gene at Xp22.2–22.3 | Hereditary persistence of fetal haemoglobin |
| Mutation in a putative gene at 6q22.3–23.1 | Hereditary persistence of fetal haemoglobin |
| Mutation in the *XPD* gene at 19q13.2–13.3, which encodes one component of the general transcription factor, TFIIH [32] | Recessive trichothiodystrophy and β thalassaemia |
| Mutation in the *GATA1* gene at Xp11–12 [33] | X-linked thrombocytopenia and β thalassaemia |

haemoglobin. For example, the α chain variant, G-Philadelphia, has arisen twice, from an AAC to AAG change in an α2α1 fusion gene and from an AAC to AAA change in an α2 gene [34]. There are more than 900 known variant haemoglobins resulting from point mutations. Some point mutations are 'nonsense' mutations in which the new codon is one of the three that do not code for an amino acid. A nonsense mutation thus functions as a 'stop' or 'termination' codon, leading to termination of chain synthesis. If this type of mutation is near the 3′ end of the gene, an abnormal but functional globin chain is produced; however, if it is more proximal, the chain produced is likely to be not only short but very unstable, leading to a dominant thalassaemia phenotype. Point mutations can also convert a stop codon to a coding sequence, so that an elongated mRNA and elongated globin chain are produced. A variant haemoglobin with two amino acid substitutions resulting from two point mutations can be produced either from a new mutation occurring in the gene encoding a variant globin chain, e.g. in a parental germ cell, or from cross-over between two variant alleles.

An unusual result of a point mutation is the production of an abnormal amino acid that is converted to a different amino acid by post-translational modification. This may be the result of deamidation, acetylation or oxidation. There are six reported variant haemoglobins in which the abnormal DNA sequence codes for asparagine, but this is subsequently deamidated to aspartic acid [11]; of these, the most common is haemoglobin J-Sardegna (α50(CD8)$^{\text{His}\rightarrow\text{Asn}\rightarrow\text{Asp}}$), which has a prevalence of

0.25% in northern Sardinia. Post-translational acetylation occurs in haemoglobin Raleigh, which has a β1$^{\text{Val}\rightarrow\text{Ala}}$ substitution; proteins with an N-terminal alanine are often acetylated and this is the case with this variant haemoglobin [35]. The presence in one individual of haemoglobins with three different β chains may be attributable to post-translational modification. For example, the replacement of leucine by hydroxyleucine that characterizes haemoglobin Coventry is not encoded by genomic DNA and is found only in the presence of an unstable haemoglobin, either haemoglobin Atlanta or haemoglobin Sydney. Some mutations affecting the haem pocket and leading to haemoglobin instability permit the oxidation of leucine to isoleucine [36]. Haemoglobin Bristol also shows post-translational modification. It is an unstable haemoglobin resulting from conversion of the β67 valine codon to a codon for methionine; however, the final haemoglobin has aspartic acid rather than methionine as a consequence of post-translational modification [11].

In a slightly different mechanism, the abnormal structure of a variant haemoglobin resulting from a point mutation leads to post-translational modification of a normal amino acid, in three cases leucine being modified to hydroxyleucine [11] and in one case asparagine adjacent to the abnormal residue being deamidated to aspartic acid [35].

Mutations in the codon for the N-terminal valine may mean that a different amino acid is encoded, with resultant retention of the initiator methionine and full acetylation of the N-terminal residue (e.g. the glutamate of the α chain variant haemoglobin

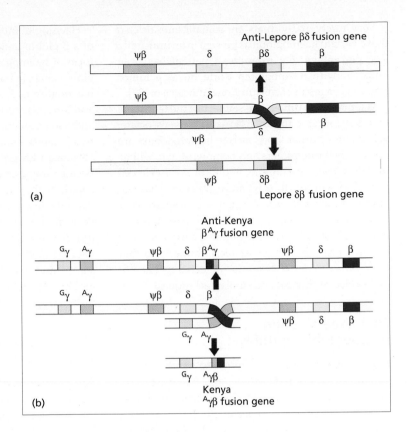

**Fig. 1.14** Some examples of fusion genes produced by non-homologous cross-over: (a) formation of genes encoding Lepore and anti-Lepore haemoglobins; (b) formation of genes encoding Kenya and anti-Kenya haemoglobins.

Thionville) or normal cleavage of methionine but full acetylation of the N-terminal residue (e.g. the alanine of the α chain variant haemoglobin Lyon-Bron) [19]. Similarly, a histidine to proline change in position β2 leads to retention of the initiator methionine [35]. If methionine is retained, the globin chain is extended by one residue.

Deletions and insertions can lead to a frame shift, i.e. unless the deletion or insertion involves three nucleotides or multiples of three, the nucleotide sequences beyond the mutation will be in a different reading frame and will be 'read' during translation as coding for a completely different sequence of amino acids. Frame shift mutations can lead to a premature stop codon, so that both mRNA and the resultant globin chain are shorter than normal. Unless this occurs, a frame shift mutation is likely to lead to elongated mRNA and an elongated globin chain. The original stop codon is no longer in the reading frame and transcription continues until another stop codon is encountered.

Small deletions and large deletions and insertions can result from non-homologous cross-over between a pair of chromosomes during meiosis. These are usually in-frame. Non-homologous cross-over can involve not only a single pair of allelic genes (e.g. two α genes), but also two structurally similar but non-allelic genes (e.g. a β gene and a δ gene); in the latter instance, there may be a loss of the two normal genes and the production of a fusion gene which has 5' sequences of one gene and 3' sequences of the other gene; alternatively, the two normal genes may be retained with part of both genes being reduplicated in the fusion gene. Some examples of non-homologous cross-over are shown in Fig. 1.14. Non-homologous cross-over can also result in the reduplication of genes; for example, some individuals, instead of having two α genes on each chromosome 16, have three or even four α genes on one chromosome. Duplicated α genes occur in many populations and in some are quite frequent. For example, 2% of Sri Lankans have ααα.

Very rarely, individuals are somatic mosaics, so that a variant haemoglobin is present in an unusually low percentage. For example, a patient has been reported with haemoglobin Korle Bu as a minor fraction as a result of constitutional mosaicism [37].

Haemoglobin dimers are stable, but the tetramers that they form are able to dissociate and re-associate. When both normal and variant haemoglobins are present, heterotetramers and homotetramers will be found *in vivo*; for example, in the case of sickle cell trait, there will be $\alpha_2\beta_2$, $\alpha_2\beta^S_2$ and $\alpha_2\beta\beta^S$. When haemoglobins are studied *in vitro*, e.g. by electrophoresis or chromatography, the heterotetramers dissociate and re-associate as homotetramers. Some variant haemoglobins have abnormally stable tetramers, so that three rather than two forms are detected by haemoglobin electrophoresis and similar techniques.

## Thalassaemias and haemoglobinopathies

Mutations can lead not only to the synthesis of a structurally abnormal haemoglobin, but also to a reduced rate of synthesis of a globin chain and therefore of the haemoglobin species of which it forms a part. The term 'thalassaemia' is used to describe disorders with a significant decrease in the rate of synthesis of one or more globin chains: $\alpha$ thalassaemia indicates a reduced rate of synthesis of $\alpha$ globin chain; similarly, $\beta$, $\delta$, $\delta\beta$ and $\gamma\delta\beta$ thalassaemias indicate a reduced rate of synthesis of $\beta$, $\delta$, $\delta + \beta$ and $\gamma + \delta + \beta$ chains, respectively. In some disorders, there is both synthesis of a structurally abnormal haemoglobin and a reduced rate of synthesis of the variant haemoglobin. This is the case, for different reasons, with the $\alpha$ chain variant haemoglobin Constant Spring (first described in a Chinese patient in Constant Spring, a district of Kingston, Jamaica) and the $\beta$ chain variant haemoglobin E. The term 'haemoglobinopathy' is sometimes used to indicate only those disorders with a structurally abnormal haemoglobin, while others use the term to include all disorders of globin chain synthesis, encompassing also the thalassaemias. If the term 'haemoglobinopathy' is used only to designate a structurally abnormal haemoglobin, variant haemoglobins, such as haemoglobin E and haemoglobin Constant Spring, can be referred to as 'thalassaemic haemoglobinopathies'.

Haemoglobinopathies may result from mutation of a $\beta$ globin gene, in which case there is a variant form of haemoglobin A, or from mutation of an $\alpha$ globin gene, in which case there are variant forms of haemoglobins F, A and $A_2$. Similarly, mutations of $\gamma$ and $\delta$ genes result in mutant forms of haemoglobin F and haemoglobin $A_2$, respectively. Because there are two $\beta$ genes, an individual can have both a $\beta$ chain variant and haemoglobin A or two $\beta$ chain variants. Because there are usually four $\alpha$ genes, an individual could, in theory, have up to four different $\alpha$ chain variants; in practice, a number of individuals have been described with both haemoglobin A and two different $\alpha$ chain variants, e.g. haemoglobin Buda, haemoglobin Pest and haemoglobin A in one instance and haemoglobin G-Philadelphia, haemoglobin J-Sardegna and haemoglobin A in several instances.

## The proportion of variant haemoglobins

The proportion of an $\alpha$ chain variant in the blood might be expected to be around 25%, as there are usually four $\alpha$ genes. However, the situation is far more complex. The variant is likely to be more than 25% if it results from mutation of the $\alpha2$ gene (as the ratio of $\alpha2$ to $\alpha1$ synthesis is normally about $3:1$) and less than 25% if it results from mutation of the $\alpha1$ gene. The percentage is raised if there is coinheritance of $\alpha$ thalassaemia and lowered if there is coinheritance of triple $\alpha$ ($\alpha\alpha\alpha$). If a gene encoding an $\alpha$ chain variant is a mutated $\alpha1$ gene in *cis* with deletion of the $\alpha2$ gene, it may be upregulated, increasing the percentage further. The percentage is reduced if the variant $\alpha$ chain is synthesized at a reduced rate, if it has a lower affinity for $\beta$ chains than does the normal $\alpha$ chain or if the variant $\alpha$ chain or the variant haemoglobin is unstable.

Similarly, it might be expected that a $\beta$ chain variant would represent about 50% of total haemoglobin in heterozygotes, as there are two $\beta$ genes. As for $\alpha$ chain variants, the situation is much more complex. The percentage may be above 50% in the case of variants with negatively charged $\beta$ chains, which have a greater affinity than normal $\beta$ chains for the positively charged normal $\alpha$ chains (e.g. haemoglobin J-Baltimore or J-Iran); if there is coexisting $\alpha$

**Table 1.5** Consequences of mutation of globin genes.

| Type of mutation and consequence | Example |
| --- | --- |
| Substitution of an external amino acid not involved in inter-chain contacts; no functional abnormality | Haemoglobin G-Philadelphia |
| Amino acid substitution leading to reduced solubility, polymerization of haemoglobin and deformation of cells into a holly leaf or sickle shape with consequent haemolysis and vascular obstruction | Haemoglobin S (sickle cell haemoglobin) |
| Amino acid substitution leading to reduced solubility, formation of straight-edged crystals and haemolysis | Haemoglobin C |
| Replacement of haem-binding or haem-related histidine residue by another amino acid leading to an increased tendency to oxidation, i.e. formation of methaemoglobin; there is cyanosis at birth if the defect is in a $\gamma$ gene, cyanosis from birth if the defect is in an $\alpha$ chain and cyanosis from approximately 6 months of age if the defect is in a $\beta$ chain; there may be associated haemoglobin instability | M haemoglobins |
| Mutation involving amino acids of the haem pocket or $\alpha_1\beta_2$ (tetrameric) contacts or mutation interfering with the helical structure of haemoglobin, leading to haemoglobin instability and Heinz body haemolytic anaemia; there may also be decreased oxygen affinity and consequent cyanosis | Haemoglobin Köln, haemoglobin Zurich (haem pocket mutation), haemoglobin Kansas (mutation affecting $\alpha1\beta2$ contacts) |
| Mutations involving $\alpha_1\beta_2$, $\alpha_2\beta_1$ tetrameric haemoglobin contacts or C-terminal end of $\beta$ chain, where there are residues involved in 2,3-DPG interaction and stability of the deoxy form of haemoglobin, leading to increased oxygen affinity and polycythaemia | Haemoglobin Chesapeake, haemoglobin Bethesda, haemoglobin Kempsey, haemoglobin J-Capetown, haemoglobin Yakima |
| Mutation leading to decreased oxygen affinity and therefore anaemia, as normal tissue delivery of oxygen is achieved with a lower concentration of haemoglobin; may cause cyanosis | Haemoglobin S, haemoglobin Seattle (also unstable), haemoglobin Kansas (also unstable), haemoglobin Beth Israel |
| Mutation in $\beta$ gene leading to markedly reduced or absent $\beta$ chain production, reduced synthesis of haemoglobin A and possibly ineffective erythropoiesis consequent on damage to developing erythroblasts by excess $\alpha$ chains | $\beta$ thalassaemia (major, intermedia or minor) |
| Mutation in $\beta$ gene leading to structurally abnormal and very unstable $\beta$ chain | (Dominant) $\beta$ thalassaemia phenotype |
| Mutation in $\alpha$ gene leading to markedly reduced or absent $\alpha$ chain synthesis and reduced synthesis of haemoglobins F, A and A$_2$ | $\alpha$ thalassaemia ($\alpha$ thalassaemia trait, haemoglobin H disease or haemoglobin Bart's hydrops fetalis) |
| Mutation in $\alpha$ gene leading to structurally abnormal $\alpha$ chain synthesized at a greatly reduced rate | $\alpha$ thalassaemia phenotype, e.g. haemoglobin Constant Spring |
| Mutation in $\delta$ gene leading to a structural abnormality or markedly reduced or absent $\delta$ chain production | Haemoglobin A$_2$ variant or $\delta$ thalassaemia; no clinical significance as haemoglobin A$_2$ is a minor haemoglobin, but complicates the diagnosis of thalassaemia trait |
| Mutation in $\gamma$ gene leading to structural abnormality or reduced rate of synthesis of $\gamma$ chain and therefore haemoglobin F | Some methaemoglobins |

2,3-DPG, 2,3-diphosphoglycerate.

thalassaemia, leading to a lack of α chains, the percentage of the variant is even higher. The converse is seen with positively charged β chains, such as $β^S$, $β^C$, $β^{O-Arab}$ and $β^{D-Punjab}$, which have a lower affinity than normal β chains for normal α chains. The percentage of the variant is thus somewhat less than 50% and, if there is coexisting α thalassaemia, is even lower. The percentage is also reduced considerably below 50% if there is a reduced rate of synthesis of the variant β (or δβ) chain (e.g. $β^E$, $δβ^{Lepore}$), if the β chain is unstable or if the variant haemoglobin is unstable (e.g. haemoglobin Köln).

An alteration in the amino acid sequence of the globin chains, i.e. an alteration in the primary structure of haemoglobin, often has no significant effect on the secondary, tertiary and quaternary structure of haemoglobin; this is the case when the substituted amino acid is of a similar size to the normal amino acid, has the same charge and the same hydrophobic or hydrophilic properties, and does not have a role in the binding of haem or 2,3-DPG or in interactions between chains. In this case, a variant haemoglobin has no consequences for the health of the individual. In other cases, an alteration in the primary structure of haemoglobin affects the secondary, tertiary or quaternary structure of the molecule, sometimes with very profound effects. Some of the effects of mutations in globin genes are shown in Table 1.5.

Over 1000 mutations of the globin genes have been recognized. Some 690 of them have been collated in a single volume [38] and this database is now available electronically, in updated form, on the World Wide Web (http://globin.cse.psu.edu/).

## Check your knowledge

One to five answers may be correct. Answers to almost all questions can be found in this chapter or can be deduced from the information given. The correct answers are given on p. 25.

1.1   The haemoglobin molecule
(a)  requires iron for its synthesis
(b)  is composed of three pairs of globin chains
(c)  alters its structure when oxygen is bound
(d)  is assembled in the cytosol
(e)  binds 2,3-diphosphoglycerate

1.2   Haemoglobin F
(a)  is the major haemoglobin present in the fetus
(b)  has a lower oxygen affinity than haemoglobin A
(c)  is absent in normal adults
(d)  percentage shows a non-Gaussian distribution in the population
(e)  is composed of two α chains and two β chains

1.3   The functions of haemoglobin include
(a)  transport of glucose
(b)  transport of $CO_2$
(c)  transport of oxygen
(d)  buffering
(e)  transport of creatinine to the kidney

1.4   The affinity of haemoglobin for oxygen is decreased by
(a)  fever
(b)  alkalosis
(c)  binding of $CO_2$
(d)  binding of 2,3-diphosphoglycerate
(e)  glycosylation

1.5   When blood circulates through the lungs, haemoglobin
(a)  is oxidized
(b)  takes up oxygen
(c)  loses $CO_2$
(d)  takes up water
(e)  dissociates into haem and globin

1.6   Structurally abnormal haemoglobins may result from
(a)  point mutations
(b)  gene fusion
(c)  frame shift mutations
(d)  mutation of a stop codon to a coding sequence
(e)  mutation of a coding sequence to a stop codon

1.7   Abnormal haemoglobins may
(a)  have increased oxygen affinity
(b)  have decreased oxygen affinity
(c)  be prone to crystallize

(d) be unstable

(e) be abnormally prone to oxidation

1.8 Mutations in globin genes

(a) can occur in $\alpha$, $\beta$, $^G\gamma$, $^A\gamma$ and $\delta$ genes

(b) always result in a structural abnormality of haemoglobin

(c) always have harmful effects

(d) can lead to a reduced rate of globin chain synthesis

(e) can convert one gene to another

1.9 Haemoglobin F

(a) is present, in adult life, in a subset of erythrocytes referred to as F cells

(b) is composed of two $\alpha$ chains and two $\gamma$ chains, encoded by two pairs of structurally similar $\alpha$ genes and two pairs of structurally similar $\gamma$ genes

(c) has a sigmoid dissociation curve

(d) constitutes a higher proportion of total haemoglobin in premature than in full-term babies

(e) on average is present at a somewhat higher level in women than in men

1.10 Cooperativity is essential for

(a) a sigmoid oxygen dissociation curve

(b) the higher oxygen affinity of haemoglobin F in comparison with haemoglobin A

(c) the Bohr effect

(d) the binding of $CO_2$ to haemoglobin

(e) conversion of haemoglobin to methaemoglobin

1.11 The proportion of a variant haemoglobin is usually

(a) greater in the case of an $\alpha$ chain variant than a $\beta$ chain variant

(b) greater in the case of an $\alpha$ chain variant if there is coexisting deletion of an $\alpha$ gene

(c) greater if the variant $\beta$ chain has a higher affinity for normal $\alpha$ chains than does the normal $\beta$ chain

(d) greater, in the case of haemoglobin S, if there is coexisting $\alpha$ thalassaemia

(e) greater if the variant haemoglobin is unstable

## Further reading

Bunn HF and Forget BG. *Hemoglobin: Molecular, Genetic and Clinical Aspects*. W. B. Saunders, Philadelphia, PA, 1986.

Huisman THJ, Carver MFH and Efremov GD. *A Syllabus of Human Hemoglobin Variants*. The Sickle Cell Anemia Foundation, Augusta, GA, 1996.

Lehmann H and Huntsman RG. *Man's Haemoglobins including the Haemoglobinopathies and their Investigation*. North Holland Publishing Company, Amsterdam, 1974.

Nienhuis AW and Benz EJ (1997) Regulation of hemoglobin synthesis during the development of the red cell. *N Engl J Med* **297**, 1318–1328, 1371–1381, 1430–1436.

Stamatoyannopoulos G and Nienhuis AW. Hemoglobin switching. In: Stamatoyannopoulos G, Nienhuis AW, Majerus PW and Varmus H, eds. *The Molecular Basis of Blood Diseases*, 2nd edn. W. B. Saunders, Philadelphia, PA, 1994, pp. 107–156.

Steinberg MH, Forget BG, Higgs DR and Nagel RL, eds. *Disorders of Hemoglobin: Genetics, Pathophysiology, and Clinical Management*. Cambridge University Press, Cambridge, 2001.

The Globin Gene Server, hosted by Pennsylvania State University, USA and McMaster University, Canada. URL http://globin.cse.psu.edu/.

Weatherall D and Clegg JB. *The Thalassaemia Syndromes*, 4th edn. Blackwell Science, Oxford, 2001.

## References

1 Gross GS and Lane P (1999) Physiological reactions of nitric oxide and hemoglobin: a radical rethink. *Proc Natl Acad Sci USA* **96**, 9967–9969.

2 Nagel RL and Jaffé ER. CO-, NO-, met-, and sulf-hemoglobinemias: the dyshemoglobinemias. In: Steinberg MH, Forget BG, Higgs DR and Nagel RL, eds. *Disorders of Hemoglobin: Genetics, Pathophysiology, and Clinical Management*. Cambridge University Press, Cambridge, 2001, pp. 1214–1233.

3 Schechter AN and Gladwin MT (2003) Hemoglobin and the paracrine and endocrine functions of nitric oxide. *N Engl J Med* **348**, 1483–1485.

4 Pauling L, Itano HA, Singer SY and Wells IG (1949) Sickle-cell anemia, a molecular disease. *Science* **110**, 543–548.

5 Kunkel HG and Wallenius G (1955) New hemoglobin in normal adult blood. *Science* **122**, 288.

6 Bunn HF and Forget BG. *Hemoglobin: Molecular, Genetic and Clinical Aspects*. W. B. Saunders, Philadelphia, PA, 1986.

7 Huehns ER, Flynn FV, Butler EA and Beaven GH (1961) Two new hemoglobin variants in the very young human embryo. *Nature* **189**, 496–497.

8 Hecht F, Jones RT and Koler RD (1967) Newborn infants with Hb Portland 1, an indicator of α-chain deficiency. *Ann Hum Genet* **31**, 215–218.

9 Fantoni A, Farace MG and Gambari R (1981) Embryonic hemoglobins in man and other mammals. *Blood* **57**, 623–633.

10 Nagel RL and Steinberg MH. Hemoglobins of the embryo and fetus and minor hemoglobins of adults. In: Steinberg MH, Forget BG, Higgs DR and Nagel RL, eds. *Disorders of Hemoglobin: Genetics, Pathophysiology, and Clinical Management*. Cambridge University Press, Cambridge, 2001, pp. 197–230.

11 Rees DC, Rochette J, Schofield C, Green B, Morris M, Parker NE *et al.* (1996) A novel silent posttranslational mechanism converts methionine to aspartate in hemoglobin Bristol (β67[E11] Val-Met→Asp). *Blood* **88**, 341–348.

12 Ponka P (1997) Tissue-specific regulation of iron metabolism and heme synthesis: distinct control mechanisms in erythroid cells. *Blood* **89**, 1–25.

13 Steinberg MH and Adams JG (1991) Haemoglobin A$_2$: origin, evolution, and aftermath. *Blood* **78**, 2165–2177.

14 Stamatoyannopoulos G and Nienhuis AW. Hemoglobin switching. In: Stamatoyannopoulos G, Nienhuis AW, Majerus PW and Varmus H, eds. *The Molecular Basis of Blood Diseases*, 2nd edn. W. B. Saunders, Philadelphia, PA, 1994, pp. 107–156.

15 Weatherall D and Clegg JB. *The Thalassaemia Syndromes*, 4th edn. Blackwell Science, Oxford, 2001.

16 Ho PJ and Thein SL (2000) Gene regulation and deregulation: a β globin perspective. *Blood Rev* **14**, 78–93.

17 Russell JE and Liebhaber SA (1996) The stability of human β-globin mRNA is dependent on structural determinants positioned within its 3′ untranslated region. *Blood* **87**, 5314–5322.

18 Jane SM and Cunningham JM (1998) Understanding fetal globin gene expression: a step towards effective Hb F reactivation in haemoglobinopathies. *Br J Haematol* **102**, 415–422.

19 Lacan P, Souillet G, Aubry M, Prome D, Richelme-David S, Kister J *et al.* (2002) New alpha 2 globin chain variant with low oxygen affinity affecting the N-terminal residue and leading to N-acetylation [Hb Lyon-Bron α1(NA1)Val→Ac-Ala]. *Am J Hematol* **69**, 214–218.

20 Bernini LF and Harteveld CL (1998) α-Thalassaemia. *Bailliere's Clin Haematol* **11**, 53–90.

21 Serjeant BE, Mason KP and Serjeant GR (1978) The development of haemoglobin A$_2$ in normal Negro infants and in sickle cell disease. *Br J Haematol* **39**, 259–263.

22 Steinberg MH (1998) Pathophysiology of sickle cell disease. *Bailliere's Clin Haematol* **11**, 163–184.

23 Huehns ER and Beaven GH. Developmental changes in human haemoglobins. In: Benson PF, ed. *The Biochemistry of Human Development*. Spastics International Medical Publications, London, 1971, p. 175. Quoted by Weatherall D and Clegg JB. *The Thalassaemia Syndromes*, 3rd edn. Blackwell Scientific Publications, Oxford, 1981.

24 Colombo B, Kim B, Atencio RP, Molina C and Terrenato L (1976) The pattern of foetal haemoglobin disappearance after birth. *Br J Haematol* **32**, 79–87.

25 Cheron G, Bachoux I, Maier M, Massonneau M, Peltier JY and Girot T (1989) Fetal hemoglobin in sudden infant death syndrome. *N Engl J Med* **320**, 1011–1012.

26 Garner C, Tatu T, Reittie JE, Littlewood T, Darley J, Cervino S *et al.* (2000) Genetic influences on F cells and other hematologic variables: a twin heritability study. *Blood* **95**, 342–346.

27 Miyoshi K, Kaneto Y, Kawai H, Ohchi H, Niki S, Hasegawa K *et al.* (1988) X-linked dominant control of F-cells in normal adult life: characterization of the Swiss type as hereditary persistence of fetal hemoglobin regulated dominantly by genes on X chromosome. *Blood* **72**, 1854–1860.

28 Merghoub T, Perichon B, Maier-Redelsperger M, Dibenedetto SP, Samperi P, Ducrocq R *et al.* (1997) Dissection of the association status of two polymorphisms in the β-globin gene cluster with variations in F-cell number in non-anemic individuals. *Am J Hematol* **56**, 239–243.

29 Craig JE, Rochette J, Sampietro M, Wilkie AOM, Barnetson R, Hatton CSR *et al.* (1997) Genetic heterogeneity in heterocellular hereditary persistence of fetal hemoglobin. *Blood* **90**, 428–434.

30 Tadmouri GO, Yuksel L and Basak AN (1998) Hb S/beta (del) thalassemia associated with high hemoglobin A$_2$ and F in a Turkish family. *Am J Hematol* **59**, 83–86.

31 Zertal-Zidani S, Ducrocq R, Weil-Oliver C, Elion J and Krishnamoorthy R (2001) A novel δβ fusion gene expresses hemoglobin A (HbA) not Hb Lepore: Senegalese δ⁰β⁺ thalassaemia. *Blood* **98**, 1261–1263.

32 Viprakasit V, Gibbons RJ, Broughton BC, Tolmie JL, Brown D, Lunt P *et al.* (2001) Mutations in the general transcription factor TFIIH result in beta-thalassaemia in individuals with trichothiodystrophy. *Hum Mol Genet* **10**, 2797–2802.

33 Yu C, Niakan KK, Matsushita M, Stamatoyannopoulos G, Orkin SH and Raskind WH (2002) X-Linked thrombocytopenia with thalassemia from a mutation in the amino finger of GATA-1 affecting DNA binding rather than FOG-1 interaction. *Blood* **100**, 2040–2045.

34 Huisman THJ (1997) Gamma chain abnormal human fetal hemoglobin variants. *Am J Hematol* **55**, 159–163.

35 Steinberg MH and Nagel RL. New and recombinant mutant hemoglobins of biological interest. In: Steinberg MH, Forget BG, Higgs DR and Nagel RL, eds. *Disorders of Hemoglobin: Genetics, Pathophysiology, and Clinical Management.* Cambridge University Press, Cambridge, 2001, pp. 1195–1211.

36 Brennan SO, Shaw J, Allen J and George PM (1992) β141 Leu is not deleted in the unstable haemoglobin Atlanta-Coventry but is replaced by a novel amino acid of mass 128 daltons. *Br J Haematol* **81**, 99–103.

37 Wild BJ, Green BN, Lalloz MRA and Layton DM (2000) When is a minor haemoglobin fraction worthy of investigation? *Br J Haematol* **108** (Suppl. 1), 40.

38 Huisman THJ, Carver MFH and Efremov GD. *A Syllabus of Human Hemoglobin Variants.* The Sickle Cell Anemia Foundation, Augusta, GA, 1996.

## Answers to questions

| 1.1 | (a) T | 1.3 | (a) F | 1.5 | (a) F | 1.7 | (a) T | 1.9 | (a) T | 1.11 | (a) F |
|---|---|---|---|---|---|---|---|---|---|---|---|
| | (b) F | | (b) T | | (b) T | | (b) T | | (b) T | | (b) T |
| | (c) T | | (c) T | | (c) T | | (c) T | | (c) T | | (c) T |
| | (d) T | | (d) T | | (d) F | | (d) T | | (d) T | | (d) F |
| | (e) T | | (e) F | | (e) F | | (e) T | | (e) T | | (e) F |

| 1.2 | (a) T | 1.4 | (a) T | 1.6 | (a) T | 1.8 | (a) T | 1.10 | (a) T |
|---|---|---|---|---|---|---|---|---|---|
| | (b) F | | (b) F | | (b) T | | (b) F | | (b) F |
| | (c) F | | (c) T | | (c) T | | (c) F | | (c) T |
| | (d) T | | (d) T | | (d) T | | (d) T | | (d) F |
| | (e) F | | (e) F | | (e) T | | (e) T | | (e) F |

# 2 Laboratory techniques for the identification of abnormalities of globin chain synthesis

The diagnosis of disorders of haemoglobin chain synthesis usually requires a combination of techniques. It is important to recognize that many of the laboratory tests in routine diagnostic use indicate only the physicochemical characteristics of a haemoglobin rather than permitting its precise identification. For clinical purposes, an adequate presumptive identification usually requires a combination of at least two techniques, with results being assessed in relation to the clinical features, the ethnic origin of the subject and the blood count and film [1]. The principles of the techniques and the selection of technique are discussed in this chapter. Some methods found to be satisfactory in the author's laboratory are given in the Appendix to this chapter (see p. 62). For precise technical details and other recommended methods, the reader is referred to references [2–4].

## Sample collection

Laboratory investigations for haemoglobinopathies are most conveniently performed on venous blood samples anticoagulated with one of the salts of ethylene diamine tetra-acetic acid (e.g. $K_2$EDTA). In the case of children, anticoagulated capillary samples obtained by skin prick, e.g. from the heel, are also suitable. Testing of neonates can be performed on cord blood, venous blood or skin prick samples. To reduce the chances of maternal contamination, cord blood samples should be obtained from an umbilical cord vessel by means of a syringe and needle after wiping away any surface blood. They should not be obtained by squeezing blood from the end of the cord. Skin prick samples from neonates can be taken into a heparinized capillary tube and sent to the laboratory as anticoagulated blood, or can be absorbed onto a filter paper and sent as a dried blood spot, usually referred to as a 'Guthrie spot' from the originator

of the technique. Anticoagulated blood is more stable than dried blood spots and the bands obtained on electrophoresis are more distinct.

Samples should be stored at 4°C and ideally should be tested within a week, as longer storage leads to denaturation of haemoglobin and less distinct bands on electrophoresis. Dried blood spots are stable for 7–10 days at room temperature.

Samples for testing should be accompanied by the full name, date of birth and ethnic origin of the individual to be tested. A knowledge of clinical features and family history is sometimes essential for adequate interpretation, and information on consanguinity is also useful. When blood is taken for genetic counselling of potential parents, identifying details of the partner should also be obtained so that the results of both partners can be assessed simultaneously and guidance on genetic risks can be given. Those responsible for requesting tests and obtaining blood samples should ensure that samples are not inadvertently obtained after a blood transfusion has been given.

## Blood count, film and reticulocyte count

A full blood count (FBC) and a blood film examination are usually indicated whenever an abnormality of globin chain synthesis is suspected. The exception is in neonatal screening for haemoglobinopathies when usually only a small sample of blood, possibly only a dried blood spot, is available for analysis.

The FBC is essential in the assessment of possible thalassaemia and in the differential diagnosis of thalassaemia and hereditary persistence of fetal haemoglobin.

A reticulocyte count is indicated if a blood film shows polychromasia or if haemoglobin H disease or an unstable haemoglobin is suspected (Fig. 2.1).

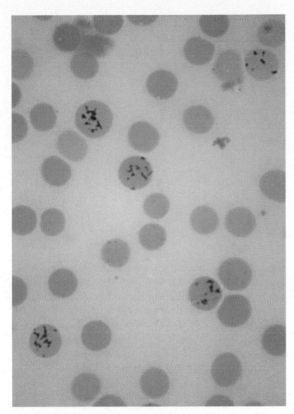

**Fig. 2.1** Reticulocyte preparation showing an increased reticulocyte count in a patient with homozygosity for haemoglobin Bushwick, a mildly unstable haemoglobin.

## Preparing a red cell lysate

A red cell lysate suitable for most purposes is most simply prepared using a lysing reagent containing tetrasodium ethylene diamine tetra-acetic acid and potassium cyanide (1 g/l of $Na_4EDTA$ in 100 mg/l of potassium cyanide). The lysate is prone to oxidation and so should be used within 1 week. If there is a requirement for long-term storage of a lysate, a solution of carbon tetrachloride or toluine is preferred. An alternative is to freeze drops of washed red cells by dropping them on to a layer of liquid nitrogen. When the drops are frozen and the liquid nitrogen has evaporated, they can be stored at −40°C. Long-term storage may be needed for control samples for routine use or to retain a reference preparation of a rare haemoglobin.

The method of preparing a red cell lysate can affect the ability of a laboratory to detect significant abnor-malities. For example, in one study, it was found that, when electrophoresis on agarose at an alkaline pH was employed, it was necessary to prepare the lysate with carbon tetrachloride if haemoglobin H was to be quantified correctly. So much less haemoglobin H was detected with lysates prepared in other ways that cases of haemoglobin H disease could have been missed [5].

## Haemoglobin electrophoresis

Haemoglobin electrophoresis [6,7] is still the most common technique for the initial detection and characterization of a variant haemoglobin, although high performance liquid chromatography (HPLC) is increasingly taking its place. Haemoglobin electrophoresis depends on the principle that, when proteins applied to a membrane are exposed to a charge gradient (Fig. 2.2), they separate from each other and can then be visualized by either a protein stain or a haem stain (Fig. 2.3). Haemoglobin electrophoresis can be carried out on filter paper, a cellulose acetate membrane, a starch gel, a citrate agar gel or an agarose gel. Haemoglobin electrophoresis is best performed on lysed packed red cells so that a consis-tent amount of haemoglobin is applied and there are no bands caused by the presence of plasma proteins. If whole blood is used, the presence of a paraprotein or a very high concentration of polyclonal im-munoglobulins may lead to a prominent band which can be confused with a variant haemoglobin (Fig. 2.4). If this is suspected in a laboratory using whole blood for lysate preparation, plasma should be removed and packed red cells should be washed before a new lysate is prepared.

### Cellulose acetate electrophoresis at alkaline pH

The most useful initial electrophoretic procedure is electrophoresis on cellulose acetate at alkaline pH (pH 8.2–8.6). This permits the provisional identifi-cation of haemoglobins A, F, S/G/D/Lepore, C/E/O-Arab, H and a number of less common variant haemoglobins (Fig. 2.3). Separation is largely but not entirely determined by the electrical charge of the haemoglobin molecule. At this pH, haemoglobin is a negatively charged protein and will move towards

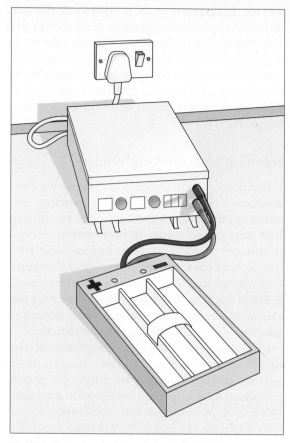

**Fig. 2.2** Diagram of apparatus for performing haemoglobin electrophoresis.

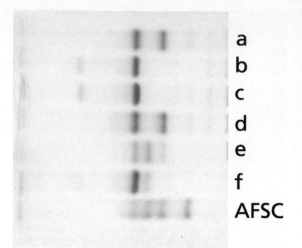

**Fig. 2.3** Haemoglobin electrophoresis on cellulose acetate at pH 8.3 showing: (a) haemoglobins A and S (sickle cell trait); (b) haemoglobins A and H (haemoglobin H disease); (c) haemoglobins A and H (haemoglobin H disease); (d) haemoglobins A and S (sickle cell trait); (e) haemoglobins A, F and S (sickle cell trait in a baby); (f) haemoglobins A and F (normal baby); AFSC, control sample containing haemoglobins A, F, S and C.

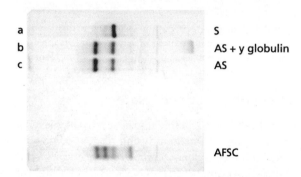

**Fig. 2.4** Haemoglobin electrophoresis on cellulose acetate at pH 8.3 showing an abnormal band caused by the presence of a paraprotein: (a) patient with sickle cell anaemia; (b) patient with sickle cell trait and a paraprotein band; (c) patient with sickle cell trait; AFSC, control sample containing haemoglobins A, F, S and C.

the positively charged anode. A control sample containing haemoglobins A, F, S and C should be run with each set of samples. Control samples containing haemoglobins A, F, S, C, D-Punjab, E, G-Philadelphia and N-Baltimore are commercially available. It should be noted that, if a protein stain rather than a haem stain is used, carbonic anhydrase will be apparent in addition to haemoglobin bands, moving behind haemoglobin $A_2$. With good electrophoretic techniques, haemoglobin F levels greater than 2% can be recognized visually. Good techniques also permit a split $A_2$ band and a significant elevation or reduction of the percentage of haemoglobin $A_2$ to be recognized visually. Recognition of a split $A_2$ band is useful in distinguishing α chain variants, such as haemoglobin G-Philadelphia, from β chain variants, such as haemoglobin D-Punjab. A split $A_2$ band will

be present when there is an α chain variant but not when there is a β chain variant. Recognition of a split $A_2$ band is also essential if β thalassaemia trait is to be diagnosed in individuals who also have a δ chain variant. Recognition of a split $A_2$ band on cellulose acetate electrophoresis requires a fairly heavy appli-

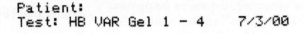

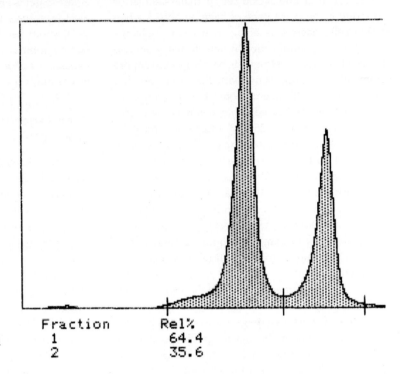

**Fig. 2.5** Scanning densitometry of a cellulose acetate electrophoretic strip showing the quantification of haemoglobin S in a patient who had received an exchange transfusion for sickle cell anaemia; there is approximately 64% haemoglobin A and approximately 36% haemoglobin S.

cation of haemolysate and can be difficult; HPLC (see below) is more reliable. Recognition of increased haemoglobin F on an electrophoretic strip should be followed by precise quantification whenever this is necessary for diagnosis. A visual estimation of the proportion of haemoglobin $A_2$ can be used as a supplement to precise measurement by an appropriate technique.

If a variant haemoglobin with the mobility of haemoglobin S is detected, haemoglobin electrophoresis should be followed by a sickle solubility test. If this is negative or if abnormal bands with other mobilities are present, a supplementary alternative technique (e.g. electrophoresis at acid pH or HPLC) should be used. If bands are very faint or if haemoglobin A appears to be absent (e.g. in a neonatal sample), a supplementary alternative technique should also be used, as both HPLC and electrophoresis on agarose gel at acid pH are more sensitive techniques for the detection of a low concentration of a

variant or normal haemoglobin. A supplementary alternative procedure is also indicated in patients with a positive sickle solubility test and a single band with the mobility of S, in order to distinguish homozygosity for haemoglobin S from compound heterozygosity for S and β chain D or G variants, haemoglobin Korle Bu and haemoglobin Lepore. Flow charts indicating the sequential application of appropriate tests are given in Chapter 7.

Haemoglobin electrophoresis on cellulose acetate can be used for the quantification of normal or variant haemoglobins, either by scanning densitometry (Fig. 2.5) or by elution followed by spectrophotometry. Scanning densitometry requires that the cellulose acetate membrane be rendered transparent by use of a clearing solution, a procedure which some laboratories use routinely, even when scanning is not intended. Scanning densitometry is sufficiently precise to quantify haemoglobins that are present as a large percentage of total haemoglobin. For example, this technique is adequate to determine the percentage of haemoglobin S to permit a distinction between sickle cell trait and sickle cell/β thalassaemia, or to monitor the percentage of haemoglobin S when sickle cell anaemia is being treated by exchange transfusion. Quantification by densitometry can also be used to help distinguish haemoglobin Lepore from other haemoglobins with the same mobility as haemoglobin S; haemoglobin Lepore comprises about 10% of total haemoglobin, whereas haemoglobins D and G comprise 25–50%. Quantification of the haemoglobin $A_2$ percentage by scanning densitometry is not sufficiently precise for the diagnosis of β thalassaemia trait. When cellulose acetate electrophoresis is used for the quantification of haemoglobin $A_2$, elution and spectrometry are required. This is a labour-intensive technique and, when large numbers of samples require testing, microcolumn chromatography or HPLC (see below) is preferred.

Typical mobilities of normal and variant haemoglobins on cellulose acetate electrophoresis at alkaline pH are shown diagrammatically in Fig. 2.6. It should be noted that haemoglobin $A_2$ has the same electrophoretic mobility as haemoglobins C, E, O-Arab and the S–G-Philadelphia hybrid and therefore cannot be quantified by cellulose acetate electrophoresis when any of these variant haemoglobins is present. There are subtle differences in the mobility of haemoglobins D-Punjab and Lepore, in comparison with haemoglobin S; they are both slightly anodal (i.e. slightly faster). Nevertheless, various D and G haemoglobins cannot be reliably distinguished from haemoglobin S by the use of this technique in isolation, and haemoglobin Lepore can be easily distinguished only because it is present in a much lower amount. There are also subtle differences between the mobilities of C and E, with haemoglobin C moving slightly more slowly than haemoglobin E (i.e. being more cathodal) and usually constituting a higher percentage. Nevertheless, a second confirmatory technique is obligatory.

Other characteristics of haemoglobins that have the same mobility as haemoglobin S or haemoglobin C on cellulose acetate electrophoresis are shown in Tables 2.1 and 2.2.

## Agarose gel electrophoresis at alkaline pH

Agarose gel is an alternative to cellulose acetate for electrophoresis at alkaline pH (Fig. 2.7). It is somewhat more sensitive for the detection of variant haemoglobins present in small amounts, but is more expensive and less convenient than cellulose acetate electrophoresis.

## Citrate agar or agarose gel electrophoresis at acid pH

If a variant haemoglobin is detected by electrophoresis on cellulose acetate or agarose at alkaline pH, it is necessary to confirm its identity by an alternative technique. This is often electrophoresis on a citrate agar (Fig. 2.8) or agarose gel (Fig. 2.9) at acid pH (e.g. pH 6.0–6.2). Separated haemoglobins are stained with a haem stain such as o-dianisidine or o-toluidine. With this technique, separation of haemoglobins is dependent not only on their electrical charge, but also on their interaction with various components in the agar or agarose. Agar contains both agarose and agaropectin, a sulphated polysaccharide [8]. Agarose polymerizes and is immobile, but agaropectin is able to complex with some of the amino acids of haemoglobin; the haemoglobin–agaropectin complex then migrates towards the anode, whereas any non-complexed haemoglobin is carried towards the cathode by endo-osmotic flow [8]. There are some differences in the relative mobilities of variant haemoglobins between agarose gel (Fig. 2.6) and citrate agar (Fig. 2.10). Both techniques distinguish S from D/G, but do not distinguish between most types of D and G. Electrophoresis at acid pH will distinguish haemoglobin C from E, C-Harlem and O-Arab and will help to distinguish the latter three variant haemoglobins from each other. Acid agar and agarose gel electrophoresis do not resolve haemoglobin $A_2$ from haemoglobin A. Electrophoresis at acid pH is indicated in the investigation of suspected high-affinity haemoglobins even when electrophoresis at alkaline pH is normal, as some high-affinity haemoglobins have abnormal mobility only at acid pH.

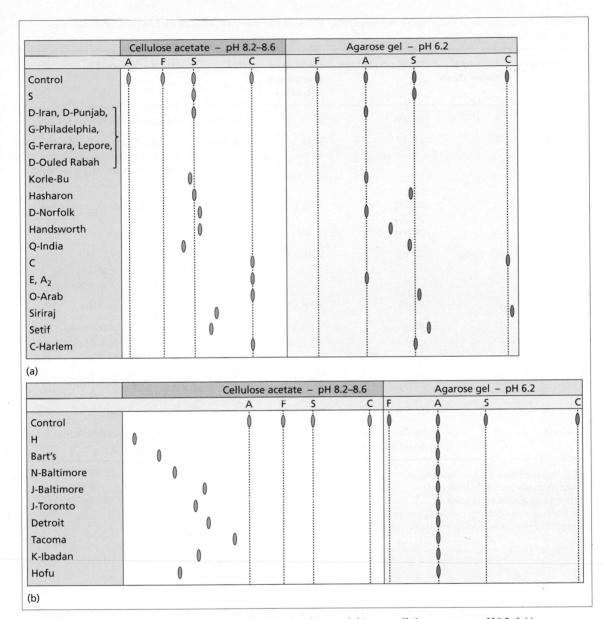

**Fig. 2.6** Diagram showing the mobility of normal and variant haemoglobins on cellulose acetate at pH 8.2–8.6 in comparison with the mobility on agarose gel at pH 6.0–6.2: (a) haemoglobins with mobility close to A, S or C; (b) fast haemoglobins.

**Table 2.1** Characteristics of some variant haemoglobins with the same mobility as haemoglobin S on cellulose acetate electrophoresis at alkaline pH.

| Haemoglobin | Abnormal globin chain | Usual percentage | Mobility on agarose gel at acid pH | HPLC | Usual ethnic origin |
|---|---|---|---|---|---|
| S | β | 40–45* | S | S window | African ancestry, Arab, Indian |
| D-Punjab | β | 40–45* | With A | D window | Punjabi, Northern European, Greek, Turkish, Yugoslav, Afro-American, Afro-Caribbean, Chinese |
| G-Philadelphia | α | 20–25‡ 25–35‡ 35–45‡ | With A | D window† | African ancestry, Chinese, Italian |
| Lepore | δβ fusion | 7–15 | With A | $A_2$ window | Greek, Italian, Turkish, Cypriot, Eastern European, English, Spanish, Afro-Caribbean |
| Korle Bu | β | 40–45 | With A§ | $A_2$ window | West African ancestry |
| G-Coushatta | β | 40–45 | With A | $A_2$ window | Native American, Chinese, Korean, Japanese, Thai, Italian, Turkish, Algerian |
| D-Iran | β | 36–45 | With A | $A_2$ window | Iranian, Pakistani, Italian, Jamaican |
| Zurich | β | 22–35 | With A | $A_2$ window | Swiss, Japanese |
| Hasharon | α | 15–20 (if Jewish) or 30–35 (if Italian) | With S | Between S and C† | Ashkenazi Jewish, Italians from Ferrara district |

HPLC, high performance liquid chromatography.
* Lower if coexisting α thalassaemia trait.
† Variant haemoglobin $A_2$ also present.
‡ Depending on the number of normal α genes present.
§ Or slightly on the S side of A; if present with S, gives a broader band than S alone.

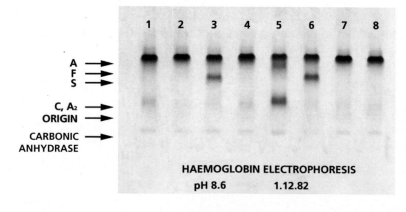

**Fig. 2.7** Haemoglobin electrophoresis on agarose gel at alkaline pH (pH 8.6): (1) haemoglobin A and increased $A_2$ (β thalassaemia trait); (2) haemoglobins A and $A_2$ (normal); (3) haemoglobins A and S (sickle cell trait); (4) haemoglobins A and $A_2$ (normal); (5) haemoglobins A, F and C (haemoglobin C trait in a baby); (6) haemoglobins A and S (sickle cell trait); (7) haemoglobins A and $A_2$ (normal); (8) haemoglobins A and $A_2$ (normal).

**Table 2.2** Characteristics of variant haemoglobins with the same mobility as haemoglobin C on cellulose acetate electrophoresis at alkaline pH.

| Haemoglobin | Relevant globin chain | Usual percentage | Mobility on agarose gel at acid pH | HPLC | Usual ethnic origin |
|---|---|---|---|---|---|
| $A_2$ | δ | 2–3.5* | With A | $A_2$ window | Normal minor haemoglobin |
| C | β | 40–45† | C | C window | West African ancestry |
| E | β | 30–35 | With A | $A_2$ window | South-east Asian |
| O-Arab | β | 40–45 | Slightly on C side of S‡ | Between S and C windows but closer to C window | Eastern European, Afro-American, Afro-Caribbean |
| C-Harlem | β | 40–45† | With S‡ | Between S and C but closer to C window | West African ancestry |
| E-Saskatoon | β | 35–40 | With A | S window | Scottish, Turkish |

HPLC, high performance liquid chromatography.

*3.5–8% in most β thalassaemia trait.

†Lower if coexisting α thalassaemia trait.

‡O-Arab and C-Harlem are more readily distinguished from each other on citrate agar than on agarose; on citrate agar at acid pH, C-Harlem moves with S and O-Arab is between S and A but closer to A.

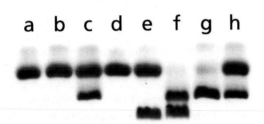

**Fig. 2.8** Haemoglobin electrophoresis on citrate agar at pH 6.0–6.2 showing from left to right: (a) normal (haemoglobin A); (b) normal (haemoglobin A); (c) sickle trait (haemoglobins A and S) with coinheritance of G-Philadelphia; (d) haemoglobins A and J; (e) haemoglobins A and C; (f) haemoglobins S and C; (g) haemoglobin S; (h) haemoglobins A and S. (By courtesy of Dr Barbara Wild.)

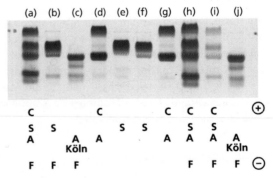

**Fig. 2.9** Haemoglobin electrophoresis on agarose gel at pH 6.0–6.2 showing from left to right: (a) control sample with haemoglobins F, A, S and C; (b) haemoglobins F and S (sickle cell anaemia); (c) haemoglobins F, Köln and A (heterozygosity for haemoglobin Köln); (d) haemoglobins A and C (haemoglobin C trait); (e) haemoglobin S (sickle cell anaemia); (f) haemoglobin S (sickle cell anaemia); (g) haemoglobins A and C (haemoglobin C trait); (h) control sample with haemoglobins F, A, S and C; (i) control sample with haemoglobins F, A, S and C; (j) haemoglobins F, Köln and A (heterozygosity for haemoglobin Köln).

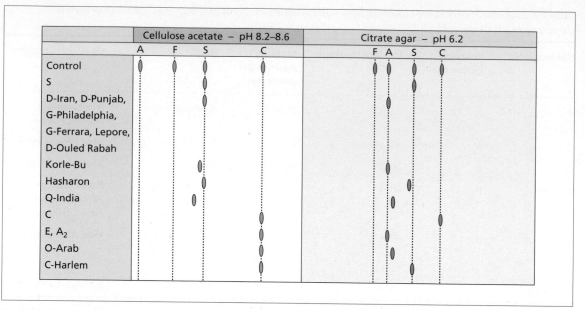

| | Cellulose acetate – pH 8.2–8.6 | | | | Citrate agar – pH 6.2 | | | |
|---|---|---|---|---|---|---|---|---|
| | A | F | S | C | F | A | S | C |
| Control | ● | ● | ● | ● | ● | ● | ● | ● |
| S | | | ● | | | | ● | |
| D-Iran, D-Punjab, G-Philadelphia, G-Ferrara, Lepore, D-Ouled Rabah | | | ● | | | | ● | |
| Korle-Bu | | | ● | | | | | |
| Hasharon | | | ● | | | | ● | |
| Q-India | | ● | | | | ● | | |
| C | | | | ● | | | | ● |
| E, A₂ | | | | ● | | ● | | |
| O-Arab | | | | ● | | ● | | |
| C-Harlem | | | | ● | | | | ● |

**Fig. 2.10** Diagram showing the mobility of normal and variant haemoglobins on cellulose acetate at pH 8.2–8.6 in comparison with the mobility on citrate agar gel at pH 6.0–6.2; the fast haemoglobins shown in Fig. 2.6(b) have the same mobility as haemoglobin A on citrate agar at acid pH.

## Capillary electrophoresis

This term includes capillary zone electrophoresis and capillary isoelectric focusing and refers to electrophoresis or isoelectric focusing carried out in a capillary tube, permitting higher voltages and shorter running times to be used. These methods have the further advantage of a small sample size. Capillary isoelectric focusing can be automated.

## Isoelectric focusing

Isoelectric focusing (IEF) depends on the fact that the net charge of a protein depends on the pH of the surrounding solution. At a low pH, the carboxylic acid groups of proteins are generally uncharged and their N-containing basic groups are fully charged ($NH_3^+$), giving a net positive charge. At high pH, the converse occurs; the carboxylic acid groups are negatively charged ($COO^-$) and the basic groups are uncharged, giving a net negative charge. In IEF, various haemoglobins are separated in a gel (e.g. an agarose gel) ac-

cording to their isoelectric points (pI), i.e. the point at which they have no net charge. Commercially available prepared plates of polyacrylamide or cellulose acetate contain carrier amphoteric molecules with various pI values, establishing a pH gradient across the plate. When a haemolysate is applied to the prepared plate in a strong electric field, the haemoglobin molecules migrate through the plate until they reach the point at which the pH corresponds to the pI of the haemoglobin. Because the haemoglobin molecule then has no net charge, it remains at that point. The various haemoglobin bands are stained (Fig. 2.11) and can be quantified by densitometry (Fig. 2.12). Densitometric traces can be superimposed on traces of known variants to aid in their identification.

Bands on IEF are sharper than those obtained with cellulose acetate electrophoresis. In addition, some haemoglobins that cannot be distinguished from each other by electrophoresis can be separated by IEF. For example, some D and G variants (such as D-Punjab/Los Angeles and G-Philadelphia) can be separated from haemoglobin S and from each other

(Fig. 2.13) [9]. Haemoglobins that can be distinguished from each other by IEF differ between different instrument/reagent systems. Although quantification by densitometry is possible, the precision at low concentrations is poor and this method is therefore not suitable for the quantification of haemoglobin $A_2$. IEF is a more expensive procedure than electrophoresis on cellulose acetate, both because of greater capital costs and because the cost per test is greater. It has a role in diagnosis in neonates when the ability to use a small sample volume or an

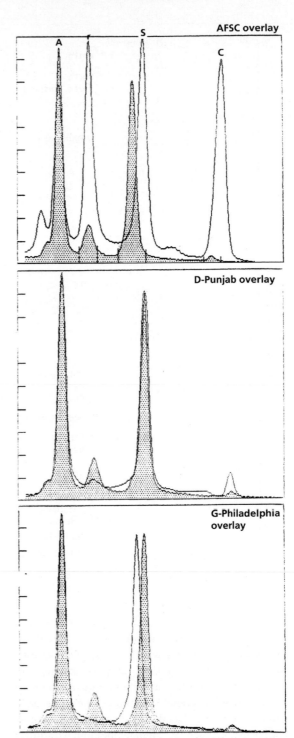

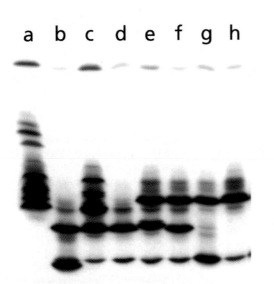

**Fig. 2.11** Photograph of isoelectric focusing plate showing from left to right: (a) haemoglobins F, A and Bart's; (b) haemoglobins S and C; (c) haemoglobins S and F; (d) haemoglobin S; (e) haemoglobins A and D; (f) haemoglobins A and S; (g) haemoglobins A and E; (h) normal (haemoglobins A and $A_2$). (By courtesy of Dr Barbara Wild.)

**Fig. 2.12** Densitometric scanning of one lane of an isoelectric focusing (IEF) plate from a sample showing bands with the mobilities of haemoglobins A and S on cellulose acetate electrophoresis at alkaline pH. The patient's IEF scan is stippled; comparison with an A, F, S, C control sample shows that the variant haemoglobin is not S; comparison with control results for haemoglobin D-Punjab and haemoglobin G-Philadelphia identifies the variant as haemoglobin D-Punjab.

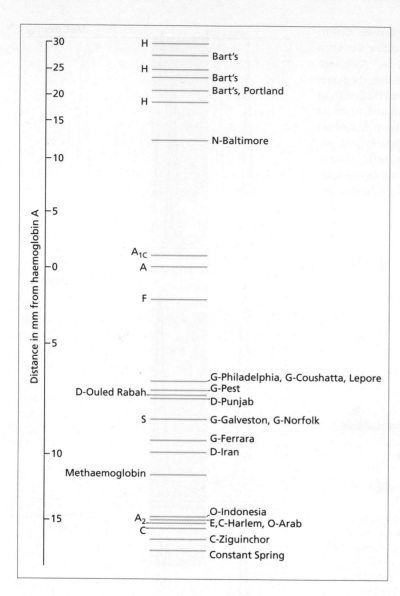

**Fig. 2.13** Diagram showing the mobilities of various haemoglobins on an isoelectric focusing (IEF) plate. Haemoglobins with similar mobility on haemoglobin electrophoresis can be distinguished from each other: haemoglobins $A_2$, C and E can be distinguished from each other (but E cannot be distinguished from C-Harlem and O-Arab); haemoglobins S, D-Punjab and G-Philadelphia can be distinguished from each other (and also from D-Iran and G-Galveston, but G-Philadelphia has the same pI as G-Coushatta and Lepore). (Modified from reference [9].)

eluate from a dried blood spot, together with the ability to obtain good separation of bands, is particularly important. In dealing with samples from adults, the advantages of IEF over cellulose acetate electrophoresis are less important, although the ability to characterize haemoglobins D and G more precisely can be useful. IEF has the disadvantage that minor components, such as methaemoglobin (resulting from ageing of the sample) and glycosylated haemoglobins, are resolved as separate bands and this adds to the complexity and difficulty in interpretation. For routine use in adults, HPLC is a much more useful technique.

## High performance liquid chromatography

Cation-exchange high performance liquid chromatography (CE-HPLC or HPLC) is a process in which a mixture of molecules (such as normal and variant haemoglobins) with a net positive charge is separated into its components by their adsorption onto a negatively charged stationary phase in a chromatography column, followed by their elution by a mobile phase. The mobile phase is a liquid with an increasing concentration of cations flowing through the column; the cations in the mobile phase compete with the adsorbed proteins for the anionic binding sites. Thus the adsorbed positively charged haemoglobin molecules are eluted from the column into the liquid phase at a rate related to their affinity for the stationary phase. When separated in this way, they can be detected optically in the eluate, provisionally identified by their retention time and quantified by computing the area under the corresponding peak in the elution profile. There is some correlation between HPLC retention times and mobility on cellulose acetate electrophoresis at alkaline pH. The more positively charged haemoglobins (e.g. haemoglobins S and C) have a longer retention time, correlating with a slower mobility on cellulose acetate at alkaline pH.

The application of HPLC to the identification of variant haemoglobins depends on the fact that, for each normal or variant haemoglobin on a specified system, there is a characteristic period of time, referred to as the retention time, before the haemoglobin appears in the eluate. Many variant haemoglobins can be separated from each other, although there are some that overlap with others. Some haemoglobins can be resolved by HPLC that are not resolved by cellulose acetate electrophoresis at alkaline pH, e.g. haemoglobins D-Punjab/Los Angeles and G-Philadelphia can be resolved from haemoglobin S and from each other. A slower rate of flow of buffer improves the separation of different haemoglobins with a similar retention time, but increases the time taken to process each sample. Haemoglobins eluted from the column are represented graphically and automatically quantified by spectroscopy; the retention time is stated in relation to that expected for a known normal or abnormal haemoglobin (usually in relation to haemoglobin A, F, S, C or D).

The automated HPLC instruments currently in use are of a high precision and are moderately rapid; they use specially designed microbore columns, high precision gradient-forming liquid pumps and optical detectors. There is computer control and data handling and sometimes computer/intranet-assisted interpretation.

HPLC can be used not only for the detection, provisional identification and quantification of variant haemoglobins, but also for the quantification of haemoglobins A, $A_2$ and F. Control materials for monitoring the precision of measurements of haemoglobins F and $A_2$ are commercially available. HPLC has the following advantages over haemoglobin electrophoresis:

- the technique is less labour intensive;
- a very small sample is adequate;
- quantification of normal and variant haemoglobins is available for each sample;
- as haemoglobin $A_2$ is quantified, β thalassaemia trait can be diagnosed in a single procedure, replacing the combination of haemoglobin electrophoresis and microcolumn chromatography (see below);
- a larger range of variant haemoglobins can be provisionally identified;
- a haemoglobin $A_2$ variant can be detected easily, thus facilitating the differentiation of α and β chain variants (even those with identical retention times) and making the diagnosis of β thalassaemia trait when a δ chain variant is present more accurate.

The main disadvantages are the higher capital and reagent costs. However, if the greater labour costs of electrophoresis are considered, in developed countries with high wages the overall costs are comparable [10].

Considerable skill and experience are needed in interpreting the results of HPLC as the data produced are quite complex. Glycosylated variant haemoglobins have different elution times from non-glycosylated forms and acetylated haemoglobins from non-acetylated forms (haemoglobin F is partially acetylated). In addition, a variant haemoglobin may have the same retention time as either a normal haemoglobin or another variant. For example, haemoglobin E, haemoglobin Korle Bu and haemoglobin Lepore may overlap with haemoglobin $A_2$, and haemoglobin $A_2$ may be falsely elevated in the presence of haemoglobin S. Glycosylated haemoglobin S may have a retention time the same as, or very similar to, that of haemoglobin A, so that patients with sickle cell anaemia may be thought to have a small amount of haemoglobin A (Fig. 2.14). With some instruments and programmes, haemoglobin F may merge with the peak resulting from glycosylated haemoglobin A and may not be detected

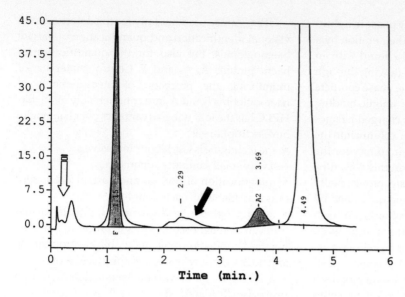

**Fig. 2.14** Bio-Rad Variant II HPLC chromatogram from a patient with sickle cell anaemia showing glycosylated haemoglobin S with the same retention time as haemoglobin A (black arrow) and haemoglobin F including acetylated form (white arrow).

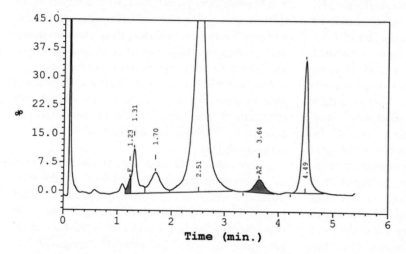

**Fig. 2.15** Bio-Rad Variant II HPLC chromatogram from a patient with a bilirubin of 970 mmol/l showing a peak in the same region as haemoglobin Bart's; from left to right, the peaks are bilirubin, haemoglobin F, altered haemoglobin A (two peaks) and haemoglobins A, $A_2$ and S.

when it is 0.6% or less [11]. Conversely, an elevated percentage of glycosylated haemoglobin A may lead to a factitious elevation of haemoglobin F [11]. Certain artefacts need to be recognized; for example, increased bilirubin in the plasma may lead to a sharp peak in the same general area as haemoglobin H, haemoglobin Bart's and acetylated haemoglobin F (Fig. 2.15). The haemoglobins that can be distinguished from each other vary somewhat between different instruments and reagent systems. However, all systems permit the provisional identification of many more variant haemoglobins than can be distin-

guished by electrophoresis. Haemoglobins A, $A_2$, F, S, C, O-Arab, D-Punjab and G-Philadelphia can be separated from each other. However, haemoglobin E usually overlaps with haemoglobin $A_2$. The nature of any variant haemoglobin detected by HPLC should be confirmed by an alternative technique.

Evaluations of a number of the automated HPLC systems that are now commercially available have been published [11–15].

Typical elution patterns of normal and variant haemoglobins are shown in Figs 2.16–2.18, and some of the variants that may have retention times

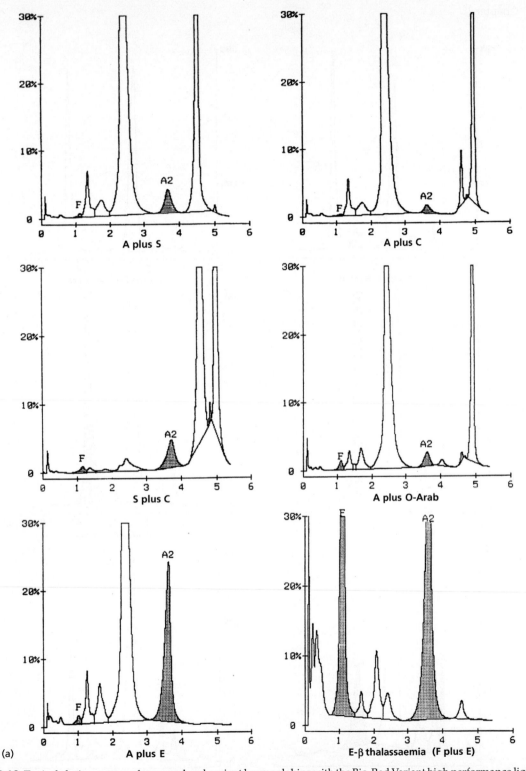

(a)

**Fig. 2.16** Typical elution patterns for normal and variant haemoglobins with the Bio-Rad Variant high performance liquid chromatography (HPLC) system. Unless specified, heterozygosity is illustrated: (a) some clinically relevant haemoglobins; (b) some haemoglobins that have the same mobility as haemoglobin S on cellulose acetate electrophoresis at alkaline pH, but can be distinguished by HPLC; (c) Q-India plus some variant haemoglobins that are 'fast' on cellulose acetate electrophoresis at alkaline pH; (d) miscellaneous variant haemoglobins including heterozygosity for Tacoma, which cannot be distinguished from haemoglobin A. Note that in the case of A plus H and A plus Korle Bu the Y axis is in volts rather than percentages as the A_2 peak was too low for the instrument to standardize. (*Continued on pp. 40–42.*)

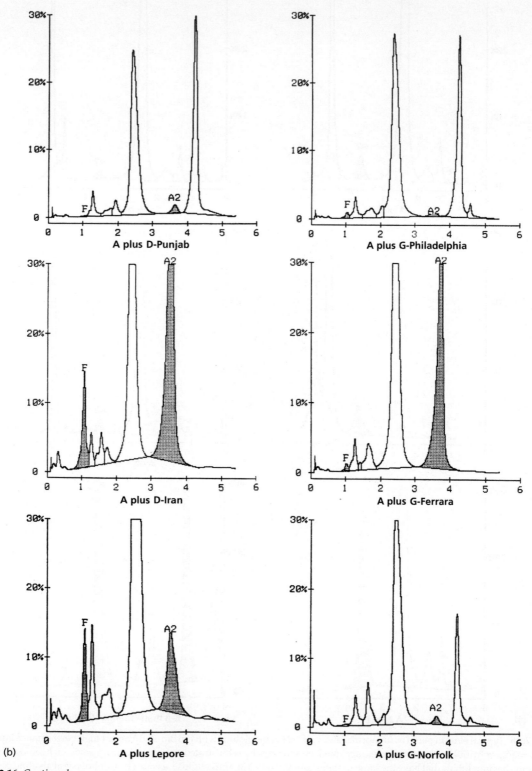

**Fig. 2.16** *Continued.*

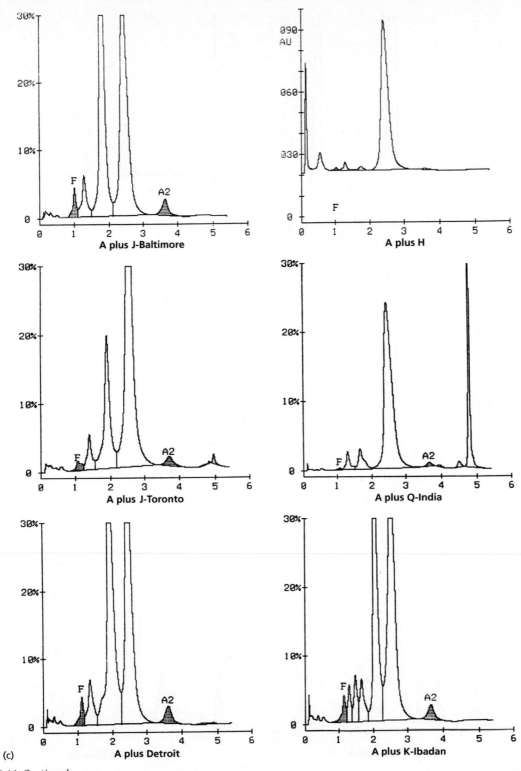

(c)

**Fig. 2.16** *Continued.*

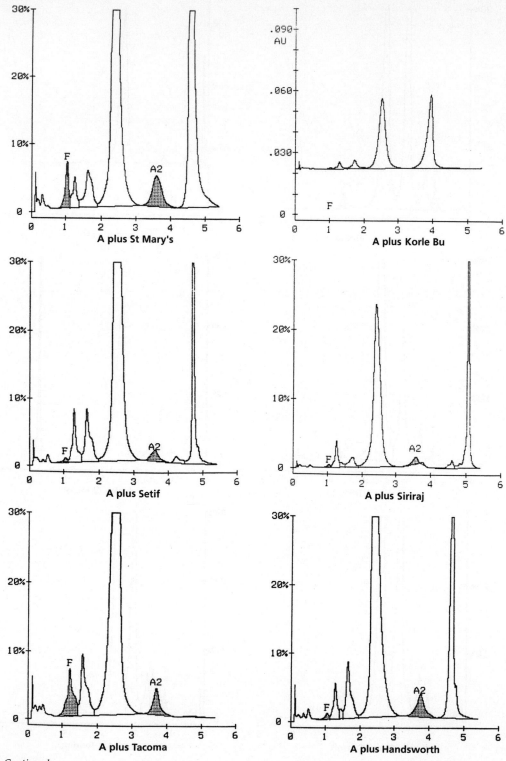

(d)

**Fig. 2.16** *Continued.*

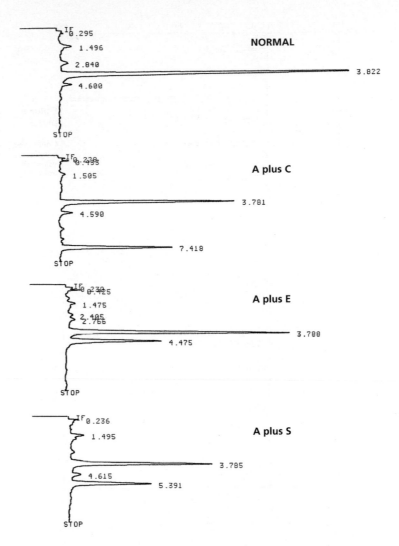

**Fig. 2.17** Typical elution patterns for normal and variant haemoglobins with the Primus Corporation CLC330 high performance liquid chromatography (HPLC) system showing a normal pattern (with haemoglobin A and haemoglobin $A_2$) and patterns from patients with haemoglobin C trait, haemoglobin E trait and haemoglobin S trait.

overlapping with those of haemoglobin $A_2$ and haemoglobin S are shown in Table 2.3.

## Sickle solubility test and other methods for the detection of haemoglobin S

### Sickle test

The presence of haemoglobin S can be demonstrated by a sickle test in which sickle cell formation is induced when blood is deoxygenated. A drop of blood is placed between a glass slide and a cover slip and is sealed with molten paraffin wax so that the metabolic activity of white cells leads to deoxygenation.

After an appropriate period of time, the preparation is observed with a microscope. In a common modification of the method, the drop of blood is first mixed with a drop of 2% sodium metabisulphite and the preparation is observed at 24 h. These methods are not very suitable for use in a routine diagnostic laboratory where their place has largely been taken by the sickle solubility test.

### Sickle solubility test

A sickle solubility test should be performed whenever a variant haemoglobin with the electrophoretic or HPLC characteristics of haemoglobin S is detected.

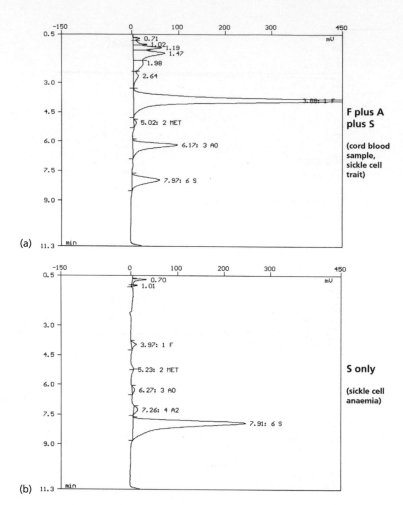

**F plus A plus S**

(cord blood sample, sickle cell trait)

**S only**

(sickle cell anaemia)

**Fig. 2.18** Typical elution patterns for normal and variant haemoglobins with the Kontron Instruments Haemoglobin System PV high performance liquid chromatography (HPLC) system showing sickle cell trait in a baby (F, A and S) (a), sickle cell anaemia (S as the only major band) (b), haemoglobin C trait (c) and haemoglobin E trait (d).

The only exception is when the quantity of the variant haemoglobin present is so low that a positive sickle solubility test would be unlikely; in this circumstance, an alternative second technique should be employed to strengthen the presumptive identification of the variant haemoglobin. It is also prudent to perform a sickle solubility test whenever a variant haemoglobin of uncertain nature is present, as there are a number of abnormal haemoglobins that have a second amino acid substitution in addition to the glutamic acid for valine substitution of haemoglobin S (see Table 4.2). These variant haemoglobins may have an electrophoretic mobility that differs from that of haemoglobin S, but nevertheless their presence leads to red cell sickling *in vitro* and *in vivo*.

A sickle solubility test can be performed by purchasing the necessary reagents or commercial kits that include the necessary reagents [3,16]. A number of kits have been evaluated and have been found to detect haemoglobin S down to a concentration of 20% and sometimes below — in some cases as low as 8% [16]. Positive and negative controls should be included whenever a patient sample is tested (Fig. 2.19). If the patient is anaemic, it is essential to correct the haematocrit to about 0.50 in order to avoid false negative tests. This can be carried out by removing some of the plasma, but it is preferable for a sickle solubility test to be performed on reconstituted packed red cells in order to avoid problems from anaemia and also to lessen the possibility of false pos-

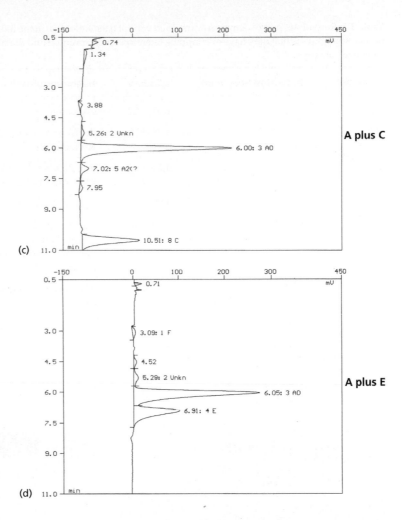

**Fig. 2.18** *Continued.*

itive tests when an abnormal plasma protein is present (Fig. 2.20) or when there is hyperlipidaemia. Other causes of false positive tests include a very high count of either white cells or nucleated red cells or a Heinz body haemolytic anaemia, see below. Most methods require that all negative or equivocal sickle solubility tests be centrifuged before reading to increase the sensitivity and reliability. It is important that this step is not omitted if samples with a relatively low percentage of haemoglobin S are to be detected reliably. It should be noted that the presence of not only a paraprotein but also large numbers of Heinz bodies can cause a false positive sickle solubility test. The latter phenomenon may lead to a false positive test in a patient with an unsta-

ble haemoglobin, particularly if the patient has been splenectomized.

Sickle solubility tests should be capable of giving positive results in all cases of sickle cell trait beyond the period of early infancy, even when there is coexisting α thalassaemia trait. However, they should not be relied on in early infancy when the percentage of haemoglobin S may be a great deal less than 20%. In this circumstance, the provisional identification of haemoglobin S should be based on two independent methods other than a sickle solubility test, e.g. IEF plus HPLC or cellulose acetate electrophoresis plus an immunoassay.

All sickle solubility tests, whether positive, negative or equivocal, should be confirmed by haemoglo-

**Table 2.3** Retention times of common normal and variant haemoglobins on the Bio-Rad Variant II system compared with other haemoglobins that may have overlapping retention times; common and diagnostically important haemoglobins are shown in bold type.

| 'Window' | Retention time (min) | Window | Haemoglobins that may overlap |
|---|---|---|---|
| F | 1.10 | 0.98–1.22 | Okayama |
| 'P2'* | 0.11 | 1.28–1.50 | Beckman, Geelong, **glycosylated A**, Hope, I-Philadelphia, K-Woolwich |
| 'P3'† | 1.70 | 1.50–1.90 | Buffalo, Camden, Fannin-Lubbock, Grady, J-Bangkok, J-Meerut, J-Baltimore, J-Norfolk, N-Baltimore |
| A | 2.50 | 1.90–3.10 | **A**, glycosylated S, New York, Köln (when not denatured) |
| $A_2$ | 3.60 | 3.30–3.90 | Deer Lodge, D-Ouled Rabah, D-Iran, **E**, G-Copenhagen, G-Coushatta, G-Ferrara, G-Honolulu, Kenya, Korle Bu, **Lepore**, M-Saskatoon‡, Osu-Cristiansborg, Spanish Town, Zurich |
| D | 4.10 | 3.90–4.30 | Alabama, **D-Punjab**, G-Norfolk, **G-Philadelphia**, Kempsey, Osler |
| S | 4.50 | 4.30–4.70 | Q-Thailand (Mahidol), $A_2'$, Manitoba |
| C | 5.10 | 4.90–5.30 | Agenogi, **C**, Siriraj, **Constant Spring** |

*A glycosylated fraction of haemoglobin A.
† A minor peak representing modified haemoglobin A.
‡ Plus a second peak in the C window.

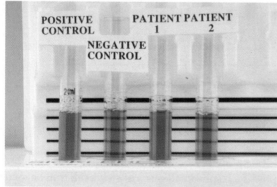

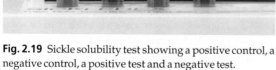

**Fig. 2.19** Sickle solubility test showing a positive control, a negative control, a positive test and a negative test.

**Fig. 2.20** False positive sickle solubility test caused by increased plasma proteins. From left to right: a negative control, a positive control (before and after centrifugation) and a false positive result caused by a myeloma protein (before and after centrifugation).

bin electrophoresis or an alternative technique in order to: (i) confirm the presence of haemoglobin S; (ii) distinguish sickle cell trait from sickle cell anaemia and from compound heterozygous states, and (iii) detect false negative results due to technical

error or an unusually low percentage of haemoglobin S. If rapid results are required, e.g. before emergency anaesthesia, the distinction between sickle cell trait and sickle cell anaemia or compound heterozygous states can be made with reasonable accuracy by combining a sickle solubility test with a blood film and a blood count (see Chapter 4).

In general, a sickle solubility test is not indicated in an infant less than 6 months of age, as a negative result may be misleading. However, a sickle solubility test can sensibly be performed before an emergency anaesthetic as, if it is negative, it is unlikely that anaesthesia will cause any clinical problems. The wording of the report on such a test must state that a negative test does not exclude the presence of a low percentage of haemoglobin S and that further testing is necessary and will follow.

## Other tests for haemoglobin S

A modification of the gel technology used for blood grouping has been designed for the detection of haemoglobin S, the principle being that cells which have sickled will not pass through the gel; this test has been found to be unreliable and cannot be recommended [17]. Haemoglobin S can also be detected by immunoassay (see below).

## Quantification of haemoglobin $A_2$

### Choice of method

Haemoglobin $A_2$ can be quantified with acceptable accuracy by:

* HPLC;
* microcolumn chromatography;
* cellulose acetate electrophoresis followed by elution and spectrophotometry;
* capillary zone electrophoresis.

Elution followed by spectrophotometry is only satisfactory for dealing with relatively small numbers of samples. Cellulose acetate electrophoresis followed by scanning densitometry is not sufficiently precise to be recommended [18,19]. This technique has a coefficient of variation (CV) of around 20%, in comparison with a CV of 3–4% for the recommended techniques [18]. Similarly, IEF is unsuitable as it has a CV of 20% or more [20]. It should be noted that, when using HPLC, the haemoglobin $A_2$ percentage is overestimated in the presence of haemoglobin S [21].

## Microcolumn chromatography

Microcolumn chromatography is an anion-exchange chromatography method. Microcolumns are prepared containing a suspension of an anion-exchange resin in buffer. The resin is composed of small particles of cellulose covalently bound to small positively charged molecules. A haemoglobin solution is applied to the column and is adsorbed on to the resin. There is then an interchange of charged groups between the positively charged resin and the negatively charged haemoglobin molecules, which retards the passage of haemoglobin through the column. The strength of the association of various types of haemoglobin molecule to the matrix can be altered by alterations in the pH and ionic strength of an eluting solution applied to the column. It is therefore possible to elute different haemoglobins selectively by using different eluting solutions (Fig. 2.21). When this method is used for the quantification of haemoglobin $A_2$, there is elution of haemoglobin $A_2$ first and then, using a second eluting solution, of haemoglobin A. The two fractions are collected separately and the absorbance of the eluate is read on a spectrophotometer, permitting the expression of the amount of haemoglobin $A_2$ present as a percentage of total haemoglobin. Alternatively, it is possible to elute only haemoglobin $A_2$ and to measure total haemoglobin in a second tube.

Microcolumn chromatography is a satisfactory technique for the quantification of haemoglobin $A_2$ when relatively large numbers of samples are to be assayed. Chromatography columns can be prepared by individual laboratories, but are more often purchased in kit form.

It should be noted that the standard column for the measurement of haemoglobin $A_2$ in suspected β thalassaemia trait is not suitable for haemoglobin $A_2$ quantification in the presence of haemoglobin S. Modified columns for this purpose can be prepared and are also available commercially.

It should, however, be noted that the measurement of haemoglobin $A_2$ in the presence of haemoglobin S is not essential for making a distinction between sickle cell/β+ thalassaemia and sickle cell trait. This distinction can be more readily made by quantifying haemoglobin S, as S is more than 50% of total

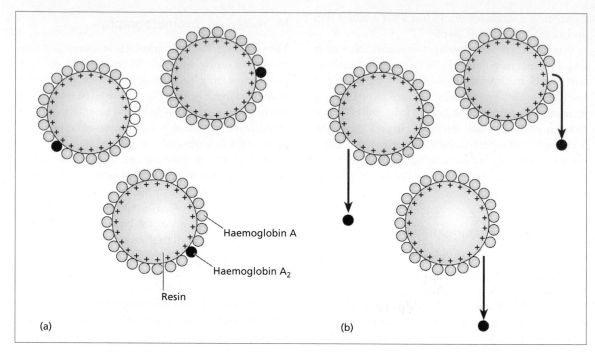

**Fig. 2.21** Diagrammatic representation of the principle of microcolumn chromatography: (a) both haemoglobin A (pink) and haemoglobin $A_2$ (dark red) are negatively charged and are bound to the positively charged beads of the anion-exchange resin; (b) with application of an eluting solution that alters the pH and ionic strength, haemoglobin $A_2$ is eluted whereas haemoglobin A remains attached to the matrix beads.

haemoglobin in sickle cell/$\beta^+$ thalassaemia and less than 50% in sickle cell trait. Expressed in another way, there is more haemoglobin A than S in sickle cell trait and more haemoglobin S than A in sickle cell/$\beta^+$ thalassaemia. Measuring haemoglobin $A_2$ in the presence of haemoglobin S is of limited value in distinguishing between sickle cell anaemia and sickle cell/$\beta^0$ thalassaemia (see pp. 160 and 172). It should be noted, in addition, that coexisting $\alpha$ thalassaemia trait will influence these values. Overlap occurs between these two conditions and interpretation should be undertaken with caution. In general, quantifying haemoglobin $A_2$ in the presence of haemoglobin S is not a test that a laboratory needs to perform.

Microcolumn chromatography should be combined with haemoglobin electrophoresis at alkaline pH in order to detect any variant haemoglobins. It should be noted that an increased haemoglobin $A_2$ percentage may occur in the presence of an unstable haemoglobin and, if there is any reason to suspect that a case is not a straightforward $\beta$ thalassaemia trait, a specific test for an unstable haemoglobin should be performed.

A reference range should be determined in each individual laboratory using blood samples from healthy subjects with a normal haemoglobin concentration and normal red cell indices. Results just above the upper limit of normal, e.g. 3.4–3.7%, should be regarded as equivocal, should be interpreted in the light of clinical and haematological features and should usually be repeated on the same sample and also on a second sample.

## Capillary zone electrophoresis

Capillary zone electrophoresis can be used to quantify haemoglobin $A_2$ and has been reported to be more satisfactory than microcolumn chromatography in patients with sickle cell trait [22].

## Immunoassay for variant haemoglobins

Haemoglobin A and certain variant haemoglobins can be detected immunologically. Kits were previously commercially available for the immuno-detection of haemoglobins S, C, E and A, known respectively as HemoCard Hemoglobin S, Hemo-Card Hemoglobin C, HemoCard Hemoglobin E and HemoCard Hemoglobin A. This technique is potentially useful and, when functioning properly, all HemoCards detect the relevant variant haemo-globins at least down to 10% and sometimes down to 5% [16,23,34]. However, there were problems with consistent availability and quality control of kits. Potential roles, if these problems could be overcome, include the confirmation of the presence of haemo-globin S in a neonate when a variant haemoglobin is detected by IEF or HPLC and confirmation of the presence of haemoglobin E or C following detection of a variant haemoglobin by HPLC or cellulose acetate electrophoresis.

## Quantification of haemoglobin F and determination of the distribution of haemoglobin F

Haemoglobin F can be quantified by HPLC or by haemoglobin electrophoresis followed by scanning densitometry or elution and spectrophotometry. Densitometry is unreliable below 10–15% and either HPLC or alkali denaturation (a modification of Betke's method [3]) is then preferred to densitometry. HPLC gives estimates somewhat higher than alkali denaturation [12,14]. For levels above 50%, scanning densitometry, elution and spectrophotometry or HPLC is preferred as alkali denaturation is inaccurate. Chromatograms should be examined carefully if haemoglobin F is apparently increased on HPLC, as an increased glycosylated haemoglobin is sometimes misidentified as haemoglobin F [4]. If haemoglobin F appears to be greater than 10% on HPLC, its nature should be confirmed by an alternative test to exclude misidentification of haemoglobin N or haemoglobin J as haemoglobin F [4]. Haemoglobin F can also be quantified by an immunoassay, using radial immunodiffusion, but this method has been found to be inaccurate [25] and therefore cannot be recommended.

The distribution of haemoglobin F between individual red cells can be determined by the Kleihauer test or, more reliably, by flow cytometry.

### Kleihauer test

A Kleihauer test is useful for confirmation whenever there appears to be an increased percentage of haemoglobin F (see Fig. 6.3). The distribution of haemoglobin F between cells can help to distinguish δβ thalassaemia trait, in which the distribution of haemoglobin F is usually heterocellular, from many cases of hereditary persistence of fetal haemoglobin, in which the distribution of haemoglobin F is pancel-lular (see Table 3.13).

### Quantification of cells containing haemoglobin F

Cells containing haemoglobin F (F cells) can be quantified by flow cytometry using permeabilized red cells and a fluorochrome-conjugated monoclonal antibody to haemoglobin F [26]. This method is applicable to the quantification of feto-maternal haemorrhage as well as to the study of patients with disorders of globin chain synthesis. By combining a labelled antibody to haemoglobin F with a fluo-rochrome that binds to nucleic acids, it is possible to quantify F cells, reticulocytes and F reticulocytes by flow cytometry [27].

## Detection of haemoglobin H inclusions

A technique for the demonstration of haemoglobin H inclusions should be performed for confirmation when haemoglobin H disease is suspected and when haemoglobin electrophoresis shows a band with a mobility similar to haemoglobin H. Whether this test should also be performed in suspected α thalas-saemia is open to debate (see p. 76).

The principle of the test is that haemoglobin H precipitates following exposure to a mild oxidant, such as brilliant cresyl blue. The appearance of haemoglo-bin H inclusions differs according to whether or not the patient has had a splenectomy. If no splenectomy has been performed, small blue-staining inclusions are evenly distributed through the cell, an appear-ance compared to a golf ball (Fig. 2.22). In patients

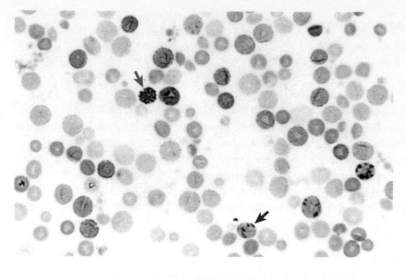

**Fig. 2.22** A haemoglobin H preparation showing haemoglobin H inclusions (blue arrow) and reticulocytes (red arrow).

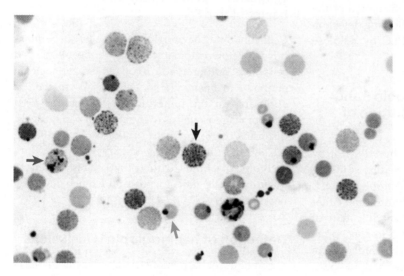

**Fig. 2.23** A haemoglobin H preparation showing haemoglobin H inclusions (red arrow), reticulocytes (blue arrow) and preformed Heinz bodies (green arrow).

with haemoglobin H disease who have had a splenectomy, haemoglobin H is present as preformed Heinz bodies and, in addition, typical 'golf-ball' inclusions appear during incubation with vital dyes (Fig. 2.23).

## Detection of an unstable haemoglobin

Unstable haemoglobins can be detected using either a heat test or an isopropanol test. Tests should be set up with a positive and a negative control. A positive result is the appearance of a precipitate at the end point of the test that is not present in a normal control (Fig. 2.24). The test should be performed promptly, as ageing of the blood can lead to a false positive result due to the formation of methaemoglobin. If any delay has occurred, the negative control should be of the same age as the test sample. An aged fetal sample is suitable as a positive control. The fact that haemoglobin F is less stable than haemoglobin A complicates testing if an unstable fetal haemoglobin is suspected. In this circumstance, a fetal sample with a similar proportion of haemoglobin F should be used as the negative control. False positive tests can result

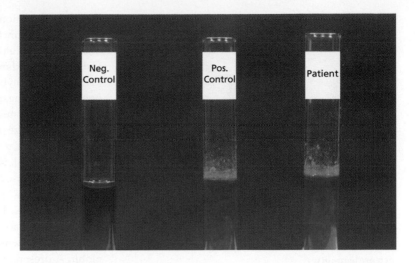

**Fig. 2.24** An isopropanol test for an unstable haemoglobin.

from the presence of haemoglobin S or an increased percentage of haemoglobin F.

The isopropanol test is less sensitive than the heat stability test and some slightly unstable haemoglobins do not give a positive result.

## Detection of Heinz bodies

Testing for Heinz bodies, by incubation with either methyl violet or brilliant cresyl blue, is relevant whenever an unstable haemoglobin is suspected, e.g. unexplained anaemia with an increased reticulocyte count, irregularly contracted cells on a blood film or blurred bands or peaks on electrophoresis and HPLC, respectively (Fig. 2.25). If Heinz bodies are not detected in a fresh specimen, they may appear after incubation at 37°C for 24 h. They are more likely to be present after splenectomy.

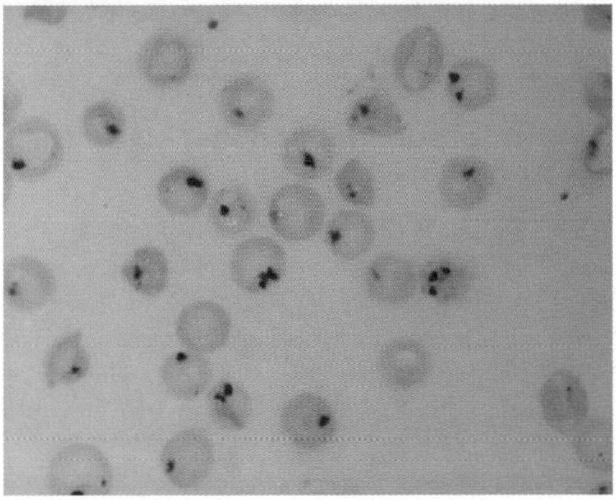

**Fig. 2.25** A Heinz body preparation (incubation with methyl violet) in a patient with haemoglobin Southampton. (With thanks to Mr D. Roper.)

## Osmotic fragility as a screening test for thalassaemia

In underdeveloped countries without easy access to automated blood counters, a simple visual one-tube osmotic fragility test has been used as a screening test for thalassaemia trait [28]. The principle is that the hypochromic cells of thalassaemia trait are osmotically resistant and, whereas normal cells lyse in buffered saline of a certain concentration, thalassaemia trait cells do not, and so there is a cloudy suspension rather than a clear solution. Cells from individuals with iron deficiency or haemoglobin E trait may also fail to lyse. The test can be performed on a finger prick sample and the number of patients requiring phlebotomy and definitive tests is thereby reduced. In one study using 0.34% saline, all samples from individuals with $\alpha^0$ thalassaemia were identified [29]. For $\beta$ thalassaemia trait, 0.34% saline is not sufficiently sensitive, 0.36%

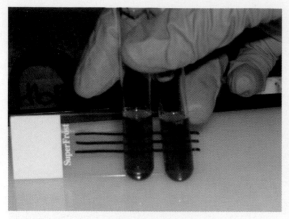

**Fig. 2.26** A 2,6-dichlorophenolindophenol (DCIP) test being read on a light box with a striped glass slide to increase legibility.

being needed [30]. False positive tests, e.g. as a result of iron deficiency, are not infrequent.

## 2,6-Dichlorophenolindophenol test for haemoglobin E screening

When resources are limited, a 2,6-dichlorophenolindophenol (DCIP) test can be used to screen for haemoglobin E [31,32] (Fig. 2.26). This reduces the number of samples that need to be referred to a central laboratory for definitive diagnosis. The test is read visually, but is harder to read than a sickle solubility test.

## Quantification of haemoglobin $A_{1c}$

Haemoglobin $A_{1c}$ is a glycosylated derivative of haemoglobin A. As haemoglobin $A_{1c}$ can be quantified by HPLC or ion-exchange microcolumn chromatography; quantification is sometimes performed by haemoglobinopathy laboratories.

The percentage of haemoglobin $A_{1c}$ is determined by the red cell life span and by the average blood glucose level during the life of the red cell. High levels are thus noted in diabetes mellitus, particularly when control is poor, and also when there has been a recent arrest of red cell production. Low levels are seen when there is a young red cell population, and this has been suggested as an aid to distinguishing haemolytic anaemia from other types of anaemia

[33]. Quantification has also been suggested in order to make a distinction between transient erythroblastopenia of childhood (increased percentage) and Diamond–Blackfan syndrome (normal percentage) [34]. The mean level is increased in iron deficiency, in one study the mean being 6.15% pre-treatment and 5.25% post-treatment [35].

The percentage of haemoglobin $A_{1c}$, measured by HPLC, may be erroneous in the presence of a variant haemoglobin [8]. Factitious elevation can be the result of an increased percentage of haemoglobin F or the presence of a 'fast' haemoglobin, such as haemoglobin I, J or N. Haemoglobin Hope and haemoglobin Raleigh also have retention times similar to glycosylated haemoglobin A. If there is no haemoglobin A present, haemoglobin $A_{1c}$ will necessarily be zero. Haemoglobin $A_{1c}$ may also appear to be low if there is a variant haemoglobin present (e.g. S, C, D, G, E) and the percentage of haemoglobin $A_{1c}$ is quantified as a percentage of total haemoglobin, ignoring the fact that there will also be a glycosylated component of the variant haemoglobin (Fig. 2.27). An alternative technique (affinity column chromatography) permits the quantification of haemoglobin $A_{1c}$ despite the presence of a variant haemoglobin.

A high glycosylated fraction may be noted during investigation of a suspected variant haemoglobin. If the patient is not known to suffer from diabetes, the presence of an elevated level should be reported and definitive testing for diabetes is then appropriate [36].

## Other more specialized tests

Some more specialized tests are required infrequently and are generally better performed in a regional centre or reference laboratory rather than in a routine diagnostic laboratory. The exception is in certain geographical areas where a high prevalence of specific disorders of haemoglobin synthesis makes it cost-effective for laboratories in large hospitals to carry out specific specialized tests. For completeness, these tests are discussed briefly in this chapter.

### Detection of high-affinity haemoglobins

An oxygen dissociation curve with the determination of $P_{50}$ (the $P_{O_2}$ at which haemoglobin is 50% satu-

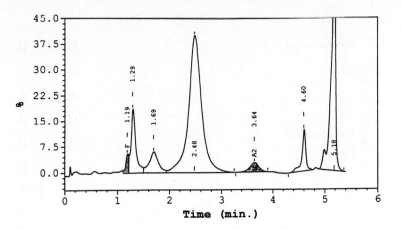

**Fig. 2.27** Bio-Rad Variant II HPLC chromatogram from a patient with haemoglobin C trait showing glycosylated haemoglobin A and glycosylated haemoglobin C; from left to right, the peaks are haemoglobin F, glycosylated haemoglobin A (retention time 1.29 min), other post-translationally modified A, haemoglobin A, haemoglobin A$_2$, glycosylated haemoglobin C (retention time 4.6 min) and haemoglobin C.

rated) should be measured if a high-oxygen-affinity haemoglobin is suspected (Fig. 2.28).

## Globin chain electrophoresis

Globin chain electrophoresis (Fig. 2.29) is carried out on a red cell lysate to which DL-dithiothreitol and urea have been added to dissociate the haem groups and globin chains. Electrophoresis is then carried out on cellulose acetate membranes using both acid and alkaline buffer systems. Globin chain electrophoresis permits a distinction between α and β chain abnormalities and, when used as a supplement to haemoglobin electrophoresis, allows a presumptive identification of a larger range of variant haemoglobins. This method has become relatively unimportant since the wider availability of HPLC has provided an alternative technique that is much more rapid and less labour intensive.

## Analysis of the rate of globin chain synthesis

The relative rates of synthesis of α and β globin chains by reticulocytes or bone marrow cells can be useful in the diagnosis of thalassaemias. This is determined by the amount of radioactivity incorporated into α and β chains after a fixed period of time. This technique is critically dependent on the blood or bone marrow sample being fresh, i.e. less than 6 h old. The results are usually expressed as a

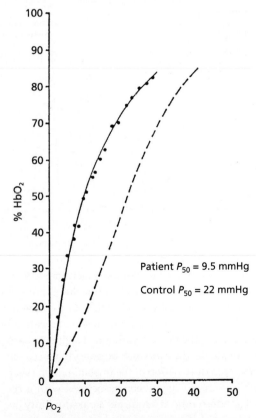

**Fig. 2.28** Oxygen dissociation curves showing haemoglobin A (broken line) and a high-affinity haemoglobin, haemoglobin Heathrow (full line). (By courtesy of Mr D. Roper.)

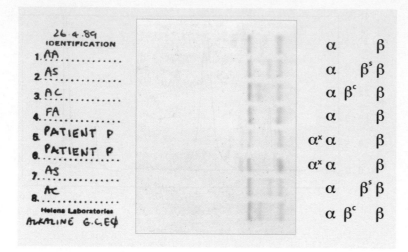

**Fig. 2.29** Results of globin chain synthesis analysis showing: (1) α and β chain (normal); (2) α, $\beta^S$ and β chain (sickle cell trait); (3) α, $\beta^C$ and β chain (haemoglobin C trait); (4) α and β chain (normal); (5) $\alpha^{variant}$, α and β chain (identifying an unknown variant as being an α chain variant); (6) $\alpha^{variant}$, α and β chain (identifying an unknown variant as being an α chain variant); (7) α, $\beta^S$ and β chain (sickle cell trait); (8) α, $\beta^C$ and β chain (haemoglobin C trait).

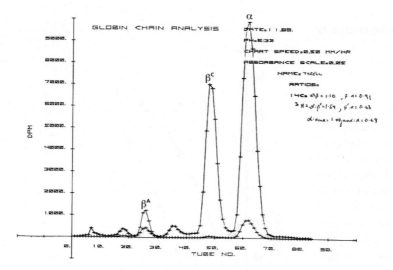

**Fig. 2.30** Globin chain synthesis studies in a patient with haemoglobin C/β thalassaemia compound heterozygosity. (By courtesy of Professor L. Luzzatto.)

ratio of α : β or α : β + γ. The results of such analysis are shown in Fig. 2.30 and typical globin chain ratios in various conditions are given in Table 2.4. An abnormal globin chain ratio does not always indicate an abnormality in the rate of synthesis. If a globin chain is very unstable, the ratio may be abnormal because of very rapid destruction of the unstable chain. Very unstable α chains have been associated with a reduced α : non-α ratio at 5 min, but a paradoxically increased ratio at 15 min and 1 h, which could lead to a misdiagnosis as β thalassaemia intermedia [37]. An abnormal ratio has also sometimes been detected in inherited disorders which do not involve the globin genes; for example, some cases of types I and III congenital dyserythropoietic anaemia have been found to have a reduced α : β ratio — 0.76 in one case of type III congenital dyserythropoietic anaemia [38].

The more ready availability of molecular techniques for the diagnosis of α thalassaemia has greatly reduced the need for the analysis of the rate of α and β globin chain synthesis.

## DNA analysis

The most important clinical applications of DNA analysis are: (i) the confirmation of the diagnosis of

**Table 2.4** The $\alpha:\beta$ globin chain ratio in normal subjects and in various thalassaemias.

| Normal or type of thalassaemia | $\alpha:\beta$ or $\alpha$:non-$\alpha$ globin chain ratio |
|---|---|
| Normal | 0.95–1.05 |
| $\alpha$ thalassaemia | |
| One gene deletion | 0.65–0.80 |
| Two gene deletion | 0.38–0.60 |
| Haemoglobin H disease | 0.20–0.30 |
| $\beta$ thalassaemia trait | 1.67–2.22 |
| $\beta$ thalassaemia major | No $\beta$ chain production, or 3.6–30 |

$\alpha^0$ thalassaemia trait, particularly for genetic counselling; (ii) the confirmation of the presence of haemoglobin D-Punjab (clinically important) rather than of any other D or G group haemoglobin; and (iii) the prenatal diagnosis of serious disorders of haemoglobin synthesis in the fetus (essential for first trimester diagnosis). In some communities in which $\alpha$, $\beta$ and $\delta$ thalassaemias and complex interactions are relatively common and in which silent $\beta$ thalassaemia occurs, there is a need for more extensive application of DNA analysis to permit accurate diagnosis prior to genetic counselling. In Thailand and Malaysia, where haemoglobin Malay represents around 15% of $\beta$ thalassaemia alleles, DNA analysis for antenatal diagnosis should include primers for the detection of this variant haemoglobin, as it is silent on electrophoresis and chromatography [39]. For fetal diagnosis, tests are usually carried out on DNA obtained by chorionic villous sampling, a procedure that can be carried out by 9–10 weeks of gestation.

Some of the techniques that can be applied are shown in Table 2.5 (updated from reference [1]). The techniques applied are modified according to the mutations expected in a given population. When the nature of a mutation is unknown, detection can be based on linkage analysis using restriction fragment length polymorphisms (RFLPs); this requires the study of family members with and without the mutation. The detection of mutations by more direct means does not require family studies; however, except for DNA sequencing, it does require a knowledge of the mutations to be expected in the population in question.

$\alpha$ thalassaemia, including $\alpha^0$ thalassaemia, can be diagnosed by Southern blot analysis of genomic DNA using $\alpha$ and $\zeta$ probes (Fig. 2.31). However, polymerase chain reaction (PCR) (Fig. 2.32) analysis is cheaper and faster, and primers have now been designed to permit the diagnosis of $--^{MED}$, $--^{FIL}$, $--^{SEA}$, $--^{THAI}$, $-\alpha^{3.7}$, $-\alpha^{4.2}$, $-(\alpha)^{20.5}$, $\alpha^{NCoI}\alpha$, $\alpha^{HphI}\alpha$ and also $\alpha\alpha\alpha^{anti3.7}$ by PCR [42–45]. $\alpha$ thalassaemia can also be diagnosed by a reverse dot blot method [46] in which membrane-bound oligonucleotide allele-specific probes are used as targets for the hybridization of amplified DNA (Fig. 2.33); filter strips are prepared with a probe for the normal $\alpha$ gene and for the variant being sought, permitting the detection of both heterozygotes and homozygotes. PCR is also the method of choice for the diagnosis of $\beta$ thalassaemia trait when the likely mutations are known. Multiplex PCR and the use of techniques such as the detection of the PCR product by an enzyme-linked immunosorbent assay (ELISA) permit automation of the process [47].

## Electrospray ionization mass spectrometry

Electrospray ionization mass spectrometry is a research technique that is now being applied to the identification of variant haemoglobins [48]. The technique depends on the measurement of the mass:charge ratio from which the mass can be deduced. It is possible to determine whether the variant is an $\alpha$ or $\beta$ chain variant, to estimate the proportion of the variant and to predict the amino acid substitution that could account for any observed change in mass. About 95% of variant haemoglobins can be

**Table 2.5** Techniques for the diagnosis of thalassaemias and haemoglobinopathies by DNA analysis [1,40,41].

| Diagnosis | Test |
| --- | --- |
| $\alpha^0$ thalassaemia | Southern blot analysis |
| | GAP PCR* |
| | PCR with allele-specific primers (ARMS)† (including multiplex PCR for deletions common in a specific region and real time (quantitative) PCR [41]) |
| | Reverse dot blot |
| | ELISA‡ for detection of embryonic $\zeta$ chains |
| | Sequencing |
| $\beta$ thalassaemia | |
|   Known mutations | PCR with allele-specific primers |
| | GAP PCR* |
|   Unknown mutations | DGGE§ or heteroduplex analysis§ |
| | RFLP linkage analysis¶ |
| | DNA sequencing |
| Haemoglobin Lepore | GAP PCR, sequencing |
| $\delta\beta$ thalassaemia | GAP PCR, sequencing |
| Deletional hereditary persistence of fetal haemoglobin | GAP PCR, sequencing |
| Haemoglobin S | PCR, *Dde*I digestion |
| Haemoglobin C | PCR with allele-specific primers |
| Haemoglobin E | PCR with allele-specific primers or restriction enzymes |
| Haemoglobin D-Punjab | PCR, *Eco*RI digestion |
| Haemoglobin O-Arab | PCR, *Eco*RI digestion |

*GAP PCR (polymerase chain reaction) indicates that there is a 'gap' in the DNA sequence (i.e. a deletion) and the primers are chosen so that, if the deletion is present, there is amplification across the 'gap'. This is useful for the diagnosis of $\alpha$ thalassaemia and the minority of cases of $\beta$ thalassaemia that are consequent on a relatively large deletion. Other haemoglobinopathies resulting from deletion are also susceptible to detection by this technique.
†ARMS (amplification refractory mutation system) is a PCR technique using two primer sets, one amplifying normal sequences and one amplifying abnormal sequences.
‡Enzyme-linked immunosorbent assay.
§DGGE (denaturing gradient gel electrophoresis) or heteroduplex analysis can be used initially to locate the mutation.
¶RFLP (restriction fragment length polymorphism) linkage analysis requires study of the family.

identified [4]. The apparatus is very expensive and considerable skill is required in the interpretation of results.

## Quality assurance

All tests should be carried out by appropriately trained personnel following standard operating procedures (SOPs) for each test. A laboratory requires clearly defined protocols for different clinical situations, e.g. for antenatal testing or for the investigation of neonates (see Chapter 7). All laboratories carrying out haemoglobinopathy testing should participate in an external quality assurance scheme.

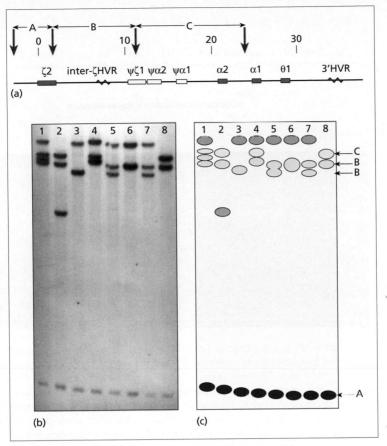

**Fig. 2.31** Southern blot analysis following hybridization of a ζ globin gene probe to *Bgl*II digests of genomic DNA, performed for the diagnosis of α thalassaemia. (a) Diagram of the α globin gene cluster showing the sites at which *Bgl*II cleaves the DNA (↓). *Bgl*II digestion of normal DNA produces three fragments (A, B and C) that will hybridize with the ζ probe: fragment A is a small fragment containing the ζ2 gene; fragments B and C are larger and each contains part of the ψζ1 gene. Fragment B is of variable length because it contains the inter-ζ hypervariable region (inter-ζHVR) and, for this reason, its position on a gel is variable, with two distinct B bands often being present. (b) Gel showing: lane 1, $\alpha\alpha/-\alpha^{3.7}$; lane 2, $\alpha\alpha/-\alpha^{4.2}$; lane 3, $-\alpha^{3.7}/-\alpha^{3.7}$; lane 4, $\alpha\alpha/-\alpha^{3.7}$; lane 5, $-\alpha^{3.7}/-\alpha^{3.7}$; lane 6, $-\alpha^{3.7}/-\alpha^{3.7}$; lane 7, $-\alpha^{3.7}/-\alpha^{3.7}$; lane 8, $\alpha\alpha/\alpha\alpha$. (By courtesy of Dr T. Vulliamy.) (c) Explanatory diagram. Lane 8, with normal α genes, shows normal A, B and C fragments. Lanes 1 and 4 show three normal fragments but, in addition, there is a larger fragment that represents an abnormal C fragment consequent on deletion of the 3' *Bgl*II cleavage site by the $-\alpha^{3.7}$ deletion; as fragments of normal size are also present, it can be seen that these individuals are heterozygous for this deletion. Lanes 3, 5, 6 and 7 show loss of the normal C fragment and replacement by a larger C fragment characteristic of $-\alpha^{3.7}$; these individuals are therefore homozygous for $-\alpha^{3.7}$. Lane 2 shows three normal fragments but, in addition, there is a fragment that is smaller than B and C; this represents a C fragment of reduced size consequent on a $-\alpha^{4.2}$ deletion; as fragments of normal size are also present, this individual must be a heterozygote.

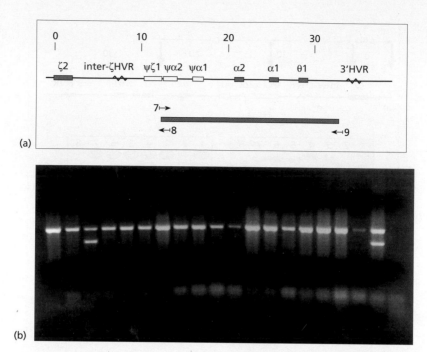

(a)

(b)

**Fig. 2.32** Polymerase chain reaction (PCR) in the diagnosis of α thalassaemia. (a) Explanatory diagram, modified from reference [43], showing an α gene cluster and the three primers (7, 8 and 9) described in this paper for the diagnosis of the $\alpha^0$ thalassaemia determinant, $--^{SEA}$. In a normal genome, primers 7 and 8 amplify a small fragment of DNA, but primers 7 and 9 are too widely separated for amplification to occur; in the presence of the large $--^{SEA}$ deletion, the sequence to which primer 8 anneals is deleted and the sequences to which primers 7 and 9 bind are brought sufficiently close together that a fragment is amplified; heterozygotes will have two fragments of different sizes, whereas a hydropic fetus with $--^{SEA}/--^{SEA}$ will have a single abnormal fragment. (b) Gel using the technique in (a) showing a control sample from a subject with $\alpha\alpha/--^{SEA}$ (far right) and 17 individuals being tested, one of whom (third from left) has $\alpha\alpha/--^{SEA}$. (By courtesy of Dr T. Vulliamy.)

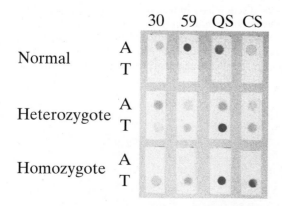

**Fig. 2.33** Reverse dot blot analysis for the detection of four non-deletional α thalassaemia determinants, codon 30 (30), codon 59 (59), $\alpha^{Quong\ Sze}$ (QS) and $\alpha^{Constant\ Spring}$ (CS). Amplified DNA samples were hybridized to strips, each containing normal (A) and mutant (T) oligonucleotide probes for the particular defect; positive signals appear as blue dots. Samples from heterozygotes show a signal with both the normal and thalassaemia probe, whereas samples from homozygotes show a signal only with the thalassaemia probe. (By courtesy of Professor V. Chan and the *British Journal of Haematology*.)

## Check your knowledge

One to five answers may be correct. Answers to almost all questions can be found in this chapter or can be deduced from the information given. The correct answers are given on p. 62.

2.1 The following variant haemoglobins have the same mobility as haemoglobin S on cellulose acetate electrophoresis at pH 8.4
 (a) haemoglobin C
 (b) haemoglobin Lepore
 (c) haemoglobin D-Punjab
 (d) haemoglobin G-Philadelphia
 (e) haemoglobin E

2.2 The following haemoglobins have the same mobility as haemoglobin A on agarose gel electrophoresis at pH 6.2
 (a) haemoglobin E
 (b) haemoglobin S
 (c) haemoglobin D-Punjab
 (d) haemoglobin C
 (e) haemoglobin G-Philadelphia

2.3 Satisfactory methods for the precise quantification of the haemoglobin $A_2$ percentage include
 (a) scanning densitometry
 (b) high performance liquid chromatography
 (c) isopropanol test
 (d) microcolumn chromatography
 (e) cellulose acetate electrophoresis followed by elution

2.4 The following variant haemoglobins have the same mobility as haemoglobin C on cellulose acetate electrophoresis at pH 8.4
 (a) haemoglobin $A_2$
 (b) haemoglobin Lepore
 (c) haemoglobin O-Arab
 (d) haemoglobin C-Harlem
 (e) haemoglobin E

2.5 A false positive sickle solubility test may be caused by
 (a) the presence of haemoglobin C
 (b) anaemia
 (c) increased plasma proteins

 (d) the presence of haemoglobin D
 (e) the presence of numerous Heinz bodies

2.6 If an unstable haemoglobin is suspected, relevant tests include
 (a) blood film
 (b) reticulocyte count
 (c) isopropanol test
 (d) heat stability test
 (e) alkali denaturation

2.7 Techniques applicable in the diagnosis of α or β thalassaemia in a fetus include
 (a) reverse dot blot analysis
 (b) polymerase chain reaction
 (c) isopropanol test
 (d) linkage studies using restriction fragment length polymorphism analysis
 (e) microcolumn chromatography

2.8 Globin chain synthesis studies are useful in the diagnosis of
 (a) sickle cell trait
 (b) sickle cell disease
 (c) α thalassaemia trait
 (d) β thalassaemia trait
 (e) haemoglobin H disease

2.9 The presence of haemoglobin S may be conclusively demonstrated by
 (a) a positive sickle test
 (b) a positive sickle solubility test
 (c) an immunoassay
 (d) polymerase chain reaction with appropriate restriction enzymes
 (e) electrophoresis on cellulose acetate at pH 8.3

2.10 A positive test for an unstable haemoglobin may result from
 (a) an aged sample
 (b) the presence of a high concentration of haemoglobin F
 (c) α thalassaemia trait
 (d) β thalassaemia trait
 (e) the presence of an unstable haemoglobin

2.11 An α:β chain synthesis ratio of 0.25:1 is compatible with
 (a) α thalassaemia trait
 (b) normal

(c) β thalassaemia trait

(d) haemoglobin H disease

(e) β thalassaemia major

## Further reading

Hoyer JD and Kroft SH, eds. *Color Atlas of Hemoglobin Disorders*. College of American Pathologists, Northfield, IL, 2003.

Wild BJ and Bain BJ. Investigation of abnormal haemoglobins and thalassaemia. In: Lewis SM, Bain BJ and Bates I, eds. *Dacie and Lewis's Practical Haematology*, 10th edn. Churchill Livingstone, London, 2005.

## References

1 Working Party of the General Haematology Task Force of the British Committee for Standards in Haematology (1998) The laboratory diagnosis of haemoglobinopathies. *Br J Haematol* **101**, 783–792.

2 International Committee for Standardization in Haematology (1988) Recommendations for neonatal screening for haemoglobinopathies. *Clin Lab Haematol* **10**, 335–345.

3 Wild BJ and Bain BJ. Investigation of abnormal haemoglobins and thalassaemia. In: Lewis SM, Bain BJ and Bates I, eds. *Dacie and Lewis's Practical Haematology*, 10th edn. Churchill Livingstone, London, 2005.

4 Wild BJ and Bain BJ (2004) Detection and quantitation of normal and variant haemoglobins: an analytical review. *Ann Clin Biochem* **41**, 355–369.

5 Lafferty J, Ali M, Carstairs K and Crawford L (1998) The effect of carbon tetrachloride on the detection of hemoglobin H using various commercially available electrophoresis products. *Am J Clin Pathol* **109**, 651–652.

6 International Committee for Standardization in Haematology (1978) Simple electrophoretic system for presumptive identification of abnormal haemoglobins. *Blood* **52**, 1058–1064.

7 International Committee for Standardization in Haematology (1978) Recommendations for a system for identifying abnormal hemoglobins. *Blood* **52**, 1065–1067.

8 Hoyer JD and Kroft SH, eds. *Color Atlas of Hemoglobin Disorders*. College of American Pathologists, Northfield, IL, 2003.

9 Basset P, Beuzard Y, Garel MC and Rosa J (1978) Isoelectric focusing of human haemoglobins: its appli-cation to screening, to characterization of 70 variants and to study of modified fractions of normal haemoglobins, *Blood* **51**, 971–982.

10 Phelan L, Bain BJ, Roper D, Jury C and Bain K (1999) An analysis of relative costs and potential benefits of different policies for antenatal screening for β thalassaemia trait and variant haemoglobins. *J Clin Pathol* **52**, 697–700.

11 Wild BJ and Stephens AD (1997) The use of automated HPLC to detect and quantitate haemoglobins. *Clin Lab Haematol* **19**, 171–176.

12 Waters HM, Howarth JE, Hyde K, Goldstone S, Kadkhodaei-Elyaderani M, Cinkotai KI and Richards JT (1996) Evaluation of the Bio-Rad Variant Beta Thalassaemia Short Program. *MDA Evaluation Report MDA/96/28*, Medical Devices Agency, London.

13 Riou J, Godart C, Didier H, Mathis M, Bimet C, Bardakdjian-Michau J *et al.* (1997) Cation-exchange HPLC evaluated for presumptive identification of hemoglobin variants. *Clin Chem* **43**, 34–39.

14 Bain BJ and Phelan L (1997) Evaluation of the Primus Corporation CLC330TM HPLC system for haemoglobinopathy screening. *MDA Evaluation Report MDA/97/53*, Medical Devices Agency, London.

15 Bain BJ and Phelan L (1997) Evaluation of the Kontron Instruments Haemoglobin System PV for haemoglobinopathy screening. *MDA Evaluation Report MDA/97/54*, Medical Devices Agency, London.

16 Bain BJ and Phelan L (1996) An evaluation of the HemoCard Hemoglobin S test and four sickle cell solubility kits (Ortho Sickledex, Dade Sickle-Sol, Microgen Bioproducts S-Test and Lorne Sickle-Check) for the detection of haemoglobin S and the HemoCard Hemoglobin A plus S test for the detection of haemoglobins A and S. *MDA Evaluation Report MDA/96/56*, Medical Devices Agency, London.

17 Balasubramaniam J, Phelan L and Bain BJ (2001) Evaluation of a new screening test for sickle cell haemoglobin. *Clin Lab Haematol* **23**, 379–383.

18 International Committee for Standardization in Haematology (1975) Recommendations for selected methods for quantitative estimation of Hb $A_2$ and for Hb $A_2$ reference preparations. *Br J Haematol* **38**, 573–578.

19 Thalassaemia Working Party of the BCSH General Haematology Task Force (1994) Guidelines for the investigation of the α and β thalassaemia traits. *J Clin Pathol* **47**, 289–295.

20 Shephard DTS (1995) An assessment of isoelectric focusing (Helena REP Hb-IEF) for the measurement of

haemoglobin $A_2$ percentage in the diagnosis of β-thalassaemia trait. BSc Project, St Mary's Hospital Medical School, London.

21 Head CE, Conroy M, Jarvis M, Phelan L and Bain BJ (2004) Some observations on the measurement of haemoglobin $A_2$ and S percentages by high performance liquid chromatography in the presence and absence of thalassaemia. *J Clin Pathol* **57**, 276–280.

22 Shihabi ZK, Hinsdale ME and Daugherty HK (2000) Haemoglobin A2 quantification by capillary zone electrophoresis. *Electrophoresis* **21**, 749–752.

23 Bain BJ and Phelan L (1996) An assessment of Hemo-Card Hemoglobin C and HemoCard Hemoglobin E kits for the detection of haemoglobins C and E. *MDA Evaluation Report MDA/96/57*, Medical Devices Agency, London.

24 Chapman C and Chambers K (1997) Neonatal haemoglobinopathy screening methods. *MDA Evaluation Report MDA/97/64*, Medical Devices Agency, London.

25 Schultz JC (1999) Comparison of radial immunodiffusion and alkaline cellulose acetate electrophoresis for quantitating elevated levels of fetal hemoglobin (HbF): application for evaluating patients with sickle cell disease treated with hydroxyurea. *J Clin Lab Anal* **13**, 82–89.

26 Hoyer JD, Penz CS, Fairbanks VF, Hanson CA and Katzmann JA (2002) Flow cytometric measurement of hemoglobin F in red cells. *Am J Clin Pathol* **117**, 857–863.

27 Mundee Y, Bigelow NC, Davis BH and Porter JB (2001) Flow cytometric method for simultaneous assay of foetal haemoglobin containing red cells, reticulocytes and foetal haemoglobin containing reticulocytes. *Clin Lab Haematol* **23**, 349–354.

28 Kattamis C, Efremov G and Pootrakul S (1981) Effectiveness of one tube osmotic fragility screening in detecting β-thalassaemia trait. *J Med Genet* **18**, 266–270.

29 Panyasai S, Sringam P, Fucharoen G, Sanchaisuriya K and Fucharoen S (2002) A simplified screening test for α-thalassaemia 1 (SEA type) using a combination of a modified osmotic fragility test and a direct PCR on whole blood lysates. *Acta Haematol* **108**, 74–78.

30 Chow J, Phelan L and Bain BJ (2005) Evaluation of single-tube osmotic fragility as a screening test for thalassemia. *Am J Hematol* **79**, 1–4.

31 Issaragrisil S, Siritanaratkul N and Fucharoen S. *Diagnosis and Management of Thalassemia: Thailand as a Model*. American Society of Hematology, Education Program Book, American Society of Hematology, Washington DC, 2001, pp 483–488.

32 Chapple L, Harris A, Phelan L and Bain BJ (2005) Reassessment of a simple chemical method using DCIP for screening for haemoglobin E. *J Clin Pathol* in press.

33 Panzer S, Kronik G, Lechner K, Bettelheim P, Neumann E and Dudczak R (1982) Glycosylated hemoglobins (GHb): an index of red cell survival. *Blood* **59**, 1348–1350.

34 Karsten J, Anker AP and Odink RJ (1996) Glycosylated haemoglobin and transient erythroblastopenia of childhood. *Lancet* **347**, 273.

35 El-Agouza I, Shahla AA and Sirdah M (2002) The effect of iron deficiency anaemia on the levels of haemoglobin subtypes: possible consequences for clinical diagnosis. *Clin Lab Haematol* **24**, 285–289.

36 Bain BJ, Beer P, Conroy M, Hughes C and Phelan L (2005) The frequency of detection of unexpected diabetes mellitus during haemoglobinopathy investigations. In preparation.

37 Traeger-Synodinos J, Papassotiriou I, Mataxotou-Mavrommati A, Vrettou C, Stamoulakatou A and Kanavakis E (2000) Distinct phenotypic expression associated with a new hyperunstable alpha globin variant (Hb Heraklion,α1cd37(C2)Pro>): comparison to other α-thalassemic hemoglobinopathies. *Blood Cell Mol Dis* **26**, 276–284.

38 Wickramasinghe SN (1998) Congenital dyserythropoietic anaemias: clinical features, haematological morphology and new biochemical data. *Blood Rev* **12**, 178–200.

39 Fucharoen S, Sanchaisuriya K, Fucharoen G and Surapot S (2001) Molecular characterization of thalassemia intermedia with homozygous Hb Malay and Hb Malay/HbE in Thai patients. *Haematologica* **86**, 657–658.

40 Galanello R, Sollaino C, Paglietti E, Barella S, Perra C, Doneddu I *et al.* (1998) α-Thalassemia carrier identification by DNA analysis in the screening for thalassemia. *Am J Hematol* **59**, 273–278.

41 Chan V, Yiop B, Lam YH, Tse HY, Wong HS and Chan TK (2001) Quantitative polymerase chain reaction for the rapid prenatal diagnosis of homozygous α-thalassaemia (Hb Barts hydrops fetalis). *Br J Haematol* **115**, 341–346.

42 Bowden DK, Vickers MA and Higgs DR (1992) A PCR-based strategy to detect common severe determinants of α-thalassaemia. *Br J Haematol* **81**, 104–108.

43 Oron-Karni-V, Filon D, Oppenheim A and Rund D (1998) Rapid detection of the common Mediterranean α-globin deletions/rearrangements using PCR. *Am J Hematol* **58**, 306–310.

44 Hunt JA, Lee L, Donlon TA and Hsia YE (1999) Determination of the breakpoint of the common α-thalassaemia deletion in Filipinos in Hawaii. *Br J Haematol* **104**, 284–287.

45 Liu YT, Old JM, Miles K, Fisher CA, Weatherall DJ and Clegg JB (2000) Rapid detection of α-thalassaemia deletions and α-globin gene triplication by multiplex polymerase chain reactions. *Br J Haematol* **108**, 295–299.

46 Chan V, Yam I, Chen FE and Chan TK (1999) A reverse dot-blot method for rapid detection of non-deletion α thalassaemia. *Br J Haematol* **104**, 513–515.

47 Ugozzoli LA, Lowery JD, Reyes AA, Lin C-IP, Re A, Locati F *et al.* (1998) Evaluation of the BeTha gene 1 kit for the qualitative detection of the eight most common Mediterranean β-thalassaemia mutations. *Am J Hematol* **59**, 214–222.

48 Wild BJ, Green BN, Cooper EK, Lalloz MRA, Erten S, Stephens AD and Layton DM (2001) Rapid identification of hemoglobin variants by electrospray ionization mass spectrometry. *Blood Cell Mol Dis* **27**, 691–704.

## Answers to questions

| | | | | | | | | | | | | |
|---|---|---|---|---|---|---|---|---|---|---|---|---|
| 2.1 | (a) F | | 2.3 | (a) F | | 2.5 | (a) F | | 2.7 | (a) T | 2.9 | (a) T |
| | (b) T | | | (b) T | | | (b) F | | | (b) T | | (b) F |
| | (c) T | | | (c) F | | | (c) T | | | (c) F | | (c) T |
| | (d) T | | | (d) T | | | (d) F | | | (d) T | | (d) T |
| | (e) F | | | (e) T | | | (e) T | | | (e) F | | (e) F |

2.11 (a) F (b) F (c) F (d) T (e) F

| | | | | | | | | | | | | |
|---|---|---|---|---|---|---|---|---|---|---|---|---|
| 2.2 | (a) T | | 2.4 | (a) T | | 2.6 | (a) T | | 2.8 | (a) F | 2.10 | (a) T |
| | (b) F | | | (b) F | | | (b) T | | | (b) F | | (b) T |
| | (c) T | | | (c) T | | | (c) T | | | (c) T | | (c) F |
| | (d) F | | | (d) T | | | (d) T | | | (d) T | | (d) F |
| | (e) T | | | (e) T | | | (e) F | | | (e) T | | (e) T |

## Appendix

The following instruments, methods and kits have been found to be satisfactory in the author's laboratory.

**Electrophoresis on cellulose acetate at alkaline pH**: Helena Laboratories/Helena BioSciences Europe, Titan III-H and supra-Heme buffer.

**Electrophoresis on agarose gel at acid pH**: Helena Laboratories/Helena BioSciences Europe, SAS-MX Acid Hb.

**High Performance Liquid Chromatography**: Bio-Rad Laboratories, Variant™ or Variant™ II.

**Sickle solubility test**: Ortho-Clinical Diagnostics, Sickledex®.

**Quantification of haemoglobin A$_2$ by microcolumn chromatography**: Helena Laboratories, HbA2 Quik Column.

For other recommended methods, see reference [3].

# 3 The α, β, δ and γ thalassaemias and related conditions

Thalassaemia is the name given to a globin gene disorder that results in a diminished rate of synthesis of one or more of the globin chains and, consequently, a reduced rate of synthesis of the haemoglobin or haemoglobins of which that chain constitutes a part. The condition was first described by Cooley and Lee in 1925 [1], with the name 'thalassaemia' from the Greek θαλασσα, sea, being given by Whipple and Bradford in 1936 [2]. In the late 1930s, the hereditary nature of thalassaemia was clearly identified in both Greece and Italy. It is probable that the failure to identify thalassaemia as a discrete entity in the Mediterranean area until after its description in the United States was because malaria, as a cause of childhood anaemia and splenomegaly, was still prevalent around the Mediterranean.

In thalassaemia, a significantly reduced rate of synthesis of one type of globin chain leads to unbalanced chain synthesis, with an excess of a normal globin chain contributing to the pathological effects, causing either damage to erythroid precursors and ineffective erythropoiesis or damage to mature erythrocytes and haemolytic anaemia. Thalassaemia can be classified according to the phenotype or the genotype. The major types of thalassaemia, classified according to the genotype, are shown in Table 3.1. Thalassaemia may result from the deletion of a large part or all of a gene (as is usual in α thalassaemia) or from a small deletion or other mutation of a gene (as is usual in β thalassaemia). Mutations of α and β genes are of potential clinical significance as there is a reduced rate of synthesis of haemoglobin A, the major haemoglobin of adult life. A serious clinical disorder usually results only when both of the β genes or either three or four of the α genes are affected. γ thalassaemia would only be of potential significance in intrauterine and early neonatal life when haemoglobin F is a major haemoglobin. However, as there are four γ genes, significant disease is

unlikely. δ thalassaemia is of no clinical significance, except that its presence may interfere with the diagnosis of coexisting β thalassaemia.

Thalassaemia usually results from the mutation of a single globin gene or from the deletion of one or more globin genes. One mechanism of deletion is unequal crossover between chromosomes at meiosis so that parts of two genes are deleted and the 5′ end of one gene fuses with the 3′ end of another gene. This is the mechanism underlying some types of α thalassaemia trait (Fig. 3.1). Another defect of this type leads to deletion of part of both a δ gene and a β gene with production of a δβ fusion gene, leading to the synthesis of haemoglobin Lepore (named after the Italian family in whom it was first described) (see Fig. 1.14a). The rate of synthesis of the abnormal δβ chain is slower than the rate of synthesis of the β chain so that the haematological features are very similar to those of β thalassaemia. As one δ gene has effectively been lost, there is also a reduced rate of synthesis of the δ chain and a reduced proportion of haemoglobin $A_2$. A thalassaemic phenotype can also result from a mutation that leads to the formation of a very unstable globin chain that precipitates before it is incorporated into haemoglobin.

Imbalance of globin chain synthesis can result from the deletion or mutation of a globin gene, leading to a reduced rate of synthesis of the relevant globin chain, but also from duplication of a globin gene, leading to an increased rate of synthesis of that globin chain. Thus there may be three or even four α genes on a single chromosome (instead of the normal two), referred to as triple α or quadruple α. Duplication of a gene is not usually of any clinical significance, but when it coexists with thalassaemia it may either lessen the chain imbalance and ameliorate the condition or aggravate the chain imbalance and thus increase the severity of the disorder. Thus if one chromosome has ααα and the other has –α, there is likely

**Table 3.1** Classification of the thalassaemias.

| Type of thalassaemia | Chain or chains synthesized at a reduced rate | Haemoglobin or haemoglobins synthesized at a reduced rate |
|---|---|---|
| Alpha: $\alpha^0$ or $\alpha^+$ | $\alpha$ | A, $A_2$ and F |
| Beta: $\beta^0$ or $\beta^+$ | $\beta$ | A |
| Gamma: $\gamma$ | $\gamma$ | F |
| Delta: $\delta^0$ or $\delta^+$ | $\delta$ | $A_2$ |
| Delta beta: $\delta\beta^0$ or $\delta\beta^+$ | $\delta$ and $\beta$ | A and $A_2$ |
| $^A$Gamma delta beta: $^A\gamma\delta\beta^0$ | $^A\gamma$, $\delta$ and $\beta$ | A and $A_2$ |
| Epsilon gamma delta beta*: $\varepsilon^G\gamma^A\gamma\delta\beta^0$ | $\varepsilon$, $^G\gamma$, $^A\gamma$, $\delta$ and $\beta$ | A, $A_2$ and F* |
| Haemoglobin Lepore | $\delta$ and $\beta$ | A and $A_2$† |

*Often referred to as γδβ thalassaemia; in fetal life, there is decreased synthesis of haemoglobins Gower 1 and 2 and Portland 1.
†Haemoglobin Lepore is synthesized at a reduced rate in comparison with haemoglobin A, but at an increased rate in comparison with haemoglobin $A_2$

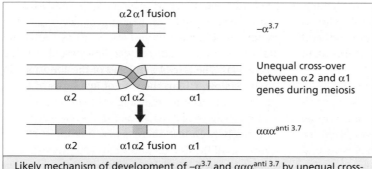

Likely mechanism of development of $-\alpha^{3.7}$ and $\alpha\alpha\alpha^{anti\ 3.7}$ by unequal cross-over between homologous sequences of the α2 and α1 genes during meiosis

**Fig. 3.1** Diagrammatic representation of the likely mechanism for the occurrence of the α gene deletion ($-\alpha^{3.7}$) and triple α ($\alpha\alpha\alpha^{anti3.7}$) by unequal cross-over between homologous sequences of the α2 and α1 genes during meiosis.

to be negligible chain imbalance and no haematological effect. However, the coexistence of ααα/αα or ααα/ααα and β thalassaemia increases the severity of the β thalassaemia.

## The α thalassaemias

The α thalassaemias are a group of conditions resulting from a reduced rate of synthesis of α globin. The severity of the defect is very variable. At one extreme is a completely asymptomatic condition, resulting from the deletion or dysfunction of one of the four α genes, which produces either a trivial abnormality in the blood count and film or no abnormality at all. At the other extreme is haemoglobin Bart's hydrops fetalis, a condition that is generally incompatible with life, usually resulting from the deletion of all four α genes and a consequent total lack of α globin synthesis. Some of the clinicopathological features of α thalassaemia syndromes result from the lack of the α globin chain, whereas others result from damage to red cell precursors and mature red cells by excess non-α chains. Excess β and γ chains may, in the absence of sufficient α chain, form haemoglobins with β or γ chain tetramers. The resultant haemoglobins are haemoglobin H with β tetramers, first described by

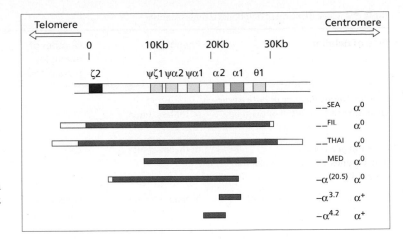

**Fig. 3.2** Diagrammatic representation of common deletions that can lead to α thalassaemia trait; the shaded blocks indicate the length of the deletion.

Rigas and colleagues in 1955 [3], and haemoglobin Bart's with γ tetramers, first described by Fessas and Papaspyrou in 1957 [4]. Haemoglobin H was so named because haemoglobin G (now known as haemoglobin Korle Bu) had been described a year earlier [5]. The current name of haemoglobin Bart's, previously designated haemoglobin Fessas and Papaspyrou or haemoglobin F and P, was given by Ager and Lehmann in 1958 [6], as the patient in whom it was observed was a patient of St Bartholomew's Hospital.

When both α genes on a single chromosome are deleted or transcriptionally completely inactive, the designation $\alpha^0$ thalassaemia (alpha zero thalassaemia) is used. When there is some residual gene function and some production of the α globin chain directed by genes on that chromosome, for example when only one of the two α genes on a chromosome is deleted, the designation $\alpha^+$ thalassaemia (alpha plus thalassaemia) is used. Function of the α globin gene cluster at 16p13.3 requires the presence of a major upstream regulatory element, referred to as HS –40 because it is 40 kilobases (kb) upstream of the ζ2 locus; thalassaemia can occur with completely normal α genes if HS –40 is deleted.

α thalassaemia can be divided broadly into deletional and non-deletional thalassaemia. Deletional α thalassaemia results in either $\alpha^0$ or $\alpha^+$ thalassaemia, depending on the length and nature of the deletion. Non-deletional α thalassaemia usually leads to $\alpha^+$ thalassaemia trait. Non-deletional α thalassaemias

can result from mutations of the α2 gene ($\alpha^T\alpha$ thalassaemia) or the α1 gene ($\alpha\alpha^T$ thalassaemia). Recognized cases of non-deletional thalassaemia are much more often caused by mutation of the α2 gene than of the α1 gene. This is likely to be, at least in part, because the former has a much more severe phenotype. Mutation in the α2 gene has a more severe phenotype than deletion of the α2 gene, as upregulation of the α1 gene occurs only in the latter instance.

Important deletions that lead to α thalassaemia are shown diagrammatically in Fig. 3.2 and deletions and mutations are summarized in Tables 3.2 and 3.3 [7–19]. Deletions and mutations causing α thalassaemia fall into seven broad categories.

1 Deletion of all or part of one or both α genes:
- deletion of an α2 gene ($\alpha^+$ thalassaemia);
- deletion of an α1 gene ($\alpha^+$ thalassaemia);
- deletion of part of an α2 gene and part of an α1 gene with formation of a fusion α gene ($\alpha^+$ thalassaemia);
- deletion of adjacent α2 and α1 genes ($\alpha^0$ thalassaemia);
- deletion of an α1 gene and more than 18 kb downstream, but with inactivation of the remaining structurally normal α2 gene by a negative positional effect, $(\alpha)^{-ZF}$ [7,17] ($\alpha^0$ thalassaemia).

There are at least 36 different deletions known, some also having deletion of the ζ gene and intervening sequences. This category includes extensive deletions or unbalanced translocations resulting in the loss of the telomere of chromosome 16, causing a

**Table 3.2** Classification of deletional $\alpha$ thalassaemia.

| Type of deletion | Phenotype | Number of examples recognized | Examples |
|---|---|---|---|
| *Deletion involving one or both $\alpha$ genes* | | | |
| Deletion of all or part of one $\alpha$ gene | $\alpha^+$ thalassaemia | 7 | $-\alpha^{4.2}$, $-\alpha^{3.7I}$, $-\alpha^{3.7II}$, $-\alpha^{3.7III}$, $-\alpha^{3.5}$, $\alpha(\alpha)^{5.3}*$, $-\alpha^{2.7}$ |
| Deletion of all or part of both $\alpha$ genes, but without deletion of HS $-40$ | $\alpha^0$ thalassaemia | 20 | $--^{SEA}$, $--^{THAI}$, $--^{MED}$, $--^{FIL}$, $--^{BRIT}$, $--^{SPAN}$, $-(\alpha)^{20.5}*$, $-(\alpha)^{5.2}*$ |
| Deletion of both $\alpha$ genes and of HS $-40$ (100–250 kb) | $\alpha^0$ thalassaemia | 8, without other phenotypic abnormality | $--^{DUTCHII}$ |
| Extensive loss of 16p13.3 (1–2 Mb) including both $\alpha$ genes and HS $-40\dagger$ | $\alpha^0$ thalassaemia | 17, with mental retardation and dysmorphism | $--^{BO}$ |
| Deletion of $\alpha 1$ gene and 18–20 kb downstream of $\alpha 1$ gene [17] | $\alpha^0$ thalassaemia | 1 | $(\alpha)-^{ZF}*$ |
| *Deletion leaving $\alpha$ genes intact* | | | |
| Deletion of upstream major regulatory element (HS $-40$) without deletion of $\alpha$ genes | $\alpha^0$ or very severe $\alpha^+$ thalassaemia | 12 | $(\alpha\alpha)^{RA}\ddagger$, $(\alpha\alpha)^{TAT}\ddagger$, $(\alpha\alpha)^{MM}\ddagger$, $(\alpha\alpha)^{IJ}\ddagger$ |

*$(\alpha)$ indicates that the gene is present but non-functional.

†Loss of 16p13.3 may be the result of deletion, inversion plus deletion, formation of a ring chromosome 16 that lacks the $\alpha$ gene cluster or unbalanced inheritance of a derivative (16) lacking 16p13.3 from a parent who had a balanced translocation, e.g. t(1;16), t(5;16) or t(16;20) [19].

‡$(\alpha\alpha)$ indicates that both $\alpha$ genes are present but non-functional.

syndrome of $\alpha$ thalassaemia trait ($\alpha^0$ thalassaemia), dysmorphism and mild to moderate mental retardation, referred to as the ATR-16 syndrome (Table 3.2).

**2** Deletion of the upstream major regulatory element, including the HS $-40$ enhancer, with marked downregulation or abrogation of expression of both structurally normal $\alpha$ genes [20] (it is estimated that $\alpha$ chain production is less than 1% of normal and so this is effectively $\alpha^0$ thalassaemia; at least 12 examples) (Table 3.2).

**3** Mutations affecting RNA splicing (Table 3.3). For example, IVS1 117 G→A in the $\alpha 1$ gene is an acceptor splice site mutation, found in India, that makes the gene non-functional. Splice site mutations such as this, as they affect only one of the two $\alpha$ genes, produce an $\alpha^+$ phenotype.

**4** Mutations affecting polyadenylation (Table 3.3). For example, $\alpha^{TSaudi}\alpha$ ($\alpha^{PA6\,A\rightarrow G}\alpha$), which is common around the Mediterranean, is one of a number of mutations affecting the highly conserved messenger RNA (mRNA) cleavage and polyadenylation signal. This mutation leads to a marked reduction in $\alpha$ chain synthesis, giving a severe $\alpha^+$ phenotype which is sometimes designated $\alpha^+$–$\alpha^0$; other mutations affecting polyadenylation may be less severe.

**5** Mutations affecting RNA translation (Table 3.3):
- initiation codon or initiation consensus sequence mutations leading to absent or reduced translation;
- frame shift mutations resulting from small deletions or deletion plus insertion or nonsense mutations acting as premature termination codons, leading to inactivation of the gene or synthesis of a very unstable $\alpha$ chain;
- mutation of a termination codon to a coding sequence, leading to an elongated $\alpha$ chain that is

**Table 3.3** Classification of non-deletional α thalassaemia.

| Type of mutation | Phenotype | Number of examples recognized | Examples |
|---|---|---|---|
| RNA splice site mutation in α1 or α2 gene (donor or acceptor site) | α⁺ thalassaemia | 3 (α2 donor site, α2 acceptor site, α1 acceptor site) | α2 IVS1 (−5 nt) donor splice site mutation in Mediterranean area and Middle East |
| RNA polyadenylation signal mutations | α⁺–α⁰ thalassaemia (i.e. severe α⁺) or α⁺ | 4 (described only for α2 gene which is likely to account for the severe phenotype) | α2 AATAAA→AATAAG ($\alpha^{PA6 A \to G}\alpha$, $\alpha^{TSaudi}\alpha$) |
| Impaired RNA translation consequent on initiation codon or initiation consensus sequence mutation | α⁺ thalassaemia, α⁺–α⁰ or, when the mutation occurs in association with deletional α thalassaemia, α⁰ thalassaemia | 5 (2 in α2 gene, 1 in α1 gene, 2 in single α gene) | α2 ATG→ACG, GTG or A–G; −α³·⁷ ATG→GTG (mutation in association with deletion gives α⁰ phenotype) |
| Impaired RNA translation consequent on a frame shift or nonsense mutation | α⁺ or α⁰ thalassaemia | 5 (4 frame shift plus 1 nonsense) | Codon 30/31 (−4 nt) frame shift and α2 CD116 GAG→TAG nonsense mutation |
| Impaired RNA translation consequent on a termination codon mutation leading to an elongated mRNA and α globin chain | α⁺ thalassaemia | 5 (all α2 gene) | Haemoglobin Constant Spring TAA→CAA ($\alpha^{CS}\alpha$), haemoglobin Icaria TAA→AAA ($\alpha^{Ic}\alpha$), haemoglobin Koya Dora TAA→TCA, haemoglobin Seal Rock TAA→GAA, haemoglobin Paksé TAA→TAT |
| Production of highly unstable α chain as a result of point mutation or a small deletion | α⁺ thalassaemia | At least 18: 14 point mutations, 4 small deletions; 11 affecting α2 gene, 4 affecting α1 gene and 3 affecting a single α gene | Haemoglobin Agrinio ($\alpha^{Agr}\alpha$), haemoglobin Petah Tikvah ($\alpha^{PT}$), haemoglobin Quong Sze ($\alpha^{QS}\alpha$), haemoglobin Suan Dok $\alpha^{SD}\alpha$) and haemoglobin Evaston (point mutations); haemoglobin Taybe (small deletion) |
| Lack of a transactivating factor encoded by the *ATRX* gene | α⁺ thalassaemia | | ATR-X syndrome |

synthesized at a reduced rate, possibly because of instability of the mRNA; examples of mutations of the termination codon leading to an elongated α chain include haemoglobin Constant Spring (found in southern China, Thailand, Cambodia, Vietnam, Laos and around the Mediterranean — e.g. Greece and Sicily), haemoglobin Koya Dora (found in India), haemoglobin Icaria, haemoglobin Seal Rock and haemoglobin Paksé; each of these α chains is elongated by 31 amino acids as translation continues into the 3′ untranslated region (UTR) until a downstream termination codon is encountered within the polyadenylation signal sequence.

**6** Mutations causing marked post-translational instability of a highly abnormal α chain, usually as the result of a defect in the haem pocket or in $\alpha_1\beta_1$ contacts [10,18]. Examples include haemoglobin Quong Sze ($\alpha^{125Leu \rightarrow Pro}\alpha$ or $\alpha^{QS}\alpha$), which is found in Kurdish Jews and in South-East Asia, and haemoglobin Agrinio ($\alpha^{29Leu \rightarrow Pro}\alpha$ or $\alpha^{Agr}\alpha$), which is found in the Mediterranean area and in South-East Asia.

**7** Transactivating abnormality resulting from mutation in the *ATRX* gene at Xq13.3 (previously known as the XH2 locus), which encodes a DNA helicase [21]. This results in a syndrome of severe mental retardation, dysmorphism and α thalassaemia in males, referred to as the ATR-X syndrome. More than 100 cases have been reported in more than 70 families.

It is likely that the two most common deletions, $-\alpha^{3.7}$ and $-\alpha^{4.2}$, are both consequent on unequal crossover during meiosis with the result that, when this mutation first arose, one chromosome was left with a single α gene while the other had a triplicated α gene. In the case of $-\alpha^{3.7}$, the single α gene and the central gene of the three α genes is a fusion gene (Fig. 3.1). Either abnormal chromosome could have passed into the gamete and thus the fetus, and thus both $\alpha\alpha\alpha^{anti3.7}$ and $\alpha\alpha\alpha^{anti4.2}$ are known to exist. It appears that both of these mutational events have occurred a number of times in a variety of ethnic groups. Further investigation of $-\alpha^{3.7}$ has established that there are in fact three slightly different deletions, occurring in different ethnic groups, which are now designated $-\alpha^{3.7I}$, $-\alpha^{3.7II}$ and $-\alpha^{3.7III}$. Only $-\alpha^{3.7I}$ is common in many ethnic groups. $-\alpha^{3.7II}$ has been described in India and Nepal, whereas $-\alpha^{3.7III}$ is confined to Oceania [22].

A variant haemoglobin may be predicted from the DNA sequence in patients with thalassaemia, but may be undetectable (e.g. haemoglobin Quong Sze) or present in very small amounts (e.g. haemoglobin Suan Dok), because of very marked instability of the α chain, the αβ dimer or the haemoglobin molecule. Sometimes a hyperunstable haemoglobin is detectable only after splenectomy. When the haematological features are those of α thalassaemia rather than of an unstable haemoglobin, classification as non-deletional α thalassaemia is appropriate. When

an α chain variant is only moderately unstable, it will constitute a larger proportion of total haemoglobin and will produce the phenotype of a Heinz body haemolytic anaemia, and classification as an unstable haemoglobin is then appropriate. An unstable haemoglobin can interact with $\alpha^0$ determinants to cause haemoglobin H disease (see Table 3.6).

The types of mutation most commonly found in different ethnic groups are shown in Table 3.4 and the incidence of $\alpha^0$ and $\alpha^+$ thalassaemia in different ethnic groups in Table 3.5 [16,23–46]. Overall, the highest prevalence of α thalassaemia is found in Oceania and the Indian subcontinent. The highest prevalence of the less common but more serious $\alpha^0$ thalassaemia is found in southern China and South-East Asia.

## α⁺ thalassaemia heterozygosity, compound heterozygosity and homozygosity

$\alpha^+$ thalassaemia trait is the most common monogenic disorder in the world. It usually results from the deletion of all or part of the α2 globin gene. The most common mutations causing $\alpha^+$ thalassaemia are $-\alpha^{4.2}$ and $-\alpha^{3.7}$. $-\alpha^{4.2}$ is a 4.2-kb deletion including the α2 gene. $-\alpha^{3.7}$ designates a group of three slightly different 3.7-kb deletions of the 3′ end of the α2 gene and the 5′ end of the α1 gene with formation of an α2α1 fusion gene. Both $-\alpha^{4.2}$ and $-\alpha^{3.7}$ result in about a 50% reduction in α chain synthesis from the affected chromosome. Although the α2 gene is usually responsible for about 70% of α chain production, there is some upregulation of the α1 gene when the α2 gene is deleted ($-\alpha^{4.2}$), whereas the α2α1 fusion gene is downregulated in comparison with the normal α2 gene. About one-quarter of individuals with African ancestry are heterozygous for $\alpha^+$ thalassaemia (having the genotype $-\alpha^{3.7}/\alpha\alpha$), while 1–2% are homozygous (having the genotype $-\alpha^{3.7}/-\alpha^{3.7}$). Other ethnic groups in which deletional $\alpha^+$ thalassaemia occurs include Greeks, Cypriots, Turks, Sardinians, Lebanese, Saudi Arabs, Indians, Thais, Filipinos, Indonesians, Melanesians and Polynesians. Less often, $\alpha^+$ thalassaemia is found to result from a mutation rather than deletion of the α2 or α1 gene, designated $\alpha^T\alpha$ or $\alpha\alpha^T$. However, many cases, particularly those affecting the α1 gene, are likely to be unrecognized so that the true frequency is unknown. Non-deletional α thalassaemia affecting the α2 gene leads to a more

**Table 3.4** Types of mutation most often responsible for α thalassaemia in different ethnic groups.

| Ethnic group | Type of thalassaemia | Designation | Nature of mutation |
|---|---|---|---|
| South-East Asia and southern China | $\alpha^0$ | $--^{SEA}$ | Deletion of both α genes |
| | | $--^{FIL}$ | Deletion of both α genes |
| | | $--^{THAI}$ | Deletion of both α genes |
| | $\alpha^+$ | $-\alpha^{4.2}$ | Deletion of α2 gene |
| | | $-\alpha^{3.7}$ | Deletion of part of both α genes with formation of an α2α1 fusion gene |
| | | $\alpha^{CS}\alpha$ | Haemoglobin Constant Spring, reduced rate of synthesis of a haemoglobin with an elongated α chain |
| | | $\alpha^{NcoI}\alpha$ | Mutation in initiation codon of α2 gene |
| | | $\alpha\alpha^{NcoI}$ | Mutation in initiation codon of α1 gene |
| | | $\alpha^{Suan\,Dok}\alpha$ | Very unstable α chain |
| | | $\alpha^{Quong\,Sze}\alpha$ | Very unstable α chain |
| Mediterranean (particularly Greece and Cyprus) | $\alpha^0$ | $--^{MED}$ | Deletion of both α genes |
| | | $-(\alpha)^{20.5}$ | Deletion of all of one α gene and part of the other |
| | $\alpha^+$ | $-\alpha^{3.7}$ | As above |
| | | $-\alpha^{TSaudi}\alpha$ | Polyadenylation signal sequence mutation |
| | | $\alpha^{Hph}\alpha$ | Small frame shift mutation of IVS1 donor site |
| Middle East | $\alpha^0$ | $--^{MED}$ | Deletion of both α genes |
| | $\alpha^+$ | $\alpha^{TSaudi}\alpha$ | Polyadenylation signal sequence mutation |
| India | $\alpha^+$ | $-\alpha^{3.7}$ | As above |
| | | $-\alpha^{4.2}$ (less common than $-\alpha^{3.7}$) | As above |
| | | $\alpha\alpha^{IVS1\,nt\,117\,G\rightarrow A}$ | Acceptor splice site mutation |
| | | $\alpha^{Koya\,Dora}\alpha$ | Mutation of termination codon resulting in an extended unstable α chain |
| Sri Lanka | $\alpha^+$ | $-\alpha^{3.7}$ | As above |
| | | $-\alpha^{4.2}$ | As above |
| African, Afro-American and Afro-Caribbean | $\alpha^+$ | $-\alpha^{3.7}$ | As above |
| Melanesia | $\alpha^+$ | $-\alpha^{3.7}$ | As above |
| | | $-\alpha^{4.2}$ (less frequent than $-\alpha^{3.7}$ except in Papua New Guinea) | As above |
| Polynesia | $\alpha^+$ | $-\alpha^{3.7}$ | As above; $-\alpha^{3.7III}$ is most characteristic of Polynesia and almost confined to this area |

**Table 3.5**  The prevalence of $\alpha^0$, $\alpha^+$ and $\beta$ thalassaemia heterozygosity in different countries and ethnic groups. (Derived from multiple sources including references [16,23–46].)

| Country or ethnic group | $\alpha^0$ thalassaemia | $\alpha^+$ thalassaemia | $\beta$ thalassaemia |
|---|---|---|---|
| Greece | About 1.5% | 7–10% | 6–28% (overall 8%) |
| Cyprus | Uncommon, averaging around 2% (both Greek and Turkish Cypriots) | 26% (including 1% $\alpha^T\alpha$) | 14–18% (incidence is similar in Greek and Turkish Cypriots; overall 15%) |
| Turkey | Rare (*c.* 0.6%) | 6% | 1–37% (high incidence confined to Eti-Turks on south-eastern coast; overall 2–3%) |
| Italy | Rare (0.5% in Sardinia, 0.2% in Sicily, even lower in southern Italy) | 10% in Sicily, 28% in Sardinia | 1–30% (highest prevalence in Po delta, southern Italy, Sicily and Sardinia (10%); overall 4%) |
| Spain | Very rare (0.2%) | 2% | 1–8% (highest in Minorca, southern Spain and Galicia); 5% in Spanish gypsies |
| Portugal | Rare | 10% | 0.5–1% |
| France — Corsica | | | 3% |
| Malta | | | 1–6% |
| Eastern Europe (Romania, Bulgaria, ex-Yugoslavia, ex-USSR) | | | Overall 2–20% (rare in ex-Czechoslovakia, Hungary, northern ex-USSR; higher in Romania, 3% in Uzbekistan, 5% in Tajikistan, 5.5% in Azerbaijan) |
| British (white) | Rare (occurs particularly in Lancashire and Cheshire; 0.05% in Wigan) | <1% | <0.5%, probably about 0.1% |
| Middle East (Iran, Iraq, Syria, Lebanon, Jordan, Bahrain, United Arab Emirates, Saudi Arabia, Israel, Palestine, Yemen) | Rare (occurs in Israel and United Arab Emirates) | <1–20% (overall 9%); 47% in Saudi Arabia, highest in Eastern province; 18–50% in United Arab Emirates; 64% in Kuwait; 89% in Oman; relatively frequent in Israeli Arabs and Yemenite Jews; 9% in Ashkenazi Jews | Overall 2–20%: Iran 1–4% (overall 3%), Iraq 2–3%, Syria 1%, Lebanon 2–6%, Jordan <1–4%, Bahrain 2–3%, Oman 1–2%, United Arab Emirates 2%, central Saudi Arabia 3–4%, eastern Saudi Arabia 13–18%, overall Saudi Arabia 1%, Yemen 1–2%, Yemenite Jews 9%, Kurdish Jews 20%, Israeli Arabs 3–25%, Israeli Jews 3–25%, Palestine (Gaza strip) 4% |
| North Africa and Horn of Africa (Morocco, Tunisia, Algeria, Libya, Egypt, Sudan, Ethiopia) | | 5–8% overall, Egypt 8% | Libya <1–11%, Algeria <1–15% (overall 2%), Morocco <1–7% (overall 3%), Tunisia 3.5%, Egypt <1–3%, Sudan 1–10% (overall 4%), Ethiopia <1–8% |

**Table 3.5** *Continued*.

| Country or ethnic group | α⁰ thalassaemia | α⁺ thalassaemia | β thalassaemia |
|---|---|---|---|
| West Africa | Nil | Gambia 8–15%, Togo 46%, Nigeria 8–58%, Senegal 22%, Benin and Burkina Faso (formerly Upper Volta) 29%, Ivory Coast 39% | Overall 1–14%: Senegal <1–5%, Liberia <1–9%, Ivory Coast 1–12%, Mali < 1%, Burkina Faso 2–12%, Ghana 1–11% (overall 1–2%), Togo <1–2%, Nigeria 1–4% (overall 0.8%), Cameroon < 1–2% |
| East Africa | Nil | Kenya 19–34%, Tanzania 2% | Rare in Kenya, Uganda and Tanzania; 2% in Mauritius and Reunion Island |
| Central Africa | Nil | Central African Republic 39% (23% of pygmy population), Republic of the Congo 36–40% (29% of pygmy population) | Central African Republic <1%, Republic of the Congo <1% (pygmy population of 6.5%) |
| Southern Africa | Nil in South African blacks | Zambia 20–27%, Malawi 39%, Namibia 11.5%, South African Cape Coloured population 7%, South African black 12% (San) to 36% (Venda), Mozambique 5–6%, Madagascar <1–3%, Comoros 2% or more | Comoros 3% |
| Africans in UK | | Probably 25–30% | 0.9% |
| Afro-Americans | | 25% | 1–2% |
| Afro-Caribbeans | Rare (but recognized in West Indians with Chinese ancestry) | Overall 25%, Jamaica 34% | 0.5–10% (overall 1%): Jamaica 4–5%, Lesser Antilles <1–10%, Guadeloupe 0.5%, 0.9% in Afro-Caribbeans in UK |
| Mexico | | | Up to 15% |
| Afghanistan | | | 3% |
| Pakistan | | 15–20% | 5%, about 4.5% in UK Pakistanis |
| Nepal | | 6–14% (but up to 97% in some tribal populations) | 13% |
| India | Rare | 5–33% (17–99%, mainly above 50%, in tribal populations) | Overall 1–16% (overall 3%, but up to 40% in some tribal populations), about 3.5% in UK Indians |
| Bangladesh | | | 3% |
| Indian subcontinent populations in Britain | | | Overall about 4.5% (from 3% in UK Bangladeshis and Punjabi Sikhs to about 6% in East African Asians) |
| Sri Lanka | | 15–16% (about 13% – α³·⁷ and about 2% –α⁴·²) | 1–5% (overall 2.2%) |
| Japan | | <1% | Rare |

*Continued on p. 72.*

**Table 3.5** *Continued.*

| Country or ethnic group | $\alpha^0$ thalassaemia | $\alpha^+$ thalassaemia | $\beta$ thalassaemia |
|---|---|---|---|
| Korea | | | Very low |
| Hong Kong | 4.5% | 0.5–1% | 3% |
| Singapore | 3–4% | 8% | |
| China | 3–9% in southern China | <1–6% in southern China | 0.5% in north and north-west, 2–6% in south, overall *c.* 1.7% |
| Chinese in UK | | | About 3% |
| Taiwan | 3.5% (higher and lower in different aboriginal populations) | 2% | 1–3% |
| Myanmar (previously Burma) | | | 0.5–6% (overall 3%) |
| Thailand | 4% in central Thailand, 14% in northern Thailand | 3–17%, 3% around Bangkok, 9% in north, 17% in north-east; 1–8% haemoglobin Constant Spring | 4–11% (overall 3%) |
| Cambodia | 1–4% | 12–28%, haemoglobin Constant Spring up to 2% | 1–5% (overall *c.* 2.8%) |
| Laos | 4% | *c.* 14%, haemoglobin Constant Spring 9% | 1–9% (overall 5%) |
| Vietnam | Significant | *c.* 8% | 1–25% (overall 4%) |
| Malaysia | 3–9% | Haemoglobin Constant Spring <1–6%, overall up to 29% | 1–5% (overall 2%) |
| Philippines | 10% | 5% | 1–2% |
| Brunei | | | 2% |
| Indonesia | Rare | 6% (2–30% on different islands) | 0–11% (overall 3%) |
| Papua New Guinea | | 10% in highlands, 62% in lowlands | 1–25% |
| Solomon Islands | | 45% | |
| Vanuatu (previously New Hebrides) | | 45% | |
| New Caledonia | | 6% | |
| New Zealand (Maori) | | 5–10% | |
| Australia (aboriginal) | | 6% | Rare |
| Indigenous Americans | | | Rare |
| Brazil | | | Overall 1% |

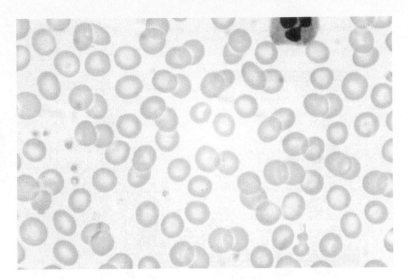

**Fig. 3.3** Blood film from an adult male α⁺ thalassaemia homozygote (genotype $-\alpha^{3.7}/-\alpha^{3.7}$). The red cell indices were red blood cell count (RBC) $5.77 \times 10^{12}$/l, haemoglobin concentration (Hb) 13.9 g/dl, haematocrit (Hct) 0.44, mean cell volume (MCV) 76 fl, mean cell haemoglobin (MCH) 24.1 pg and mean cell haemoglobin concentration (MCHC) 31.8 g/dl.

marked reduction of α globin production than does α2 deletion, as there is no upregulation of the α1 gene. Consequently, the haematological abnormality is more marked. $\alpha^T\alpha$ is most common in the Middle East, particularly in Saudi Arabia ($\alpha^{TSaudi}\alpha$), but also in Cyprus and Sardinia. Non-deletional α thalassaemia affecting the α1 gene, $\alpha\alpha^T$, is milder than $\alpha^T\alpha$, usually being intermediate in severity between $-\alpha/\alpha\alpha$ and $--/\alpha\alpha$.

Certain α chain variants give rise to the phenotype of α⁺ thalassaemia (Table 3.3). The most common non-deletional α thalassaemia is haemoglobin Constant Spring, with a frequency of 1–8% in Thailand. This results from mutation of the stop codon of the α2 gene so that a further 31 amino acids are added to the α chain; the mRNA is very unstable and the rate of α chain synthesis is reduced to about 1% of normal [47].

α⁺ thalassaemia is of little significance to the individual as it is clinically silent. The condition is of some genetic significance as compound heterozygotes for deletional α⁺ thalassaemia and $\alpha^0$ thalassaemia suffer from haemoglobin H disease (see below). Homozygotes for more severe non-deletional α⁺ thalassaemia ($\alpha^T\alpha/\alpha^T\alpha$) may also have the clinical features of haemoglobin H disease. Homozygosity for haemoglobin Constant Spring leads to more abnormality than is usual in homozygosity for α⁺ thalassaemia. There is usually anaemia and some cases have mild jaundice and hepato-splenomegaly. The deletion of HS –40 also leads to a severe phenotype, equivalent to $\alpha^0$.

*Laboratory features*

Heterozygotes for α⁺ thalassaemia ($-\alpha/\alpha\alpha$) may have a completely normal blood count and film or trivial anaemia and microcytosis with slight reduction of the mean cell volume (MCV) and mean cell haemoglobin (MCH). On average, the haemoglobin concentration is probably about 1 g/dl lower than in subjects with four α genes. All haematological variables (red blood cell count (RBC), haemoglobin concentration, haematocrit (Hct), MCV, MCH) show considerable overlap with normal values. Homozygotes ($-\alpha/-\alpha$) have more marked haematological abnormalities (Figs 3.3 and 3.4), usually comparable with those seen in β thalassaemia heterozygotes. Haemoglobin electrophoresis or high performance liquid chromatography (HPLC) is normal, with the haemoglobin $A_2$ percentage being normal or reduced.

During pregnancy, the haematological changes in women with α thalassaemia trait mirror those in normal women. On average, the haemoglobin concentration falls by about 1.4 g/dl, the MCV rises by about 5% and the MCH rises by about 7% [48].

Heterozygotes for haemoglobin Constant Spring have more marked anaemia than is usual in α⁺

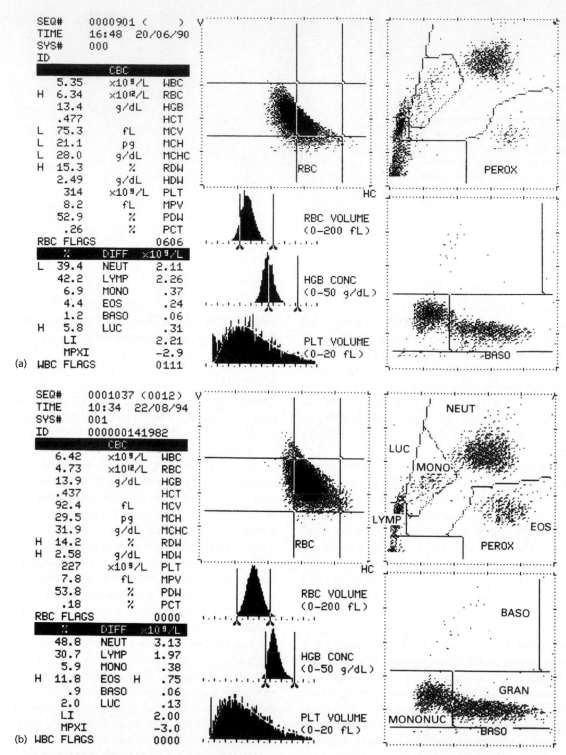

**Fig. 3.4** Red cell cytograms and histograms of (a) a male $\alpha^+$ thalassaemia trait homozygote and (b) a haematologically normal control subject; $\alpha$ thalassaemia is associated with microcytosis that is more marked than the associated hypochromia.

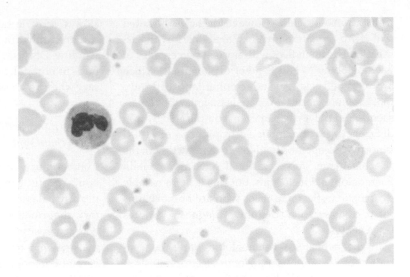

**Fig. 3.5** Blood film from a haemoglobin Constant Spring heterozygote showing basophilic stippling.

thalassaemia trait, but the MCV is not proportionately reduced [47]. Basophilic stippling is usually prominent (Fig. 3.5) [9,49]. Homozygotes for this variant haemoglobin are usually anaemic (haemoglobin concentration around 10 g/dl) with a marked reduction of the MCH (on average around 26 pg) [49]. However, the mean MCV is normal or low-normal (in one study averaging 88 fl) [49], i.e. considerably less reduced than would be expected given the degree of reduction of the MCH; this is because damage to red cell membranes by oxidized α and $\alpha^{CS}$ globin chains leads to cellular overhydration. There is a considerably shortened red cell survival and reticulocytosis (usually around 6–10%). There is usually 2–11% haemoglobin Constant Spring and 1–3% haemoglobin Bart's, but no haemoglobin H [9,49]. In occasional cases, haemoglobin Constant Spring is lower or even undetectable [50]. Haemoglobin $A_2$ tends to be low [50]. Haemoglobin F is normal.

Increased red cell protoporphyrin, which has been used as a screening test for iron deficiency, has been found in 20% of cases of α thalassaemia trait [51,52]. The elevation tends to be less than that in iron deficiency, but there is some overlap, so that this test is not reliable in distinguishing between these two conditions.

At birth, neonates with $\alpha^+$ thalassaemia trait have a lower mean haemoglobin concentration than other neonates. In one study, the mean level was 15.1 g/dl in heterozygotes and 14.1 g/dl in homozygotes, in comparison with a normal mean of 15.4 g/dl [53]. The MCV and MCH were similarly reduced. The mean MCVs were 100 and 94 fl in comparison with a normal mean of 105 fl. The MCHs were 33 and 31 pg in comparison with a normal mean of 35 pg. Using haemoglobin electrophoresis, some but not all babies with heterozygous $\alpha^+$ thalassaemia have around 1–2% of haemoglobin Bart's, in comparison with 0.5–1.0% in neonates with four α genes. However, a minority (less than 10%) of babies with four α genes have haemoglobin Bart's up to 1.2–2.6%. $\alpha^+$ thalassaemia homozygotes have around 3–10% haemoglobin Bart's, but overlap with heterozygotes occurs. When HPLC is used for quantification, there is a difference in mean haemoglobin Bart's level between heterozygotes and homozygotes for $\alpha^+$ thalassaemia — mean values of 1.8% and 6.4%, respectively, in one study [53] and a range of 0.8–2.8% in comparison with 2.5–8% in another [54], but again overlap occurs. Individuals with $\alpha^+$ thalassaemia homozygosity have a lower haemoglobin Bart's percentage than those with $\alpha^0$ thalassaemia heterozygosity, 2.5–8.0% in comparison with 7.6–12.3%, even though both have only two α genes [54]. Haemoglobin Bart's disappears by 3–6 months of age.

*Diagnosis*

The diagnosis of α thalassaemia trait is usually suspected when an individual is found to have microcytosis that is not explained by β or δβ thalassaemia trait or iron deficiency. (However, it should be noted that there are alternative explanations for 'thalassaemic' red cell indices with normal percentages of haemoglobins $A_2$ and F; other explanations, which are discussed below, include coinheritance of β and δ thalassaemia, normal-$A_2$ β thalassaemia, γδβ thalassaemia and polycythaemia vera complicated by iron deficiency.) Haemoglobin electrophoresis or HPLC is normal except for a tendency to a reduction in the $A_2$ percentage. Very occasional cells may contain haemoglobin H inclusions, but this is not a reliable diagnostic test even in those who are homozygous for $α^+$ thalassaemia. Definitive diagnosis requires DNA analysis.

In the neonate, a haemoglobin Bart's concentration of 1–2% on haemoglobin electrophoresis is suggestive of $-α/αα$, but not all neonates with this genotype have elevated haemoglobin Bart's. Elevation is more likely in association with $-α^{4.2}$ than in association with $-α^{3.7}$. A concentration of more than 2% of haemoglobin Bart's on haemoglobin electrophoresis is suggestive of either $--/αα$ or $-α/-α$ and, in an ethnic group in which $--/αα$ does not occur, provides presumptive evidence of the $-α/-α$ genotype. When the more sensitive technique of HPLC is used, the detection of increased haemoglobin Bart's in a neonate is suggestive of α thalassaemia trait but, because of the detection of haemoglobin Bart's in some normal babies, cannot be regarded as providing a definitive diagnosis.

As many individuals with $α^+$ thalassaemia trait have haematological variables falling within the normal range, the diagnosis is unlikely to be suspected in many cases unless revealed by population surveys or by family studies of a patient with haemoglobin H disease.

When an $α^+$ thalassaemia phenotype is consequent on the presence of an α chain variant synthesized at a much reduced rate, the variant haemoglobin may be detected by haemoglobin electrophoresis or, more often, HPLC, but it comprises a very low proportion of total haemoglobin (e.g. haemoglobin Constant Spring is usually 0.5–1% of total haemoglobin). Haemoglobin Constant Spring can be identified on cellulose acetate electrophoresis at alkaline pH, particularly if a heavy application is used; it moves between carbonic anhydrase and haemoglobin $A_2$, whereas haemoglobin $A_2'$ is even

slower, moving between the application point and carbonic anhydrase. On HPLC it appears in the C window. DNA sequencing can be used for the diagnosis of non-deletional α thalassaemia and is necessary when no variant haemoglobin is detected.

### Coinheritance with other abnormalities of globin chain synthesis

Coinheritance of $α^+$ thalassaemia, particularly if homozygous, can lessen the laboratory abnormalities of β thalassaemia trait and the clinical and laboratory abnormalities of homozygosity or compound heterozygosity for β thalassaemia. Coexisting α thalassaemia trait reduces the proportion of the variant haemoglobin in individuals with sickle cell trait, haemoglobin C trait and haemoglobin E trait.

### $α^0$ thalassaemia trait

$α^0$ thalassaemia usually results from the deletion of both α genes. Rarely, it results from the deletion of only the α1 globin gene and downstream sequences with inactivation of the remaining α2 gene. $α^0$ thalassaemia is relatively common in Chinese originating in south-eastern China and in other South-East Asian populations, e.g. in Thailand, Vietnam, Laos, Kampuchea, Malaysia and the Philippines. It occurs at a lower frequency in the Mediterranean area — in Greece, Cyprus, Turkey, Israel and certain parts of Italy (e.g. Sardinia). Three types of $α^0$ thalassaemia trait are common in South-East Asia, designated $--^{SEA}$, $--^{FIL}$ and $--^{THAI}$ (Fig. 3.2). Two of these, $--^{FIL}$ and $--^{THAI}$, are large deletions which also include the ζ gene. In the Mediterranean area, the most common deletion is $--^{MED}$ which does not include the ζ gene. In the heterozygous state, there are no important clinical or haematological differences between the different mutations giving rise to $α^0$ thalassaemia.

### Laboratory features

$α^0$ thalassaemia trait leads to very mild anaemia with the haemoglobin concentration overlapping the normal range. The RBC is increased and the MCV and MCH are reduced. The blood film shows microcytosis and a variable degree of hypochromia (Fig. 3.6). The reticulocyte count is elevated to 2–3%

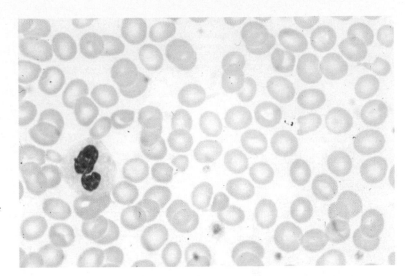

**Fig. 3.6** Blood film from a female $\alpha^0$ thalassaemia heterozygote (genotype $--^{SEA}/\alpha\alpha$). The red cell indices were RBC $5.71 \times 10^{12}/l$, Hb $11.5\,g/dl$, Hct $0.38$, MCV $66\,fl$, MCH $20.1\,pg$ and MCHC $30.4\,g/dl$.

[48]. When there is coexisting β thalassaemia trait or triple α in *trans*, the MCV and MCH are less abnormal.

At birth, haemoglobin electrophoresis shows neonates with $\alpha^0$ thalassaemia trait to have 5–10% haemoglobin Bart's. Quantification by HPLC gives values of around 7–11% [53] (Fig. 3.7); the mean value is higher than in homozygosity for $\alpha^+$ thalassaemia but overlap occurs. The haemoglobin concentration, MCV and MCH are all, on average, lower than in neonates with four α genes or with heterozygosity or homozygosity for $\alpha^+$ thalassaemia. In one study, the mean values were 13.3 g/dl, 86 fl and 29 pg, respectively [53].

*Diagnosis*

$\alpha^0$ thalassaemia should be suspected when red cell indices suggestive of thalassaemia trait are found in a patient of appropriate ethnic origin with normal percentages of haemoglobins $A_2$ and F. In this context, an MCH of less than 25 pg suggests a diagnosis of either $\alpha^0$ thalassaemia trait or homozygosity for $\alpha^+$ thalassaemia trait, rather than $\alpha^+$ thalassaemia heterozygosity. Definitive diagnosis requires DNA analysis. Because tests for the diagnosis of α thalassaemia are not readily available in many hospitals, it is usual to exclude iron deficiency, β thalassaemia and δβ thalassaemia trait (see below) and the presence of variant

haemoglobins before proceeding to DNA analysis. Iron deficiency can be excluded by measuring the serum ferritin concentration, but it should be noted that the serum transferrin receptor concentration is elevated in α thalassaemia trait [55] as well as in iron deficiency, and so is not a useful test in this context. Zinc protoporphyrin may be elevated; values tend to be lower than those in iron deficiency, although there is some overlap [52]. The detection of rare haemoglobin H inclusions in red cells is also useful in the diagnosis of $\alpha^0$ thalassaemia trait (Fig. 3.8). However, this test is time consuming and both false negative and false positive results may occur. The number of cells with haemoglobin H inclusions is reduced by concomitant β thalassaemia trait or haemoglobin E trait. It is therefore reasonable not to test for haemoglobin H inclusions, but to proceed straight to DNA analysis, if accurate diagnosis is important, e.g. in a pregnant woman and her partner with suspected $\alpha^0$ thalassaemia trait.

In the neonatal period, a significantly elevated percentage of haemoglobin Bart's (5–10%) on haemoglobin electrophoresis is compatible with a diagnosis of $\alpha^0$ thalassaemia trait, but is not diagnostic, as similar levels are seen in homozygosity for $\alpha^+$ thalassaemia trait. When quantified by HPLC, the mean percentage is higher than in $\alpha^+$ thalassaemia heterozygosity (9.2% in comparison with 6.4%), but again overlap occurs [53]. Haemoglobin Bart's

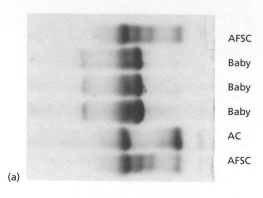

(a)

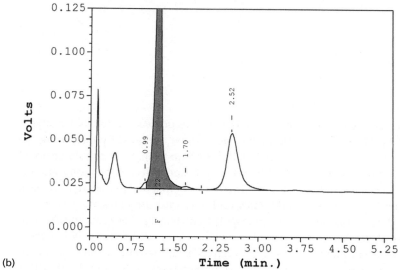

(b)

**Fig. 3.7** (a) Haemoglobin electrophoresis on cellulose acetate showing a fast band that is haemoglobin Bart's ('Baby'); AFSC, control sample containing haemoglobins A, F, S and C. (b) HPLC chromatogram showing haemoglobin Bart's, superimposed on acetylated haemoglobin F, in a baby of Filipino ancestry with $\alpha^0$ thalassaemia trait $(-\!-^{\mathrm{FIL}}/\alpha\alpha)$. HPLC was performed on washed red cells and so there is no bilirubin present. From left to right, the peaks are haemoglobin Bart's plus acetylated F, haemoglobin F (dark grey) and haemoglobin A.

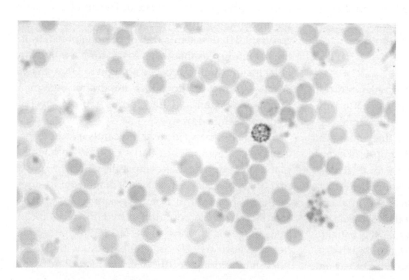

**Fig. 3.8** Haemoglobin H preparation in a patient with $\alpha$ thalassaemia trait showing a single cell containing haemoglobin H inclusions.

disappears by 3–6 months of age. $\alpha^0$ thalassaemia caused by the $-\!-^{SEA}$ mutation can be detected by demonstrating an increased percentage of $\zeta$ chains, e.g. by slot blot immunobinding or enzyme-linked immunosorbent assay (ELISA). The latter may be practicable for screening purposes in areas in which the majority of $\alpha^0$ thalassaemia is caused by this mutation [56]. This technique is only of use in countries with a significant incidence of this genotype, and DNA analysis will still be necessary if both partners appear likely to have $\alpha^0$ thalassaemia trait on the basis of red cell indices, but only one has a detectable $\zeta$ chain.

### Coinheritance with other abnormalities of globin chain synthesis

Inheritance of $\alpha^0$ thalassaemia trait has a similar effect to homozygosity for $\alpha^+$ thalassaemia on coinherited $\beta$ thalassaemia, sickle cell trait, haemoglobin C trait and haemoglobin E trait (see above). Coinheritance with $\alpha^+$ thalassaemia or with a hyperunstable $\alpha$ chain variant usually leads to haemoglobin H disease (see below), but sometimes to a more severe, transfusion-dependent condition [57].

In relation to antenatal screening of pregnant women, it should also be noted that the presence of $\beta$ thalassaemia trait does not exclude the simultaneous presence of $\alpha^0$ thalassaemia trait. Failure to detect both abnormalities may lead to a failure to predict haemoglobin Bart's hydrops fetalis when one partner has $\alpha^0$ thalassaemia trait and the other has both $\alpha^0$ and $\beta$ thalassaemia trait. In ethnic groups in which $\alpha^0$ thalassaemia occurs, DNA analysis of both partners is indicated if one partner has $\beta$ thalassaemia trait and the other has probable $\alpha^0$ thalassaemia trait [58]. The increase in the MCV and MCH if $\alpha^0$ thalassaemia trait and triple $\alpha$ are coinherited ($-\!-/\alpha\alpha\alpha$) may mean that occasional cases of $\alpha^0$ heterozygosity are missed [59].

### Haemoglobin H disease

Haemoglobin H disease is a clinical syndrome resulting from a variety of genetic abnormalities (Table 3.6). The most common causes are compound heterozygosity for $\alpha^+$ thalassaemia and $\alpha^0$ thalassaemia, e.g. $-\!-^{SEA}/-\alpha^{4.2}$ in South-East Asia and $(\alpha)^{20.5}/-\alpha^{3.7}$ or $-\!-^{MED}/-\alpha^{3.7}$ in the Mediterranean. An alternative mechanism is compound heterozygosity for $\alpha^0$ thalassaemia and a non-deletional $\alpha$ thalassaemia, such as haemoglobin Constant Spring or the Saudi type of non-deletional $\alpha$ thalassaemia, e.g. $-\!-^{SEA}/\alpha^{CS}\alpha$ or $-\!-^{MED}/\alpha^{TSaudi}\alpha$, or homozygosity or compound heterozygosity for non-deletional $\alpha$ thalassaemia, mainly $\alpha^{TSaudi}\alpha/\alpha^{TSaudi}\alpha$ or $\alpha^{TSaudi}\alpha/\alpha^{Agr}\alpha$. Rare non-deletional cases are caused by mutation of a gene on the X chromosome, designated the ATR-X syndrome.

Haemoglobin H disease is characterized by a greatly reduced rate of synthesis of the $\alpha$ chain, leading to a hypochromic microcytic anaemia. The excess of $\beta$ chain production over $\alpha$ chain production leads to the formation of an abnormal haemoglobin with $\beta$ chain tetramers, referred to as haemoglobin H. Haemoglobin H functions poorly from the point of view of oxygen delivery to tissues; it lacks haem–haem interaction, so that the oxygen dissociation curve is hyperbolic rather than sigmoid, and has a very high oxygen affinity. Haemoglobin H is soluble but is prone to oxidation; it then becomes unstable, precipitating to some extent in erythroblasts with resultant intramedullary cell death (ineffective erythropoiesis) [60]. Apoptosis of bone marrow cells is increased. When haemoglobin H disease results in part from the synthesis of a highly unstable $\alpha$ chain or haemoglobin, such as haemoglobin Quong Sze, aggregation of the hyperunstable $\alpha$ chain can also contribute to erythroblast damage [60]. Haemoglobin H is oxidized and precipitates in circulating erythrocytes, becoming attached to and damaging the red cell membrane, with resultant membrane rigidity, red cell fragmentation and chronic haemolytic anaemia [47,60]. Erythrophagocytosis by splenic macrophages is attributable in part to membrane rigidity and in part to increased binding of immunoglobulin to damaged membranes, so that the cells are then recognized by the Fc receptors of macrophages. Haemolysis is more important than ineffective erythropoiesis as a cause of anaemia.

Haemoglobin H disease presents clinically with splenomegaly and symptoms of anaemia. Jaundice is sometimes present. The anaemia is aggravated by infection, pregnancy or exposure to oxidant drugs. A sudden worsening of anaemia can also be due to superimposed folate deficiency or aplastic crisis

**Table 3.6**  Examples of genetic abnormalities leading to haemoglobin H disease.

| | |
|---|---|
| $--/-\alpha$ | Compound heterozygosity for $\alpha^0$ and $\alpha^+$ thalassaemia, e.g. $--^{SEA}/-\alpha^{4.2}$ or $--^{SEA}/-\alpha^{3.7}$ in China and South-East Asia, $-(\alpha)^{20.5}/-\alpha^{3.7}$ or $--^{MED}/-\alpha^{3.7}$ in the Mediterranean area and $--^{SA}/-\alpha^{3.7}$ or $--^{SA}/-\alpha^{4.2}$ in India |
| $--/\alpha^T\alpha$ | Compound heterozygosity for $\alpha^0$ thalassaemia and non-deletional $\alpha$ thalassaemia, e.g. $--^{MED}/\alpha^{5nt}\alpha$ or $--^{MED}/\alpha^{TSaudi}\alpha$ in the Mediterranean area |
| $\alpha^T\alpha/\alpha^T\alpha$ | Homozygosity for non-deletional $\alpha$ thalassaemia, e.g. $\alpha^{Tsaudi}\alpha/\alpha^{TSaudi}\alpha$ or $\alpha^{NCO}\alpha/\alpha^{NCO}\alpha$ in the Mediterranean area |
| $\alpha^T\alpha^T\alpha/\alpha^T\alpha$ | Rare example of haemoglobin H disease with a total of five $\alpha$ genes, three of which carry the $\alpha^{TSaudi}$ mutation |
| $\alpha^{PA-1}\alpha/\alpha^{PA-1}\alpha$ and $\alpha^{PA-1}\alpha/-\alpha^{3.7}$ | Homozygosity for non-deletional $\alpha$ thalassaemia or compound heterozygosity for non-deletional $\alpha$ thalassaemia and deletional $\alpha$ thalassaemia trait in the Middle East |
| $--/\alpha^{CS}\alpha$ or $\alpha^{CS}\alpha/\alpha^{CS}\alpha$ | Compound heterozygosity for $\alpha^0$ thalassaemia and either haemoglobin Constant Spring or haemoglobin Paksé, e.g. $--^{SEA}/\alpha^{CS}\alpha$ or $--^{SEA}/\alpha^{Paksé}\alpha$, in South-East Asia* or homozygosity for $\alpha^{CS}\alpha$ in South-East Asia or the Middle East |
| $--/\alpha^{QS}\alpha$ | Compound heterozygosity for $\alpha^0$ thalassaemia and haemoglobin Quong Sze (non-deletional $\alpha$ thalassaemia), e.g. $--^{SEA}/\alpha^{QS}\alpha$ in South-East Asia |
| Genotype not certain | Compound heterozygosity for $\alpha^0$ thalassaemia and an unstable haemoglobin, haemoglobin Petah Tikva† |
| $\alpha^{TSaudi}\alpha/\alpha^{Agrinio}\alpha$ | Compound heterozygosity for non-deletional $\alpha$ thalassaemia and haemoglobin Agrinio, a haemoglobin with an unstable or rapidly catabolized $\alpha$ chain, in Greeks and Greek Cypriots |
| $-\alpha^{3.7}(-AC)/-\alpha^{3.7}(-AC)$ | Homozygosity for ACCATG$\rightarrow$–CATG mutation superimposed on $-\alpha^{3.7}$ in North Africa and Mediterranean area |
| $--/-\alpha^Q$ | Compound heterozygosity for $\alpha^0$ thalassaemia and $\alpha^Q$ on a chromosome with a $-\alpha^{4.2}$ deletion, haemoglobin H/Q disease |
| $--/\alpha^{G-Philadelphia}-$ | Compound heterozygosity for $\alpha^0$ thalassaemia and $\alpha^{G-Philadelphia}$ occurring on a chromosome on which the other $\alpha$ gene is deleted; only haemoglobins G, $G_2$ and H are present, haemoglobin H/G-Philadelphia disease |
| $(\alpha\alpha)/-\alpha$ | Compound heterozygosity for deletion of the upstream regulatory region and $\alpha^+$ thalassaemia |
| Mutation of the *ATRX* gene at Xq13.3 encoding a *trans*-acting factor | ATR-X syndrome of mild haemoglobin H disease, mental retardation and facial and genital dysmorphism |
| Acquired somatic mutation of the *ATRX* gene | Acquired haemoglobin H disease in haematological neoplasms |

*Other termination codon mutations can also interact with $\alpha^0$ thalassaemia to cause haemoglobin H disease, e.g. haemoglobin Icaria [8].
†It is not known whether the mutation is in the $\alpha2$ or $\alpha1$ gene; other very unstable $\alpha$ chains or haemoglobins can also interact with $\alpha^0$ thalassaemia to produce haemoglobin H disease, e.g. haemoglobins Suan-Dok [14], Evanston [14], Adana [14] and Pak Num Po [60].

following parvovirus B19 infection. The incidence of gallstones and cholecystitis is increased. Some patients have leg ulcers. Sometimes the clinical features are so mild that the diagnosis is made incidentally. In other patients, the anaemia is much more severe and intermittent or, rarely, regular transfusions are required. In severely affected patients, there is growth retardation and expansion of the bone marrow cavity, leading to bony deformity affecting the facial bones, similar to that which is seen in β thalassaemia major. Clinically significant iron overload is not common, but can lead to diabetes mellitus, cardiomyopathy, hepatic fibrosis and even cirrhosis [60]. Some patients require splenectomy to relieve hypersplenism. Very rarely, the phenotype of haemoglobin H disease is more severe, with hydrops fetalis leading, in some cases, to death *in utero* or soon after birth [61]. Those who survive the perinatal period may have disease of moderate severity, but with transfusion independence, in later life, or may remain transfusion dependent. This severe phenotype of haemoglobin H disease usually results from compound heterozygosity for $\alpha^0$ and non-deletional α thalassaemia affecting the α2 gene [61,62]; however, it can also occur due to compound heterozygosity for $\alpha^0$ thalassaemia and a severe $\alpha^+$ thalassaemia phenotype resulting from a very unstable α chain, such as that designated haemoglobin Adana [63].

In general, haemoglobin H disease is most severe if there is homozygosity or compound heterozygosity for non-deletional α thalassaemia, next most severe if there is compound heterozygosity for deletional and non-deletional α thalassaemia and least severe if there is deletion of three of the four α genes [64,65]. Most of the non-deletional α chain mutations described in haemoglobin H disease have been in the α2 gene, but occasional examples are in the α1 gene [64,65]. In one study, the functional defect in nondeletional haemoglobin H disease was found to be similar whether the mutation was in the α1 or α2 gene; it was suggested that this was because transcription of the abnormal gene interfered with transcription of the normal gene [64]. In another series, both patients with a non-deletional defect of the α1 gene had mild disease, whereas those with a non-deletional defect of the α2 gene generally had severe disease [65].

In the case of the ATR-X syndrome, haemoglobin H disease is relatively mild and the clinical presentation is with dysmorphism and mental retardation in young boys. There is short stature, microcephaly, facial dysmorphism and abnormalities of the external genitalia. Most patients with this syndrome have been Caucasian, but five Japanese cases have also been reported [66–68].

*Laboratory features*

There is a moderately severe hypochromic microcytic anaemia with the haemoglobin concentration varying in the range 3–11 g/dl (usually 7–10 g/dl) (Fig. 3.9). The MCV is of the order of 50–65 fl and the MCH is usually 15–20 pg. MCHC is reduced, usually to between 25 and 30 g/dl. The reduction in the MCHC reflects not only reduced haemoglobin synthesis, but also cellular overhydration resulting from membrane damage; this is particularly so in patients with haemoglobin Constant Spring [47,60]. When one of the genetic abnormalities leading to haemoglobin H disease is a non-deletional α thalassaemia (e.g. $\alpha^{\text{Constant Spring}}$ or $\alpha^{\text{Quong Sze}}$), the anaemia, reticulocytosis and hypochromia are more marked, the MCHC is lower and the MCV and MCH are significantly higher [47,60]. The RBC is increased.

The blood film (Fig. 3.10) shows striking anisocytosis, poikilocytosis, hypochromia and microcytosis. Poikilocytes may include target cells, fragments and teardrop poikilocytes. Basophilic stippling may be present. Nucleated red blood cells may be present but often they are not. The percentage and absolute reticulocyte count are increased. Serum soluble transferrin receptor and erythropoietin concentration are increased.

The bone marrow aspirate (Fig 3.11) shows erythroid hyperplasia and micronormoblastic maturation. Ultrastructural examination shows abnormal cytoplasmic inclusions that are likely to represent precipitated β chain (Fig. 3.12).

The serum bilirubin concentration and urinary urobilinogen are increased. The bilirubin is unconjugated. Serum lactate dehydrogenase (LDH) may also be increased. Serum haptoglobin is reduced.

Haemoglobin electrophoresis (Fig. 3.13), HPLC (Fig. 3.14) and isoelectric focusing (IEF) show that haemoglobin H comprises 1–40% of total haemoglobin (usually 8–10%). The haemoglobin H percentage is higher when one of the genetic defects is a non-deletional α thalassaemia and lower when there is coexisting heterozygosity for $\beta^S$, $\beta^C$ or $\beta^E$ [60]. Haemoglobin Bart's is present in some patients, usually comprising around 5% of total haemoglobin; at birth it may be 20–40% [60]. The percentage of haemoglobin $A_2$ is usually reduced to 1–2%. Haemoglobin F may be increased to 1–3%. A

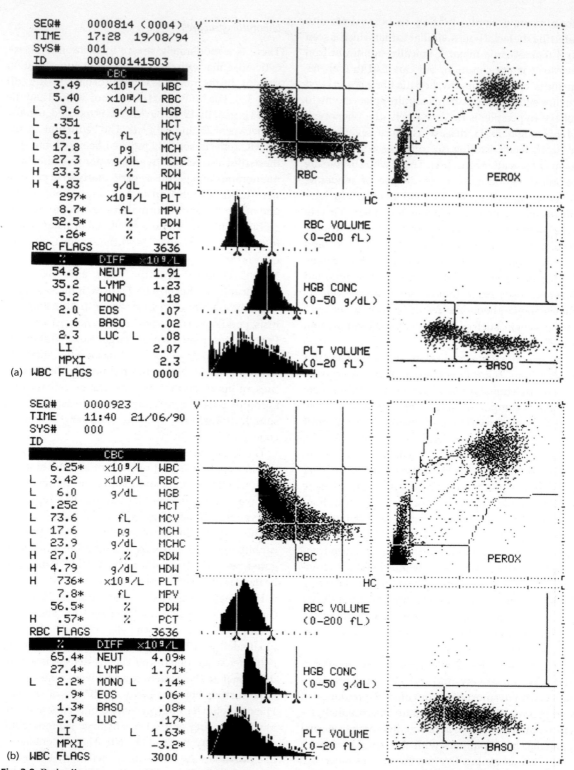

**Fig. 3.9** Red cell cytograms and histograms from two patients with haemoglobin H disease: (a) a patient with disease of average severity showing moderately severe anaemia and marked microcytosis and hypochromia; (b) a patient with disease severe enough to have required splenectomy showing marked microcytosis and an extreme degree of hypochromia.

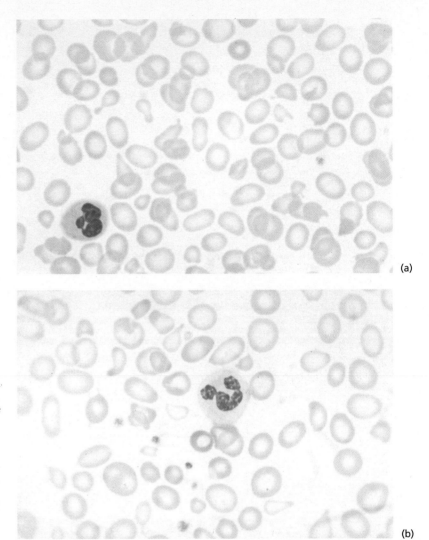

(a)

(b)

**Fig. 3.10** Blood films from four patients with haemoglobin H disease showing the range of abnormality observed. (a) The red cell indices were RBC $4.95 \times 10^{12}$/l, Hb 9.6 g/dl, Hct 0.30, MCV 60.5 fl, MCH 19.4 pg, MCHC 32.1 g/dl and reticulocytes $237 \times 10^{9}$/l. (b) The red cell indices and haemoglobin H percentage were RBC $5.34 \times 10^{12}$/l, Hb 9.3 g/dl, Hct 0.34, MCV 63 fl, MCH 17.5 pg, MCHC 27.7 g/dl and haemoglobin H 5%. (*Continued on p. 84.*)

haemoglobin H preparation in which red cells are exposed to a mildly oxidant dye, such as brilliant cresyl blue or new methylene blue, shows characteristic 'golf-ball' haemoglobin H inclusions in a large proportion, usually 35–90%, of red cells (Fig. 3.15). These inclusions, which form *in vitro* during incubation with vital dyes, are shown on ultrastructural examination to be attached to the red cell membrane (Fig. 3.16). In patients who have been splenectomized, there are, in addition, larger preformed Heinz bodies, also attached to the red cell membrane (Fig. 3.17). Both the percentage of haemoglobin H

and the proportion of cells containing haemoglobin H inclusions are lowered by concomitant iron deficiency; haemoglobin H formation may even be completely suppressed [69]. A similar temporary suppression of haemoglobin H synthesis has been reported in one patient with anaemia of chronic disease and in another with alcohol-induced sideroblastic anaemia [70]. When haemoglobin H disease is caused by non-deletional α thalassaemia, haemoglobin H is not always detectable on haemoglobin electrophoresis and haemoglobin H inclusions may be infrequent; it has been postulated that this may be

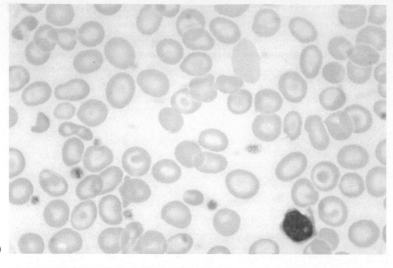

(c)

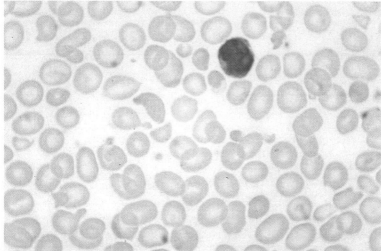

(d)

**Fig. 3.10** *Continued.* (c) The red cell indices were RBC $5.65 \times 10^{12}/l$, Hb 9.2 g/dl, Hct 0.33, MCV 58.2 fl, MCH 16.4 pg and MCHC 28.1 g/dl. (d) The red cell indices were RBC $5.34 \times 10^{12}/l$, Hb 10.4 g/dl, Hct 0.34, MCV 63.6 fl, MCH 19.5 pg and MCHC 30.6 g/dl.

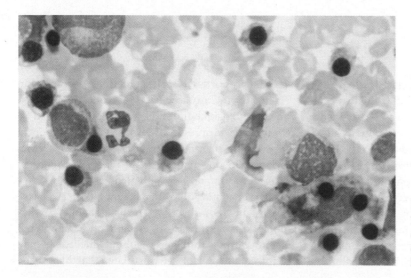

**Fig. 3.11** Bone marrow aspirate in haemoglobin H disease; there is erythroid hyperplasia and some erythroblasts show defective haemoglobinization.

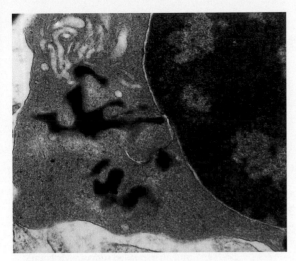

**Fig. 3.12** Ultrastructural examination of bone marrow erythroblast from a patient with haemoglobin H disease showing an electron-dense stellate inclusion, probably consisting of precipitated β chain. (By courtesy of Professor S. N. Wickramasinghe.)

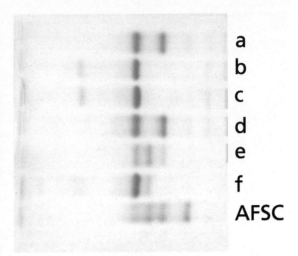

**Fig. 3.13** Haemoglobin electrophoresis on cellulose acetate at alkaline pH in a patient with haemoglobin H disease showing a fast band to the left of haemoglobin A (strips b and c); AFSC, control sample containing haemoglobins A, F, S and C.

**Fig. 3.14** HPLC chromatograms in two patients with haemoglobin H disease; the double peak to the left is haemoglobin H, while the major peak to the right is haemoglobin A.

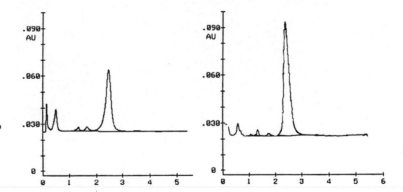

because β chains and an abnormal α chain are forming transitory and unstable dimers that are rapidly destroyed [14].

Globin chain synthesis studies show an α:non-α ratio of the order of 0.26–0.60 [65]. The oxygen dissociation curve is abnormal. As haemoglobin H comprises a relatively low percentage of total haemoglobin, the $P_{50}$ (the $P_{O_2}$ at which haemoglobin is 50% saturated) may be normal or only slightly reduced; however, the lower part of the dissociation curve is displaced to the left giving a biphasic curve.

Haemoglobin H disease occurring as part of the ATR-X syndrome is relatively mild. Not all patients are anaemic and the MCH and MCV are sometimes normal. The percentage of haemoglobin H is lower than is usual in haemoglobin H disease and, in some cases, none is detected on electrophoresis. Haemoglobin H inclusions are detectable in the great majority of cases, but in a relatively low proportion of cells, e.g. 0.5–15%.

In occasional cases of haemoglobin H disease, the single remaining α gene codes for a structurally

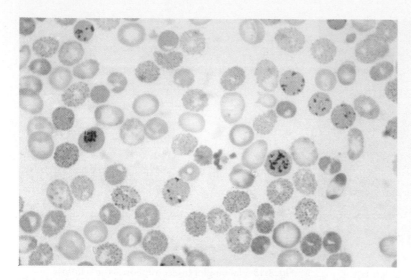

**Fig. 3.15** Haemoglobin H preparation in a patient with haemoglobin H disease showing both 'golf-ball' haemoglobin H inclusions and an increased reticulocyte count.

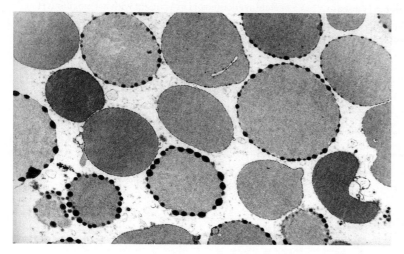

**Fig. 3.16** Ultrastructural examination of erythrocytes from a patient with haemoglobin H disease following incubation with brilliant cresyl blue; haemoglobin H inclusions are apparent, attached to the red cell membrane. (By courtesy of Professor S. N. Wickramasinghe.)

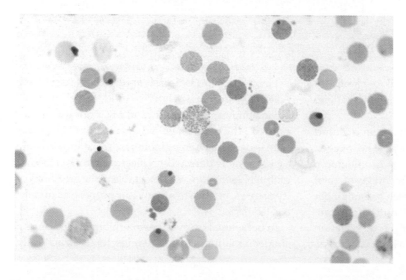

**Fig. 3.17** Haemoglobin H preparation in a patient with haemoglobin H disease who has been splenectomized showing 'golf-ball' haemoglobin H inclusions, preformed Heinz bodies and an increased reticulocyte count.

abnormal α chain so that no haemoglobin A is synthesized. There is haemoglobin H, a significant proportion of an α chain variant (e.g. haemoglobin G-Philadelphia or haemoglobin Q) and small amounts of a haemoglobin $A_2$ variant (e.g. G-Philadelphia$_2$ or Q$_2$). Less rare is haemoglobin H disease caused by compound heterozygosity for $\alpha^0$ thalassaemia and non-deletional $\alpha^+$ thalassaemia consequent on an α chain variant that is synthesized at a greatly reduced rate (e.g. haemoglobin Constant Spring or haemoglobin Icaria). In this case, small amounts of the variant (e.g. 1.5–2% of haemoglobin Constant Spring) will be present in addition to haemoglobin A and haemoglobin H. Genes coding for very unstable α chains can also lead to haemoglobin H disease, either when there is homozygosity or when they are coinherited with other α thalassaemia variants [10]. Examples include haemoglobin Quong Sze and haemoglobin Suan Dok.

Neonates with haemoglobin H disease have a lower haemoglobin concentration than other neonates, usually of the order of 12–14 g/dl, and a markedly lower MCV and MCH (e.g. 73 and 74 fl and 22 pg in two reported cases [71]). Haemoglobin Bart's comprises 5–40% (usually 20–25%) of total haemoglobin. Haemoglobin H is present at a low percentage.

*Coinheritance with other abnormalities of globin chain synthesis*

Coexisting β thalassaemia trait often makes haemoglobin H disease milder than would otherwise be the case, but some instances of transfusion dependency have been reported [72]. Usually, the haemoglobin concentration and the degree of microcytosis are similar to those seen in uncomplicated haemoglobin H disease, but the degree of haemolysis is less. The reticulocyte count and bilirubin concentration may be normal [72] or the reticulocyte count may be mildly elevated [73]. Serum soluble transferrin receptor is elevated, indicating increased (but ineffective) erythropoiesis [73]. Significant iron overload can occur [72]. The percentage of haemoglobin F and the proportion of cells containing haemoglobin H inclusions are reduced in comparison with those of uncomplicated haemoglobin H disease [71] and sometimes no haemoglobin H can be detected [72]. A trace of haemoglobin Bart's is sometimes detected.

The haemoglobin $A_2$ percentage is sometimes normal and sometimes elevated, but to a lesser extent than is usual in β thalassaemia trait. The α:non-α chain synthesis ratios are of the order of 0.5–0.7, similar to those seen in α thalassaemia heterozygosity [73].

Atypical phenotypes occur when the genotype of haemoglobin H disease is coinherited with haemoglobin S trait (see p. 148), haemoglobin C trait (see p. 194), heterozygosity for deletional hereditary persistence of fetal haemoglobin (see p. 124), non-deletional hereditary persistence of fetal haemoglobin (see p. 127) and haemoglobin E heterozygosity or homozygosity (see p. 208). Coinheritance of heterozygosity for β$^{New York}$ leads to more severe disease, as the β$^{New York}$ chain has greater affinity than the normal β chain for the available α chains and haemoglobin New York is unstable [60].

## Haemoglobin Bart's hydrops fetalis and related conditions

Homozygosity for $\alpha^0$ thalassaemia leads to a total failure of α chain synthesis so that no synthesis of haemoglobin F, A or $A_2$ can occur. The result is the clinical syndrome known as haemoglobin Bart's hydrops fetalis, first described in Indonesia in 1960 [74]. This condition is most often seen in South-East Asia, including China, but there is a low but significant incidence in Greece, Turkey and Cyprus. Rare cases have been observed in Sardinia (two cases) and in families of Indian ethnic origin. Haemoglobin Bart's hydrops fetalis is usually incompatible with extrauterine life. Some fetuses die *in utero* and others within a short time of birth. Rarely, there is survival for a few days, even in the absence of treatment. A few fetuses have been 'rescued' by intrauterine or post-delivery transfusion [16], but sometimes with significant brain damage having already occurred. Hypospadias has also been noted in survivors [75], one infant had deformity of a foot [76] and a number have had a patent ductus arteriosus.

The deletion of all four α genes, but with one or both ζ genes being intact (e.g. $-\!-^{SEA}/-\!-^{SEA}$, $-\!-^{MED}/-\!-^{MED}$, $-\!-^{SEA}/-\!-^{THAI}$ or $-\!-^{SEA}/-\!-^{FIL}$), leads to haemoglobin Bart's hydrops fetalis (Fig. 3.18). Almost all the haemoglobin present is haemoglobin Bart's, a haemoglobin with γ tetramers, which is

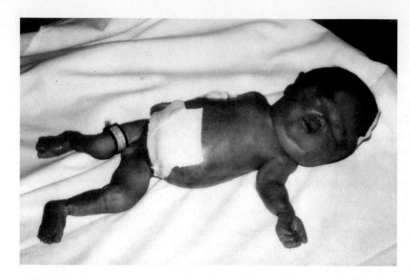

**Fig. 3.18** Fetus with haemoglobin Bart's hydrops fetalis. (With thanks to Dr R. Rodwell and Professor H. Smith.)

unable to deliver oxygen to tissues as, like haemoglobin H, it has a very high oxygen affinity and lacks haem–haem interaction, leading to a hyperbolic rather than sigmoid oxygen dissociation curve. The remainder of the haemoglobin is largely haemoglobin Portland 1 ($\zeta_2\gamma_2$) which is capable of oxygen delivery to tissues and can keep the fetus alive into the third trimester. There may be small amounts of haemoglobin Portland 2 ($\zeta_2\beta_2$) and haemoglobin H. There is severe anaemia (consequent on a reduced rate of haemoglobin synthesis together with ineffective haemopoiesis and a shortened red cell life span caused by precipitation of haemoglobin Bart's) and extramedullary haemopoiesis leading to hepatosplenomegaly. Because haemoglobin Bart's is a high-affinity haemoglobin, the functional effects of the anaemia are much greater than would be expected from the haemoglobin concentration. The combination of severe anaemia, failure of oxygen delivery to tissues and hypoalbuminaemia (likely to be related to the marked extramedullary haemopoiesis in the liver) leads to cardiac failure and abnormal organogenesis. There is gross placental enlargement and oedema. There may be congenital cardiac abnormalities, genital abnormalities (ambiguous genitalia, hypospadias, undescended testes), terminal transverse limb defects, pulmonary hypoplasia and retarded brain growth [8]. At birth, the neonate is pale, faintly jaundiced, growth retarded and usually hydropic. There may

be subcutaneous blue nodules of haemopoietic tissue.

When there is homozygosity for a large deletion, including the $\zeta$ genes as well as both $\alpha$ genes, no functional haemoglobin can be produced. The only haemoglobins synthesized are haemoglobin Bart's and a haemoglobin with tetrameric $\varepsilon$. The fetus dies early in gestation with consequent miscarriage. This syndrome can result from homozygosity for $--^{\mathrm{FIL}}$ and $--^{\mathrm{THAI}}$.

Rarely, the phenotype of hydrops fetalis can result from heterozygosity for $\alpha^0$ thalassaemia and severe non-deletional $\alpha^+$ thalassaemia (e.g. $--/\alpha^{\mathrm{TSaudi}}\alpha$, $--/\alpha^{\mathrm{QS}}\alpha$ or $--/\alpha^{59\mathrm{Gly}\rightarrow\mathrm{Asp}}\alpha$). The disease phenotype may be more severe if the $\zeta\zeta$ locus is deleted as well as the $\alpha\alpha$ locus; this can be designated by the notation $----/\zeta\zeta(\alpha\alpha)^{\mathrm{T}}$. Haemoglobin A and F are present in addition to haemoglobin Bart's, haemoglobin Portland 1 and haemoglobin H [77]. The proportions of the various haemoglobins are similar to those in haemoglobin H disease, but the haemoglobin concentration during intrauterine life and at birth is lower. The genotype $--/\alpha^{\mathrm{T}}\alpha$ more often results in haemoglobin H disease.

Women carrying a fetus with haemoglobin Bart's hydrops fetalis have an increased rate of pregnancy-related hypertension and hydramnios and usually have a difficult delivery, with an increased rate of antepartum and postpartum haemorrhage and retained placenta. If a molecular diagnosis of $\alpha^0$

thalassaemia is precluded by economic constraints, consideration should be given to ultrasound examination commencing early in pregnancy in potentially at-risk pregnancies in order to detect hydrops fetalis and offer termination of pregnancy before maternal complications occur. Increased placental thickness and an increased cardiothoracic ratio are the earliest ultrasound signs.

*Laboratory features*

A fetus with haemoglobin Bart's hydrops fetalis has severe anaemia (haemoglobin concentration usually 3–8 g/dl, occasionally up to 10 g/dl or even higher) and striking anisocytosis and poikilocytosis (including target cells and elongated cells). Erythrocytes appear large but markedly hypochromic. There is a reticulocytosis. Circulating nucleated red cells are greatly increased, a condition designated erythroblastosis fetalis (Fig. 3.19). The MCH and MCHC are greatly reduced, but the MCV may be normal.

Haemoglobin electrophoresis (Fig. 3.20) and HPLC (Fig. 3.21) show haemoglobin Bart's (70–100%) and sometimes smaller amounts of haemoglobin Portland 1 (usually around 10–20%), haemoglobin Portland 2 and haemoglobin H.

*Diagnosis*

Following the delivery of a hydropic fetus, the diagnosis of haemoglobin Bart's hydrops fetalis can be made from the haematological and electrophoretic characteristics. Sometimes the condition is diagnosed *in utero* as a result of ultrasound examination. It is desirable that this condition be predicted early in pregnancy by the identification of all women at risk of $\alpha^0$ thalassaemia trait, followed, when both partners are at risk of $\alpha^0$ thalassaemia trait, by DNA analysis. When both parents are found to have $\alpha^0$ thalassaemia trait, DNA analysis on the fetus is required. Fetal tissue for diagnosis can be obtained by chorionic villous sampling in the first or second trimester, from amniotic fluid obtained by amniocentesis in the second trimester and by fetal blood sampling in the second trimester.

## The β thalassaemias

The β thalassaemias are a group of conditions resulting from a reduced rate of synthesis of β globin. More than 200 β thalassaemia mutations have been recognized, occurring in a wide range of ethnic groups (Table 3.5). β thalassaemia is common around the Mediterranean, in the Indian subcontinent and in South-East Asia and relatively common in those of African ancestry. It is recognized but rare in the indigenous British population [78] and in other Northern European populations. The severity of the defect is very variable. As normal individuals have two allelic β globin genes, β thalassaemia may exist in a heterozygous or homozygous state. As there are a large number of β thalassaemia mutations, compound heterozygosity may also occur with the individual having two mutant genes but no normal β gene. β thalassaemia mutations are divided into two broad categories: $\beta^0$ (beta zero) thalassaemia and $\beta^+$ (beta plus) thalassaemia. In $\beta^0$ thalassaemia, there is either an abnormal gene that is not expressed or, less often, gene deletion. If $\beta^0$ thalassaemia occurs in the homozygous or compound heterozygous state ($\beta^0\beta^0$), there is a total lack of β chain production and a total failure to produce haemoglobin A. In $\beta^+$ thalassaemia, there is reduced but not absent expression of the abnormal β gene so that, in homozygotes, there is some production of haemoglobin A. There are a large number of different $\beta^+$ thalassaemia mutations with the severity of the defect in chain synthesis varying from mild to severe. Homozygotes thus have disease varying from mild to very severe. Compound heterozygotes for β thalassaemia may have two different $\beta^0$ thalassaemia genes, two different $\beta^+$ thalassaemia genes or both a $\beta^0$ and a $\beta^+$ thalassaemia gene.

β thalassaemia usually results from mutation in or near the β gene. A smaller proportion of cases result from deletion, either of the β gene itself or of controlling sequences 5′ to the gene (i.e. upstream from the gene). Disorders with the phenotype of β thalassaemia may also result from mutations that lead to structural abnormalities of the β globin chain; the mechanism may be either a reduced rate of β chain production, production of a very unstable β chain or production of a very unstable haemoglobin. Haemoglobin E is the most prevalent example of a structurally abnormal haemoglobin in which the mutated β globin is synthesized at a reduced rate as a result of activation of a cryptic splice site. It can be regarded as a thalassaemic haemoglobinopathy. Similarly,

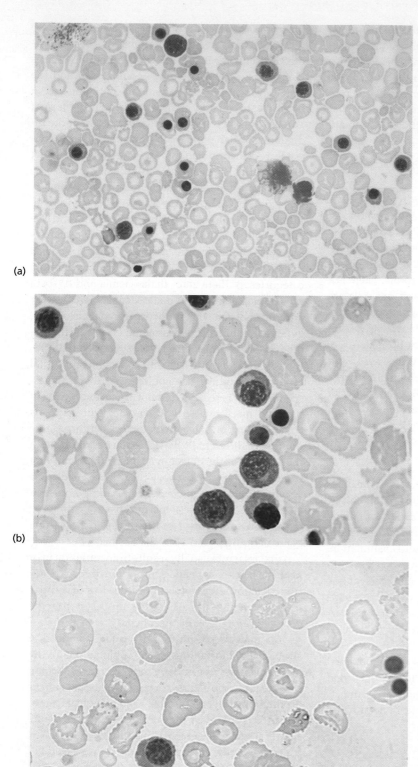

(a)

(b)

(c)

**Fig. 3.19** Blood film in two cases of haemoglobin Bart's hydrops fetalis showing a striking increase in nucleated red cells: (a) ×40; (b) ×100 (with thanks to Dr M. F. McMullin); (c) ×100 (with thanks to Professor H. Smith).

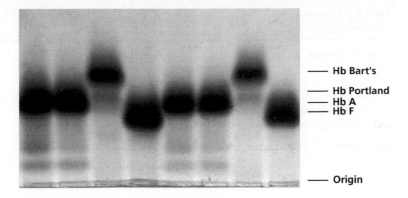

**Fig. 3.20** Haemoglobin electrophoresis in haemoglobin Bart's hydrops fetalis: third and seventh patterns from left. (With thanks to Dr H. Dodsworth.)

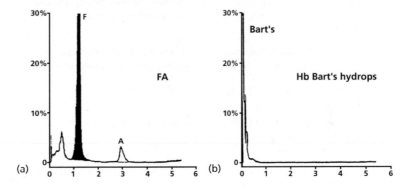

**Fig. 3.21** HPLC chromatogram in (a) a normal neonate showing post-translationally modified haemoglobin F, haemoglobin F and haemoglobin A and (b) a neonate with haemoglobin Bart's hydrops fetalis showing haemoglobin Bart's only. (Derived from reference [53].)

haemoglobin Malay, another variant haemoglobin with activation of a cryptic splice site, represents 15% of thalassaemia alleles in Malaysia and 16% in southern Thailand and also occurs in China and Indonesia [79]; it is likely to be frequently unidentified as it cannot be distinguished from haemoglobin A by electrophoresis or chromatography. Haemoglobin North Shore and haemoglobin Vicksburg are less common variant haemoglobins associated with a β thalassaemia phenotype [80]. Mutations that can result in β thalassaemia and the phenotype usually associated with each are summarized in Table 3.7 [9,81–88], and the sites of mutations leading to β⁰ and β⁺ thalassaemia are summarized in Figs 3.22 and 3.23, respectively. Rarely, there are two thalassaemia mutations on the one chromosome, as in a patient with both IVS2 654 C→T and 3′ UTR nt 1570 T→C [89]. The great majority of cases of β thalassaemia result from mutations in or near the β gene. However, there are occasional cases with no detectable abnormality in the β globin cluster and in which inheri-

tance is not linked to the β globin gene cluster [90,91]; in such cases, it may be postulated that the mutation is in a *trans*-acting gene coding for a protein that interacts with regulatory elements of the β globin gene. In one such defect, the gene responsible mapped to Xp11–12 and was identified as *GATA1*; with this mutation, the β thalassaemia trait is associated with thrombocytopenia [88].

β thalassaemia heterozygosity, also referred to as β thalassaemia trait, is usually clinically asymptomatic, a condition which may also be referred to as β thalassaemia minor. Homozygosity or compound heterozygosity for β thalassaemia usually leads to a clinically severe phenotype, referred to as β thalassaemia major, in which the individual is dependent on blood transfusion. The term 'thalassaemia intermedia' indicates that the clinical features of a case are intermediate between those of β thalassaemia minor and β thalassaemia major; the individual is symptomatic, but although he or she may need occasional blood transfusions, these are not essential to

**Table 3.7** Types of mutation that can result in the phenotype of β thalassaemia (the numbers of mutations given should be regarded as approximate as new mutations continue to be described) [9,81–88].

| Type of mutation | Consequence | Phenotype |
| --- | --- | --- |
| *Deletional* | | |
| Large deletion involving the β gene (14 known, only that occurring in Sind and Punjabi populations is common) | Absent transcription, unusually high haemoglobin A$_2$ in heterozygotes | β$^0$ thalassaemia |
| Small deletion 5′ of the β gene (three known) | Reduced transcription | β$^+$ thalassaemia |
| *Non-deletional* | | |
| Insertion into IVS2 (one known) | Reduced transcription | β$^+$ thalassaemia |
| Mutations in promoter sequences, proximal or distal CACCC box or TATA box (20 known) | Reduced transcription, increased transcription of γ and δ | Silent β, mild (β$^{++}$) thalassaemia or β$^+$ thalassaemia |
| Mutation in 5′ untranslated region near CAP site (six known) | Reduced transcription and translation and instability of mRNA | Silent or mild (β$^{++}$) thalassaemia |
| Mutation of initiation codon (six known) | Absent transcription | β$^0$ thalassaemia (more severe than most other β$^0$ thalassaemias) |
| RNA splicing mutations — involving invariant nucleotides of either donor or acceptor site (21 known) | Absence of properly spliced mRNA | β$^0$ thalassaemia |
| RNA splicing mutations — involving nucleotides flanking splice junctions (consensus sequences) (at least 12 known) | Inefficient splicing of mRNA | Silent, mild (β$^{++}$) thalassaemia, β$^+$ thalassaemia or, occasionally, β$^0$ thalassaemia |
| RNA splicing mutations — activation of cryptic splice site in an intron or an exon with or without an alteration in the coding sequence (11 known) | Aberrant mRNA is produced in addition to normal mRNA; sometimes a structurally abnormal β chain is produced, which may be highly unstable | Mild (β$^{++}$) thalassaemia, β$^+$ thalassaemia, β$^0$ thalassaemia or, occasionally, dominant β thalassaemia; haemoglobin E, haemoglobin Malay or haemoglobin Knossus |
| Mutation interfering with polyadenylation and therefore mRNA cleavage (four nucleotide substitutions and two small deletions known) | Unstable elongated RNA transcript (plus some normal transcript) | β$^+$ or mild (β$^{++}$) thalassaemia |
| Other mutations interfering with mRNA processing (four known) | Abnormal processing of mRNA | Silent, mild (β$^{++}$) or β$^+$ thalassaemia |
| Premature termination codon consequent on alteration of a single nucleotide (15 known) or on a frame shift mutation (69 known, including one large insertion in exon 2 and other deletions and insertions) | Absent translation (exon 1 and 2 mutations) or translation of aberrant mRNA (exon 3 mutations) leading to a very unstable truncated β chain | β$^0$ thalassaemia (exon 1 and 2 mutations) or dominantly inherited β thalassaemia (exon 3 mutations) |
| Other 'thalassaemic haemoglobinopathies' caused by a single nucleotide change | Reduced transcription of an abnormal mRNA<br>Transcription of abnormal RNA coding for a very unstable β chain | Haemoglobin North Shore, haemoglobin Vicksburg<br>Haemoglobin Indianapolis, haemoglobin Geneva |

**Table 3.7** *Continued.*

| Type of mutation | Consequence | Phenotype |
|---|---|---|
| 'Thalassaemic haemoglobinopathies' associated with mutation of the termination codon to a coding sequence ('anti-termination' mutation) | Synthesis of an elongated mRNA and β chain | Haemoglobin Tak, haemoglobin Cranston, haemoglobin Saverne |
| Haemoglobin Lepore* | δβ fusion gene with reduced rate of synthesis of aberrant δβ chain | Haemoglobin Lepore Boston, haemoglobin Lepore Baltimore, haemoglobin Lepore Hollandia |
| Certain unstable haemoglobins | Marked instability of haemoglobin leading to rapid post-translational degradation | Haemoglobin Showa-Yakushigi, haemoglobin K-Woolwich |
| Mutation in the *GATA1* gene, a gene at Xp11–12 encoding an erythroid transcription factor | Reduced transcription | Thalassaemia with thrombocytopenia |
| Mutation in the *XPD* gene at 19q13.2–13.3, which encodes a component of the general transcription factor, TFIIH | Reduced transcription | Thalassaemia with trichothiodystrophy |
| No abnormality of β gene demonstrable and segregating independently of β gene | Unknown but assumed to result from a mutation in a gene coding for a *trans*-acting factor | |

mRNA, messenger RNA.
*Haemoglobin Lepore can be regarded as a δβ+ thalassaemia.

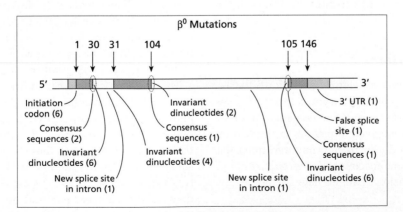

**Fig. 3.22** Sites of mutations giving rise to β⁰ thalassaemia, including dominant thalassaemia. The numbers above the chromosome represent the codons. Introns are shown in blue and the 5′ and 3′ untranslated regions (UTR) in green. The dotted lines are a diagrammatic indication of the consensus sequences flanking the invariant nucleotides at the splice sites. In addition to the mutation sites shown, there are 14 nonsense mutations (three dominant), 69 frame shift mutations (12 dominant), 10 unstable variants (nine dominant) and eight insertions or deletions of triplet codons (six dominant).

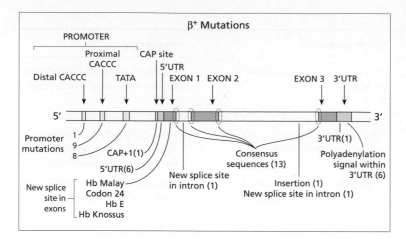

**Fig. 3.23** Sites of mutations giving rise to β⁺ thalassaemia. Introns are shown in blue, the 5′ and 3′ untranslated regions (UTR) in green and important promoter sequences in yellow. The dotted lines are a diagrammatic indication of the consensus sequences flanking the invariant nucleotides at the splice sites.

maintain life. The clinical conditions designated as thalassaemia intermedia cover a genetically heterogeneous group of disorders of very variable severity, including homozygosity or compound heterozygosity for mild β⁺ thalassaemia and heterozygous β thalassaemia aggravated by coexisting heterozygosity or homozygosity for ααα. β thalassaemia mutations that are characteristically associated with clinical abnormalities in heterozygotes are referred to as dominant β thalassaemia (see p. 103). Although, by definition, blood transfusion is not essential to maintain life in thalassaemia intermedia, patients with more severe disease may be treated electively with blood transfusion in order to improve the quality of life.

## β thalassaemia trait

β thalassaemia trait or heterozygosity for β thalassaemia is usually completely asymptomatic and may therefore be referred to as β thalassaemia minor. In conditions of haemopoietic stress, for example during pregnancy or during intercurrent infections, the patient may become anaemic and even require blood transfusion. Occasional patients have splenomegaly.

### Laboratory features

The blood count characteristically shows a normal or slightly reduced haemoglobin concentration, elevation of the RBC and reduction of the MCH and MCV.

The MCHC is usually normal when measured by impedance counters (e.g. Coulter or Sysmex instruments), but may be reduced when measured by Bayer light scattering instruments. The red cell distribution width (RDW), a measurement that reflects red cell anisocytosis, is usually normal. Mean values for haematological variables (haemoglobin concentration, MCV and MCH) differ significantly between β⁺ and β⁰ thalassaemia trait, but there is considerable overlap [92]. The haematological abnormality is less if there is coinheritance of α thalassaemia. The haemoglobin concentration falls in pregnancy as the plasma volume rises normally but the rise in red cell mass is less than normal [93]. However, a haemoglobin concentration of less than 8–9 g/dl suggests a complicating factor [93]. The MCV rises, on average, by about 2 fl, in comparison with a rise averaging about 4 fl in haematologically normal subjects [94].

The characteristic red cell indices have been used in a number of formulae designed to separate cases of iron deficiency from cases of β thalassaemia trait [95–105]; these were tabulated in the first edition of this book [106]. Although these formulae may be of some value in separating uncomplicated cases into two diagnostic categories, they are unreliable in children and during pregnancy and are of no help in patients who have *both* β thalassaemia trait *and* iron deficiency. Patients who are under treatment for iron deficiency and those who have polycythaemia vera complicated by iron deficiency may also have results more suggestive of thalassaemia trait than of iron deficiency. In a study in randomly selected adult patients with mild microcytosis, none of the four most popular formulae was found to be more effective than the MCV (cut-off point <72 fl) in distinguishing thalassaemia trait from other conditions [105]. These various formulae may be helpful in indicating the most likely diagnosis, but are not of use when it is necessary to make a definite diagnosis of β thalassaemia trait or to exclude this diagnosis. Their use is therefore not recommended.

It should be noted that, when a patient with β thalassaemia trait develops megaloblastic anaemia or significant liver disease, the MCV and MCH may rise into the normal range. The same will occur with the administration of drugs such as zidovudine or hydroxycarbamide, but in these patients there is usually a pre-treatment blood count showing characteristic red cell indices.

The blood film varies from almost normal, with only mild microcytosis, to markedly abnormal (Fig. 3.24). Abnormal features, in addition to microcytosis, include anisocytosis, hypochromia and poikilocytosis. Individuals with a more severe phenotype may have prominent basophilic stippling,

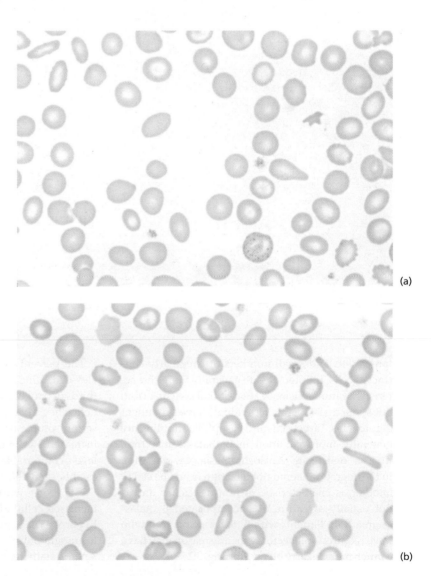

(a)

(b)

**Fig. 3.24** Blood films from three patients with β thalassaemia trait showing the range of abnormalities observed. (a) Blood film showing microcytosis, anisochromasia, a teardrop poikilocyte and basophilic stippling; the red cell indices were RBC $4.41 \times 10^{12}/l$, Hb 14 g/dl, Hct 0.42, MCV 69 fl, MCH 23.2 pg and MCHC 33.4 g/dl. (b) From the same patient showing unusually prominent elliptocytosis. (*Continued on p.96.*)

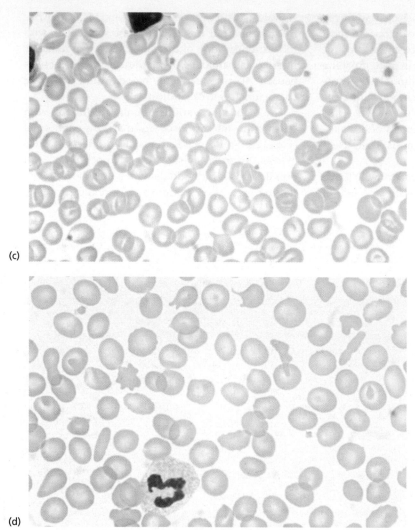

(c)

(d)

**Fig. 3.24** *Continued.* (c) From a patient with RBC $7.3 \times 10^{12}/l$, Hb 14.3 g/dl, Hct 0.43, MCV 59 fl, MCH 19.9 pg, MCHC 32.8 g/dl, haemoglobin $A_2$ 5.6%, haemoglobin F 0.6%. (d) From a patient with $\beta^0$ thalassaemia trait demonstrated by family studies.

target cells and small numbers of irregularly contracted cells. Elliptocytes are generally more characteristic of iron deficiency than of thalassaemia trait, but some thalassaemic individuals have prominent elliptocytes. Target cells and basophilic stippling are generally more common in $\beta$ thalassaemia than in iron deficiency. Anisochromasia, i.e. variation in the degree of haemoglobinization from one cell to another, is characteristic of iron deficiency and is not usually a feature of uncomplicated $\beta$ thalassaemia trait. Patients with $\beta$ thalassaemia trait who have required splenectomy for any reason may have a much more bizarre blood film (Fig. 3.25).

The percentage of reticulocytes may be slightly elevated. Zinc protoporphyrin is elevated in two-thirds of patients; values tend to be lower than in iron deficiency, although there is some overlap [52]. The serum soluble transferrin receptor concentration is increased. Pyrimidine 5′ nucleotidase 1 is reduced to levels comparable with those seen in heterozygotes for inherited deficiency [107].

The bone marrow aspirate (Fig. 3.26) shows increased cellularity as a consequence of erythroid hyperplasia. Some erythroblasts show defective haemoglobinization and cytoplasmic vacuolation. An iron stain may show heavy siderotic granulation.

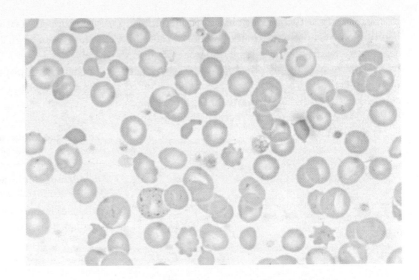

**Fig. 3.25** Blood film from a patient with β thalassaemia trait, who had been splenectomized because of a lymphoma involving the spleen, showing very abnormal red cell morphology.

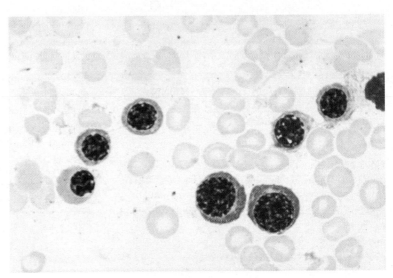

**Fig. 3.26** Bone marrow aspirate in β thalassaemia trait.

Incubation of bone marrow with methyl violet shows small numbers of erythroblasts with α chain inclusions [93].

In the neonatal period, babies with β thalassaemia trait, in contrast with those with α thalassaemia trait, have a normal haemoglobin concentration and normal red cell indices. Differences from normal start to appear around the age of 3 months.

*Diagnosis*

Diagnosis rests on the detection of an increased haemoglobin $A_2$ percentage (Fig. 3.27; see also Fig. 2.7) [108,109]. The increased haemoglobin $A_2$ percentage is due to an absolute rather than merely a relative increase in δ chain synthesis [93]. Other inherited and acquired causes of a high haemoglobin $A_2$ percentage that should be considered in the differential diagnosis are shown in Tables 3.8 and 6.3. The relatively frequent occurrence of a variant haemoglobin $A_2$, designated $A_2'$ (or $B_2$), must be considered when seeking to diagnose β thalassaemia trait. This variant $A_2$ has the same retention time on HPLC as haemoglobin S and thus, if haemoglobin S is absent, it is readily identified (Fig. 3.28). In one study, haemoglobin $A_2'$ was found in *c.* 4% of samples [114].

In individuals with haemoglobin G-Philadelphia, haemoglobin $G_2$ also elutes in the S window [114]. In seeking to make a diagnosis of β thalassaemia trait, haemoglobin $A_2'$ and any other variant $A_2$ (whether resulting from a variant δ chain or from a variant α chain) must be added to normal haemoglobin $A_2$ and the total used to determine whether 'haemoglobin $A_2'$' is elevated.

A proportion of cases, around one-third to one-half, also have an increased proportion of haemoglobin F.

In screening populations for β thalassaemia, it is possible either to measure the haemoglobin $A_2$ per-

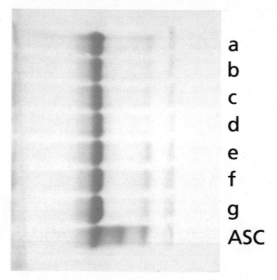

**Fig. 3.27** Haemoglobin electrophoresis on cellulose acetate at alkaline pH showing increased haemoglobin $A_2$ in two patients with β thalassaemia trait (strips e and f); ASC, control sample containing haemoglobins A, S and C.

**Table 3.8** Some inherited causes of an increased percentage of haemoglobin $A_2$.

**Disorders of globin genes**

β thalassaemia trait (almost all cases)

Vietnamese/South-East Asian type of deletional hereditary persistence of fetal haemoglobin (which spares the δ gene)

Hereditary high haemoglobin $A_2$ with autosomal dominant inheritance [110]

Hereditary high haemoglobin $A_2$ resulting from a mutation in the promoter of the δ gene [111]

Unstable haemoglobin

Sickle cell trait

Sickle cell anaemia, particularly if there is coexisting α thalassaemia

Sickle cell/$β^0$ thalassaemia

Heterozygosity for certain other β chain variants, e.g. haemoglobin Leslie [112]

**Disorders unrelated to globin genes**

Congenital dyserythropoietic anaemia (some cases amongst Israeli Bedouins) [113]

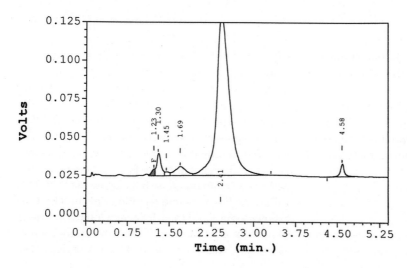

**Fig. 3.28** HPLC chromatogram in a patient with homozygosity for haemoglobin $A_2'$; normal haemoglobin $A_2$ is absent, indicating that the patient has no normal δ gene; the haemoglobin $A_2'$ was 2.2% and was in the 'S window' with a retention time of 4.58 min; from left to right, the peaks are haemoglobin F, post-translationally modified haemoglobin A (two peaks), haemoglobin A and haemoglobin $A_2'$.

centage in everyone or, alternatively, to screen by the red cell indices and test only those with an MCV or MCH below a certain cut-off point. An MCH of less than 27 pg is an indication to quantify haemoglobin $A_2$. Screening by the MCV may be less satisfactory as there is more variation in values between different instruments and, with some instruments, the measured MCV rises with storage of the blood sample [115]. In developing countries, where well-calibrated automated instruments suitable for the measurement of red cell indices may not be available, osmotic fragility can be used for initial screening. The cells of β thalassaemia trait (and of α thalassaemia trait, iron deficiency and some haemoglobinopathies) are more resistant to lysis in hypotonic solutions than are normal cells (see p. 51). The use of a one-tube visual osmotic fragility test reduces the number of samples that have to be referred to a central laboratory for definitive diagnosis.

Suitable methods for the quantification of haemoglobin $A_2$ include haemoglobin electrophoresis followed by elution and spectrophotometric estimation (only suitable when a laboratory is dealing with small numbers of samples), microcolumn chromatography and HPLC. Quantification of haemoglobin $A_2$ by scanning densitometry (Fig. 3.29) is not sufficiently precise to be used in the diagnosis of β thalassaemia trait and IEF has not been validated for this purpose.

The percentage of haemoglobin $A_2$ is dependent on the precise mutation present. In most cases of heterozygosity for $β^0$ or severe $β^+$ thalassaemia, the haemoglobin $A_2$ is between 4% and 5%, whereas when there is heterozygosity for mild $β^+$ thalassaemia there is usually 3.6–4.2% of haemoglobin $A_2$ [116]. Higher percentages are seen in β thalassaemia trait consequent on deletion of the 5' part of the β globin gene (Table 3.7). In addition, promoter mutations (such as −88 C→T and −29 A→G) and mutations of the initiation codon, such as initiation codon A→G, are associated with higher levels [116]. By definition, in silent β thalassaemia, the haemoglobin $A_2$ percentage is normal. For example, with a C→G mutation at position 6, 3' to the termination codon, the mean level is 2.4% [116].

When haemoglobin F is elevated, it usually comprises between 2% and 7% of total haemoglobin. A further rise occurs in pregnancy, paralleling the rise that takes place in haematologically normal pregnant women [93]. Elevation is usual when β thalassaemia trait is caused by deletion of the 5' part of the β globin gene. The level of haemoglobin F is influenced not only by the nature of the mutation causing the β thalassaemia, but also by coinheritance of non-deletional hereditary persistence of fetal haemoglobin mutations, some of which are quite common. A Kleihauer test shows that the distribution is heterogeneous. Quantification of haemoglobin F is not essential for the diagnosis of β thalassaemia, which is dependent on the detection of an increased concentration of haemoglobin $A_2$. However, if a patient has red cell indices suggestive of thalassaemia, but has a normal haemoglobin $A_2$ percentage, it is essential to exclude elevation of haemoglobin F as δβ thalas-

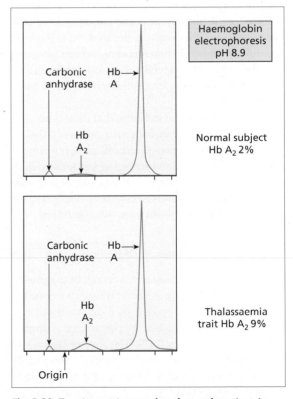

**Fig. 3.29** Densitometric scan of an electrophoretic strip in β thalassaemia trait and in a haematologically normal subject showing increased haemoglobin $A_2$ in β thalassaemia trait. This technique is not sufficiently precise to be used for reliable diagnosis, but is used here for illustrative purposes.

saemia is an alternative diagnosis. Quantification of haemoglobin F will be automatically available if haemoglobin $A_2$ is quantified by HPLC. If cellulose acetate electrophoresis and microcolumn chromatography are employed as the routine diagnostic techniques, the electrophoretic strip should be carefully inspected for a prominent haemoglobin F band. A concentration above 2% can usually be detected visually and it is then possible to select samples for quantification, e.g. by alkali denaturation. Similarly, the presence of haemoglobin Lepore should be excluded by cellulose acetate electrophoresis, IEF or HPLC. If β and δβ thalassaemia and 'thalassaemic haemoglobinopathies', such as haemoglobins E and Lepore, have been excluded, the most likely explanation of 'thalassaemic' red cell indices, in most ethnic groups, is α thalassaemia. γδβ thalassaemia is also a possible explanation, but is very rare. Other patients will have iron deficiency anaemia with atypical red cell indices. Children, in particular, may have iron deficiency anaemia with an elevated red cell count. In adults with polycythaemia vera and complicating iron deficiency, the red cell indices are very similar to those of thalassaemia trait, although the RDW tends to be higher.

A low serum ferritin indicates that there is iron deficiency, but does not exclude a diagnosis of β thalassaemia trait. An increased red cell protoporphyrin, which has been used as a screening test for iron deficiency, has been found in 51% of cases of β thalassaemia trait [51]. This test is therefore of limited value in distinguishing between these two conditions.

### Problems in the diagnosis of β thalassaemia trait

*Neonatal period.* β thalassaemia cannot be diagnosed from the haemoglobin $A_2$ percentage in neonates as levels are low. However, by 6–12 months of age, the average haemoglobin $A_2$ percentage is higher than in other infants [117]. The rate of decline in haemoglobin F is slower than in haematologically normal infants and adult levels are not reached until well into childhood [93].

*Silent and almost silent β thalassaemia.* There are β gene mutations that cause minor or no haematological abnormalities in heterozygotes, but which nevertheless can cause clinically significant disease in homozygotes and compound heterozygotes. It is convenient to divide these mutations into two groups designated 'silent β thalassaemia trait' and 'almost silent β thalassaemia trait'. In silent β thalassaemia trait, both the red cell indices and the haemoglobin $A_2$ percentage are normal. It is inevitable that most of these cases will be missed in the routine diagnostic laboratory. In almost silent β thalassaemia trait, the red cell indices are abnormal but the haemoglobin $A_2$ percentage is not increased. The haematological phenotype thus resembles that of α thalassaemia trait. Both silent and almost silent β thalassaemia trait can be detected by studies of the rates of globin chain synthesis and by molecular genetic analysis. Silent and almost silent β thalassaemia trait can also be referred to as 'normal $A_2$ β thalassaemia', although it should be noted that there are other causes of β thalassaemia trait with a normal haemoglobin $A_2$ concentration. Some mutations are so mild that they are always silent, e.g. the +1480 C→G mutation in Greeks [116,118]. In other mutations with a greater reduction in β chain synthesis, the phenotype in heterozygotes varies from silent or almost silent to mild β thalassaemia trait. For example, less than one-half of heterozygotes for −101 C→T are truly silent [118]. In one study of 45 heterozygotes, 17 (38%) were completely silent, the same number had a normal MCH but an elevated haemoglobin $A_2$, four (9%) had an abnormal MCH but a normal haemoglobin $A_2$ and four (9%) had both an abnormal MCH and an abnormal haemoglobin $A_2$ [119]. The others had only a modest elevation of haemoglobin F. Amongst individuals identified only because of a child with β thalassaemia intermedia, half were completely silent, suggesting ascertainment bias in the larger group [119].

Some of the mutations that may lead to a silent or almost silent β thalassaemia phenotype, and the ethnic groups in which they occur, are shown in Table 3.9 [9,83,87,90,116,118–124]. The most common mutations responsible for silent β thalassaemia are −101 C→T and −92 C→T. The mean values reported for individuals carrying the latter mutation are an MCV of 83.9 fl, an MCH of 28.6 pg and a haemoglobin $A_2$ of 3.4% [125]. Almost silent β thalassaemia trait results from a small group of mild β thalassaemia mutations, such as CAP +1 A→C in South Asians (Indians) and, occasionally, IVS1 6 T→C in Mediterranean

**Table 3.9** Causes of normal haemoglobin A$_2$ β thalassaemia.

| Mutation | Origin | Usual haemoglobin A$_2$ (mean or range) (%) | Usual MCH (mean or range) (pg) | Usual MCV (mean or range) (fl) |
|---|---|---|---|---|
| *Silent β thalassaemia trait (normal MCV, MCH and haemoglobin A$_2$ percentage)* | | | | |
| −101 C→T | Mediterranean | 3.3 | 28 | 85 |
| −92 C→T | Mediterranean | 3.5 | 28 | 82 |
| CAP +8 C→T [87] | Chinese | 3.0 | 33.7 | 98 |
| CAP +10 −T [87,120] | Greek | 2.5–2.7 | 30–33 | 94–102 |
| IVS2 844 C→G | Mediterranean (Italian) | 3.5 | 28–29 | 85 |
| CAP +33 C→G [121] | Mediterranean (Greek Cypriot) | 3.0 | 29 | 86 |
| CAP +1480 C→G (termination codon +6 C→G) [87,116,118] | Mediterranean (Greek) | 1.9–3.4 | 20–31 | 79–95 |
| *Almost silent β thalassaemia trait (reduced MCV and MCH, normal haemoglobin A$_2$ percentage)* | | | | |
| IVS1 6 T→C | Mediterranean* | 3.5 | 23 | 71 |
| Codon 27 G→T (haemoglobin Knossus†) | Mediterranean and Middle Eastern | 2.1 | 25 | 71 |
| IVS1 5 G→A Corfu δβ‡ | Mediterranean | | | |
| IVS1 128 T→G | Saudi | 3.5 | 25 | 70 |
| CAP +1 A→C | South Asian | 3.4 | 25 | 80 |
| Mutation not linked to β globin gene cluster [90] | Italian | 1.6§ | 23.5§ | 76§ |
| CAP +22 G→A [122] | Turkish, Bulgarian | 3.9 | 23.5 | 79 |
| Poly A T→C | African | | | |
| Other β thalassaemia mutations with a defective δ gene in *cis* or in *trans* | Mediterranean including Sardinian | | | |
| *Indices typical of thalassaemia trait, but haemoglobin A$_2$ percentage normal* | | | | |
| β thalassaemia caused by deletion of the locus control region | Various | Normal | Typical of β thalassaemia | Typical of β thalassaemia |
| γδβ thalassaemia | Various | Normal | Typical of β thalassaemia | Typical of β thalassaemia |

MCH, mean cell haemoglobin; MCV, mean cell volume.

Dr John Old from the National Haemoglobinopathy Reference Laboratory, Oxford, kindly provided some of the data on which this table is based. Further information from references [9,83,87,90,116,118,121–124].

*Sometimes referred to as the Portuguese mutation, but is common throughout the Mediterranean area. Most common mutation in Malta where one-half of heterozygotes for this mutation were demonstrated to have a haemoglobin A$_2$ percentage below that usually used for the diagnosis of β thalassaemia heterozygosity [123].

†Has a δ$^0$ thalassaemia mutation in *cis*, this being the explanation of the almost silent phenotype.

‡Actually represents δ$^0$ with β$^+$ thalassaemia in *cis*.

§One case only; compound heterozygotes with this mutation and β$^0$ thalassaemia had thalassaemia intermedia or major.

**Table 3.10** Genotypes that can produce the phenotype of β thalassaemia intermedia.

**With two β thalassaemia alleles**

Homozygosity or compound heterozygosity for mild or very mild $\beta^+$ thalassaemia alleles, e.g. CAP +1 A→C, IVS1 6 T→C, +33 C→G, −101 C→T, −88 C→T, −87 C→G, −29 A→G*, particularly if coinherited with α thalassaemia trait ($\alpha^0$ thalassaemia trait or homozygous $\alpha^+$ thalassaemia trait)

Compound heterozygosity for a mild or very mild $\beta^+$ thalassaemia allele and a severe $\beta^+$ or $\beta^0$ thalassaemia allele, particularly when ameliorated by coinheritance of α thalassaemia trait or non-deletional hereditary persistence of fetal haemoglobin (either −158 $^{G}\gamma$C→T mutation, $^{G}\gamma$ or $^{A}\gamma$ promoter mutations or enhanced synthesis of γ chain not linked to the β globin locus†)

Homozygosity or compound heterozygosity for $\beta^+$ thalassaemia if ameliorated by $\alpha^0$ thalassaemia heterozygosity, $\alpha^+$ thalassaemia homozygosity, non-deletional α thalassaemia or the genotype of haemoglobin H disease; compound heterozygosity for $\beta^+$ and $\beta^0$ thalassaemia if ameliorated by the genotype of haemoglobin H disease

Homozygosity or compound heterozygosity for severe $\beta^+$ or $\beta^0$ alleles when ameliorated by coinheritance of non-deletional hereditary persistence of fetal haemoglobin, particularly if homozygous (e.g. −158 $^{G}\gamma$C→T mutation, −196 $^{A}\gamma$C→T or enhanced synthesis of γ chain not linked to the β globin locus†), or α thalassaemia (deletion of two or three α genes or non-deletional α thalassaemia)

Homozygosity for $\beta^0$ thalassaemia caused by 5′ deletions of the β promoter leading to enhanced haemoglobin F synthesis

Homozygosity for Spanish δβ thalassaemia

Homozygosity for 'Corfu δβ thalassaemia' (coinheritance of δ and β thalassaemia in *cis* with consequent increased haemoglobin F synthesis)

Compound heterozygosity for δβ and $\beta^+$ or $\beta^0$ thalassaemia or homozygosity for δβ thalassaemia

Homozygosity for haemoglobin Lepore

Homozygosity or compound heterozygosity for $\beta^0$ or $\beta^+$ thalassaemia with no detectable ameliorating factors

Homozygosity for haemoglobin Malay or compound heterozygosity for haemoglobin Malay and haemoglobin E [79]

**With one β thalassaemia allele and a variant haemoglobin or hereditary persistence of fetal haemoglobin**

Compound heterozygosity for haemoglobin E or haemoglobin Knossus and β thalassaemia or haemoglobin Lepore

Compound heterozygosity for $\beta^0$ thalassaemia and haemoglobin D-Punjab, haemoglobin C, haemoglobin O-Arab, haemoglobin City of Hope, haemoglobin Siriraj, haemoglobin Beograd or the unstable haemoglobins, haemoglobin Acharnes, haemoglobin Arta or haemoglobin Lulu Island [137,144,150–152]

Compound heterozygosity for β or δβ thalassaemia and deletional hereditary persistence of fetal haemoglobin

**With one β thalassaemia allele**

$\beta^+$ thalassaemia or $\beta^0$ thalassaemia coinherited with heterozygosity or homozygosity for triple α or quadruple α, i.e. ααα/ααα or ααα/αα or αααα/αα

Dominant β thalassaemia due to a very unstable β globin chain [139] or an initiator codon mutation [146]

---

* In blacks, because the same chromosome carries −158 $^{G}\gamma$ C→T; in Chinese, it is associated with thalassaemia major [83].
† For example, X linked or 6q linked.

elongated β globin chain that is very unstable and may coprecipitate with normal α chains [140,141]. These mutations have a dominant negative effect consequent on the presence of this abnormal protein, in comparison with the haploinsufficiency recessive effect of other mutations. Haemopoiesis is not only ineffective but also dysplastic. Molecular mechanisms include the following [83,139,141–145]:

- nonsense mutations in the third exon leading to a truncated unstable β chain;
- mis-sense mutations, particularly in the third exon but occasionally in the first or second exon;
- frame shift mutations (e.g. small deletions or, less often, insertions or a combination of deletion and insertion) in the third exon leading to a truncated or elongated β chain;

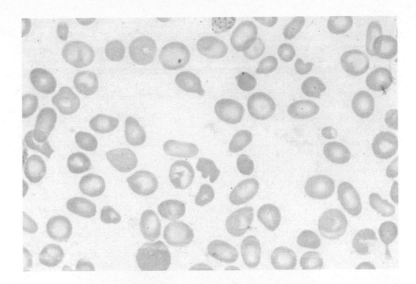

**Fig. 3.30** Blood film in dominant β thalassaemia. (By courtesy of Dr A. Eden.)

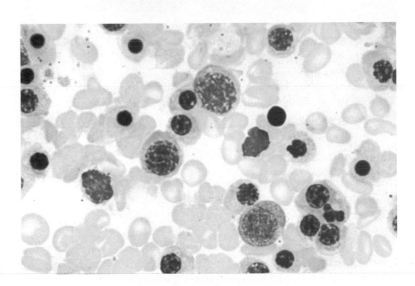

**Fig. 3.31** Bone marrow aspirate in dominant β thalassaemia. (By courtesy of Dr A. Eden.)

• deletion or insertion of complete codons in the second or third exons leading to destabilization;
• deletion within the 5′ consensus splicing region of the second intron leading to aberrant splicing.

One possible explanation for the particular association between dominant β thalassaemia and exon 3 mutations is that the abnormal globin chain that is synthesized is sufficiently long to bind haem (binding sites being mainly encoded by exon 2), but lacks the residues necessary for αβ dimer formation (encoded by exon 3) [139]; the aberrant chains are more slowly degraded than the shorter globin chains encoded by more truncated genes. There is therefore damage to red cell precursors. Some of the abnormal β chains produced when there is deletion or insertion of an entire codon may likewise be unable to form αβ dimers [139].

Many dominant β thalassaemias have been designated 'haemoglobin variants', although it is rare to be able to detect the variant haemoglobin predicted from the DNA sequence. These can be regarded as hyperunstable haemoglobins [144].

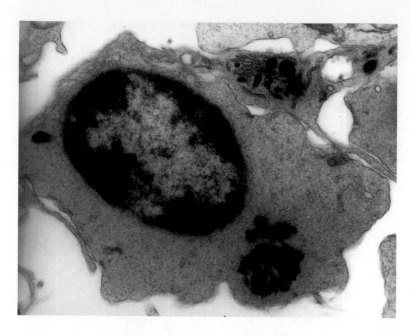

**Fig. 3.32** Ultrastructural examination in dominant β thalassaemia. (By courtesy of Professor S. N. Wickramasinghe.)

Mutations of the initiator codon can also lead to an unusually severe phenotypic abnormality in heterozygotes with significant anaemia and splenomegaly [146].

## Haemoglobin Lepore trait

Unequal cross-over during meiosis with deletion of the 3′ part of the δ gene and the 5′ part of the β gene leads to the formation of a δβ fusion gene. The fusion gene encodes a variant δβ fusion chain that is synthesized at a much reduced rate in comparison with the normal β chain. The variant haemoglobin produced is designated haemoglobin Lepore (from the family name of the first patient in whom this variant haemoglobin was recognized). As the extent of the deletion varies, there are several different haemoglobins designated 'haemoglobin Lepore' of which the most common is haemoglobin Lepore Boston/Washington. Others include haemoglobin Lepore Baltimore and haemoglobin Lepore Hollandia. Haemoglobin Lepore Boston occurs with a low frequency in a variety of ethnic groups, including Italians (particularly from around Naples), Greeks (particularly Macedonians), Turks, Spaniards, Balkan populations and individuals with African ancestry (Cubans, Caribbeans, Afro-Americans and Afro-Caribbeans

in the UK). Haemoglobin Lepore Baltimore is found in Brazil, Portugal and Italy. Haemoglobin Lepore Hollandia is rare, having been reported in isolated families in Papua New Guinea, Bangladesh and Thailand. Haemoglobin Lepore is important because of the possibility of interaction with haemoglobin S and with β thalassaemias. From the functional point of view, it can be regarded as a δβ+ thalassaemia.

### Laboratory features

The blood count and blood film (Fig. 3.33) features cannot be distinguished from those of β thalassaemia trait.

Haemoglobin electrophoresis shows 5–15% of haemoglobin Lepore with haemoglobin $A_2$ being reduced, on average, to about half of the normal level. The percentage of haemoglobin Lepore Baltimore in heterozygotes is slightly but significantly higher than the percentage of haemoglobin Lepore Boston [147]. The haemoglobin $A_2$ percentage tends to be lower with haemoglobin Lepore Baltimore than with haemoglobin Lepore Boston [147]. Haemoglobin F is sometimes mildly increased; this may be because of linkage to a polymorphism that determines haemoglobin F percentage [147]. At least in Spaniards, the haemoglobin F percentage tends to be higher in asso-

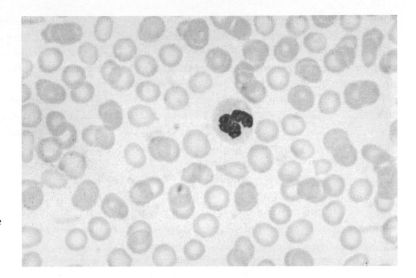

**Fig. 3.33** Blood film in haemoglobin Lepore trait. The red cell indices were RBC $5.36 \times 10^{12}$/l, Hb 12 g/dl, Hct 0.351, MCV 66 fl, MCH 22.2 pg and MCHC 33.8 g/dl.

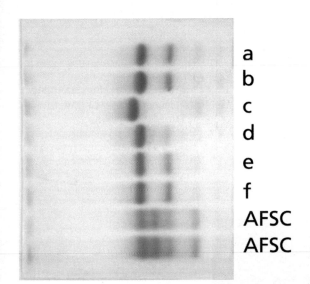

**Fig. 3.34** Haemoglobin electrophoresis on cellulose acetate at alkaline pH in haemoglobin Lepore trait (lane d); AFSC, control sample containing haemoglobins A, F, S and C.

ciation with haemoglobin Lepore Baltimore than in association with haemoglobin Lepore Boston [147]. Haemoglobin Lepore has the same mobility as haemoglobin S on cellulose acetate electrophoresis at alkaline pH (Fig. 3.34) and moves with haemoglobin A at acid pH. On HPLC, it has the same retention time as haemoglobin $A_2$ (Fig. 3.35).

## Haemoglobin Lepore homozygosity and compound heterozygosity

Haemoglobin Lepore homozygotes have the clinical and haematological picture of thalassaemia major or thalassaemia intermedia. Haemoglobin electrophoresis shows haemoglobins F and Lepore only. Similarly, compound heterozygotes for haemoglobin Lepore and β thalassaemia can have the clinical and haematological features of either thalassaemia major or thalassaemia intermedia. Haemoglobin electrophoresis shows haemoglobins F, Lepore and $A_2$ with or without some haemoglobin A.

## β thalassaemia intermedia

β thalassaemia intermedia refers to a clinical phenotype with diverse genetic explanations. In comparison with a typical patient with β thalassaemia trait, there are significant clinical problems, such as anaemia, splenomegaly, leg ulcers and bony deformity. The condition differs from thalassaemia major in that the patient is not dependent on regular blood transfusions for survival, although transfusions may be needed occasionally, e.g. during intercurrent infection, or may become necessary later in life. The severity of β thalassaemia intermedia varies from a condition in which survival without transfusion is barely possible, and there is growth retardation and bony deformity, to a much milder condition that resembles β thalassaemia trait, but has a greater degree of anaemia and splenomegaly. The incidence of gallstones is increased. Iron overload and gonadal failure can occur. Some patients develop symptoms resulting from pressure on vital organs when extramedullary haemopoietic tissue forms tumour-like masses; these are often in the mediastinum or pleura or within the spinal canal, causing spinal cord compression. In one reported patient, extramedullary haemopoietic tissue in the liver formed a tumour-like mass, detectable on computed tomography (CT) scanning (Fig. 3.36) [148]. Bone complications include expansion of the medullary cavity,

osteoporosis (related in part to gonadal failure) and fractures. Cardiovascular complications are common and include congestive cardiac failure, acute pericarditis, chronic pericardial thickening, incompetence of mitral and aortic valves and pulmonary hypertension [149]. Patients with thalassaemia intermedia may develop hypersplenism; splenic sequestration has also been recognized.

The causes of thalassaemia intermedia are summarized in Table 3.10 [79,83,137,139,144,146, 150–155]. The condition can occur in patients with either one or two abnormal β genes. Those who are homozygotes or compound heterozygotes for β thalassaemia alleles either show mutations that are

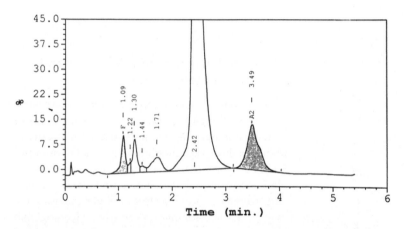

**Fig. 3.35** HPLC chromatogram in haemoglobin Lepore trait; haemoglobin Lepore was 13.4% and its retention time was 3.49 min; from left to right, the peaks are haemoglobin F, post-translationally modified haemoglobin A (two peaks), haemoglobin A and haemoglobin Lepore.

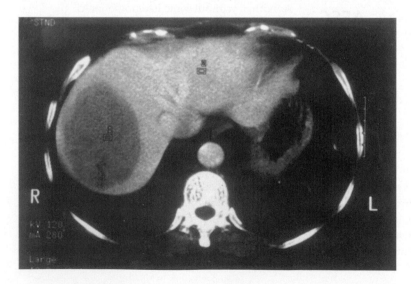

**Fig. 3.36** Computed tomography scan of the abdomen showing a tumour-like mass of haemopoietic tissue in the liver in a patient with β thalassaemia intermedia. (By courtesy of Dr S. K. Ma and W. Y. Au and the *British Journal of Haematology*.)

usually associated with mild or very mild β⁺ thalassaemia or have ameliorating factors, such as coinheritance of α thalassaemia trait or of a mutation which leads to enhanced γ chain synthesis in conditions of haemopoietic stress. Those who have only a single abnormal β gene either have 'dominant β thalassaemia' or have coinherited mutations which aggravate the chain imbalance, such as homozygosity or heterozygosity for triple α or quadruple α. A rare cause of β thalassaemia intermedia is the occurrence of a somatic mutation during development with the loss of one β gene from a proportion of haemopoietic cells in an individual who is heterozygous for a β thalassaemia mutation [156]. In some patients, the explanation for a thalassaemia intermedia rather than a thalassaemia major or thalassaemia minor phenotype is not clear. Some genotypes are consistently associated with thalassaemia intermedia, whereas others are sometimes associated with thalassaemia major and sometimes with thalassaemia intermedia.

In some communities, β thalassaemia intermedia is not uncommon. For example, in Sardinia, 10% of patients who are homozygotes or compound heterozygotes for β⁰ thalassaemia have a thalassaemia intermedia phenotype, as a result of coinheritance of homozygous α⁺ thalassaemia, non-deletional α thalassaemia or heterocellular hereditary persistence of fetal haemoglobin [157]. In countries in which haemoglobin E is common, compound heterozygosity for haemoglobin E and β thalassaemia makes thalassaemia intermedia a common phenotype.

### Laboratory features

The blood film shows features similar to those of typical β thalassaemia trait, but the abnormalities are more severe (Fig. 3.37). In addition to hypochromia, microcytosis, anisocytosis, poikilocytosis and basophilic stippling, there may be polychromasia and circulating erythroblasts. The findings on haemoglobin electrophoresis or HPLC are dependent on the precise underlying genetic defect (Table 3.10). The haemoglobin $A_2$ percentage is likely to be elevated somewhat more than in β thalassaemia trait and the haemoglobin F is elevated. The bone marrow aspirate shows abnormalities of erythropoiesis that are more severe than those of β thalassaemia trait (Fig. 3.38).

The haematological features may be altered by therapy. Response to hydroxycarbamide may be associated with a rise of haemoglobin concentration, a rise of MCV, a rise of haemoglobin F percentage and a fall in the number of circulating erythroblasts [158].

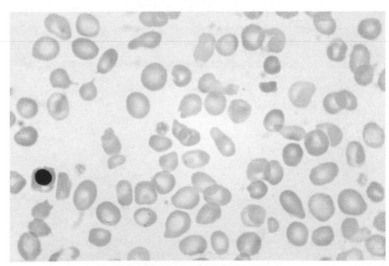

**Fig. 3.37** Blood films from four patients with thalassaemia intermedia. (a) Adult female with heterozygosity for β thalassaemia and triple α; Hb 7.9 g/dl (ββ IVS1 nt 5 mutation, ααα/αα). (By courtesy of Dr N. Jackson.) (*Continued on p. 110.*)

(a)

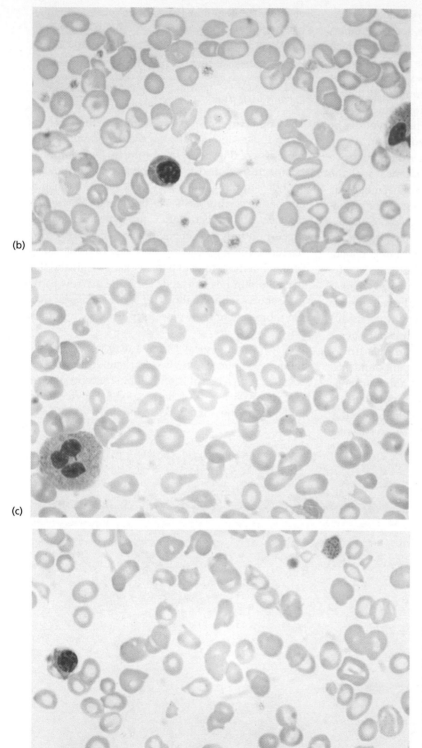

(b)

(c)

(d)

**Fig. 3.37** *Continued.* (b) A 6-year-old girl with 8 cm splenomegaly and Hb 8.6 g/dl with compound heterozygosity for $\beta^0$ thalassaemia and type 2 deletional hereditary persistence of fetal haemoglobin. (c) Adult female with compound heterozygosity for $\beta^0$ and silent $\beta$ thalassaemia trait; Hb 8.9 g/dl, haemoglobin F 23%, haemoglobin $A_2$ 6.3% (genotype $\beta39$ C→T, $\beta$ –101 C→T). (d) Adult female with homozygosity for very mild $\beta^+$ thalassaemia, the –29 A→G mutation.

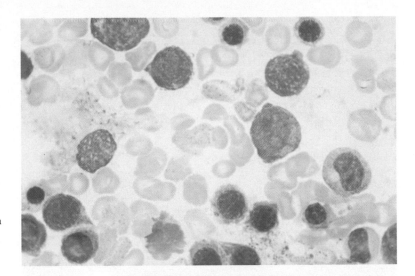

**Fig. 3.38** Bone marrow film from a patient with thalassaemia intermedia (same patient as in Fig. 3.37a) showing erythroid hyperplasia and scanty ragged cytoplasm.

## β thalassaemia major

β thalassaemia major refers to patients with homozygosity or compound heterozygosity for β thalassaemia who are dependent on blood transfusions to maintain life beyond early childhood. Very rarely, heterozygotes for β thalassaemia have the clinical phenotype of β thalassaemia major as a result of coinheritance of extra copies of the α gene; one such patient was homozygous for ααα and another was homozygous for αααα [159]. The phenotype of β thalassaemia major can also result from compound heterozygosity for a β thalassaemia allele and a 'thalassaemic haemoglobinopathy', such as haemoglobin E or the less common haemoglobin Malay [79].

Patients with β thalassaemia major have both ineffective erythropoiesis and a considerably shortened red cell life span (20 days or less), leading to severe anaemia. The disease usually presents in the first year of life, from the age of 3 months onwards. There is markedly increased erythropoiesis, both in an expanded bone marrow compartment and at extramedullary sites. The expansion of haemopoietic bone marrow leads to bony deformity, particularly in the skull and facial bones, with frontal bossing, deformity of the facial bones, displacement of the teeth and a 'hair-on-end' appearance on skull radiography (Figs 3.39 and 3.40). There is bone pain and tenderness and an increased incidence of fractures consequent on thinning of cortical bone. Erythropoiesis at

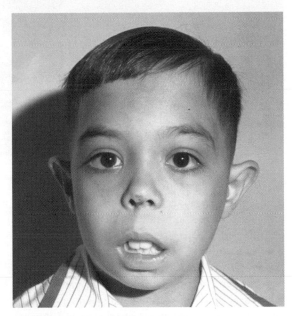

**Fig. 3.39** The face of a child with β thalassaemia major showing frontal bossing, prominence of the maxilla and displacement of the teeth. (By courtesy of Professor H. Smith.)

extramedullary sites leads to gross hepatomegaly and splenomegaly (Fig. 3.41). The splenomegaly is aggravated by trapping of cells in the spleen. The splenomegaly may, in turn, lead to hypersplenism. Ineffective haemopoiesis and shortened red cell life span lead to mild jaundice and an increased incidence of gallstones. There is wasting of the limbs

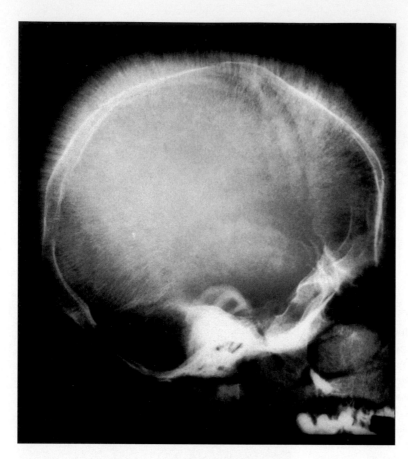

**Fig. 3.40** Skull X-ray of a child with β thalassaemia major showing a 'hair-on-end' appearance as a consequence of marked erythroid hyperplasia. (Reproduced from Hoffbrand AV and Pettit JE. *Essential Haematology*, 3rd edn. Blackwell Scientific Publications, Oxford, 1993, by kind permission of Professor A.V. Hoffbrand.)

and stunting of growth. Some patients develop pulmonary hypertension. Many of the adverse effects of β thalassaemia major can be largely avoided by an appropriate blood transfusion programme. This, however, leads to serious iron overload unless chelation therapy is given. Iron overload, in turn, can lead to cardiac and hepatic damage and delayed puberty.

In the absence of treatment, children with homozygosity for $\beta^0$ thalassaemia usually die at 3–4 years of age, whereas those with $\beta^+$ homozygosity may survive to late childhood [133].

### Laboratory features

The haemoglobin concentration, RBC, Hct, MCV, MCH and MCHC are reduced and RDW is increased. The haemoglobin is usually in the range 3–7 g/dl, the MCV 50–60 fl and the MCH 12–18 pg. The blood film (Fig. 3.42) shows marked anisocytosis, poikilocytosis (including fragments and teardrop poikilocytes), hypochromia and microcytosis. Basophilic stippling, Pappenheimer bodies and target cells may be noted. Circulating nucleated red cells showing defective haemoglobinization and dyserythropoietic features are present. The total white cell count and the neutrophil count are increased. In children with massive splenomegaly, hypersplenism leads to aggravation of the anaemia and leucopenia, neutropenia and thrombocytopenia. The absolute reticulocyte count is stated to be rarely high, although it tends to increase after splenectomy [93].

If the spleen has been removed, the usual features of hyposplenism are present — Howell–Jolly bodies, target cells, lymphocytosis, thrombocytosis and giant platelets. Pappenheimer bodies are very prominent and nucleated red cells are markedly increased. After splenectomy the red cells may show inclusions with the same staining characteristics as haemoglobin; these stain supravitally with methyl violet. They represent α chain precipitates. Such in-

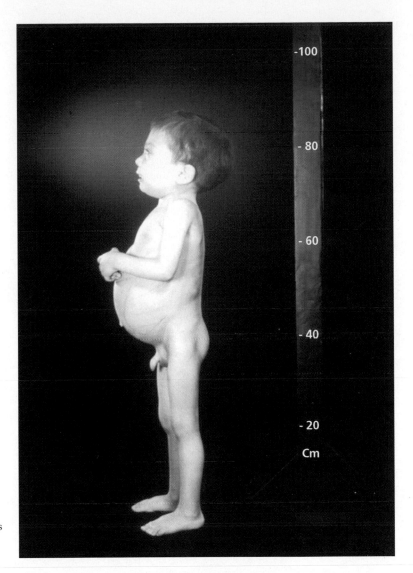

**Fig. 3.41** An undertransfused child with β thalassaemia major showing abdominal distension caused by gross hepatosplenomegaly; there is also wasting of the limbs.

clusions are present in much smaller numbers in patients who have not been splenectomized. These α chain precipitates may also be detectable in circulating nucleated red cells. Following splenectomy, the blood film may show leptocytes, very flat cells with little reduction in cell diameter but striking hypochromia.

The bone marrow aspirate (Fig. 3.43) shows gross erythroid hyperplasia. There is quite severe dyserythropoiesis with nuclear lobulation and fragmentation, basophilic stippling, defective haemoglobinization and the presence of α chain precipitates. Actively phagocytic macrophages are prominent and pseudo-Gaucher cells are present. Iron stores are increased.

In the case of homozygotes or compound heterozygotes for $\beta^0$ thalassaemia ($\beta^0\beta^0$), techniques such as haemoglobin electrophoresis, IEF and HPLC show only haemoglobin F and haemoglobin $A_2$ (Fig. 3.44). When there is homozygosity for $\beta^+$ thalassaemia ($\beta^+\beta^+$) or compound heterozygosity for $\beta^0$ and $\beta^+$ thalassaemia ($\beta^0\beta^+$), haemoglobin A is also present, in variable amounts, sometimes up to 35% of total haemoglobin. In β thalassaemia major, the

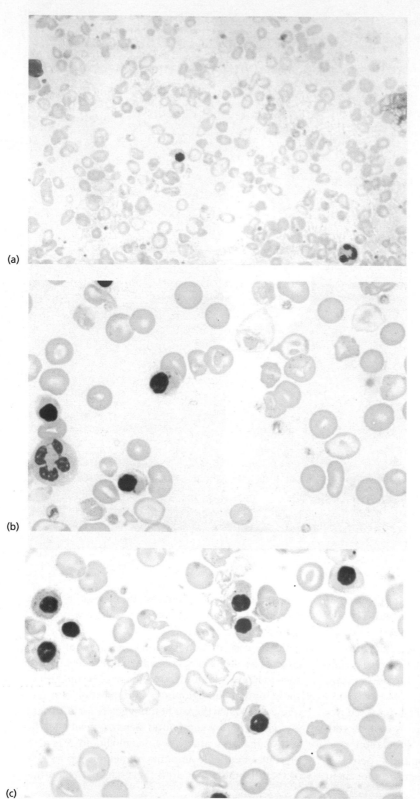

(a)

(b)

(c)

**Fig. 3.42** Blood films of four patients with thalassaemia major: patients (a) and (b) were being transfused; patient (c) had not been transfused for the previous 3 months because of the development of red cell alloantibodies; all patients had been splenectomized; α chain precipitates are clearly seen in all patients; patient (d) was a baby of 4 months of age who had never been transfused.

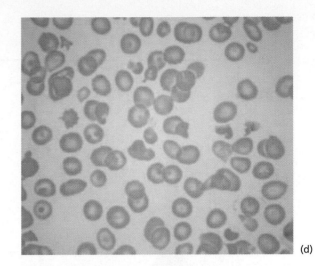

**Fig. 3.42** *Continued.*

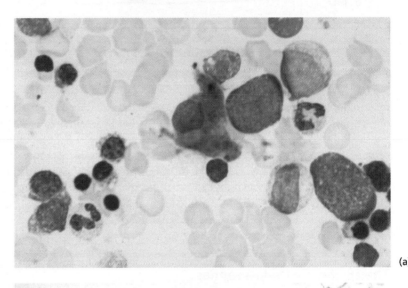

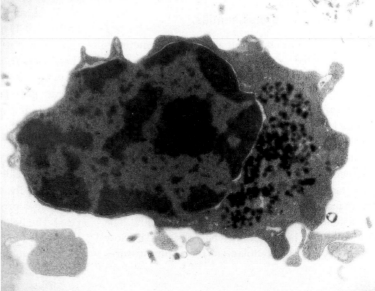

**Fig. 3.43** Bone marrow aspirates from two patients with β thalassaemia major: (a) a May–Grünwald–Giemsa (MGG)-stained film showing erythroid hyperplasia and a debris-laden macrophage; (b) ultrastructural examination showing α chain deposits. (b, By courtesy of Professor S. N. Wickramasinghe.)

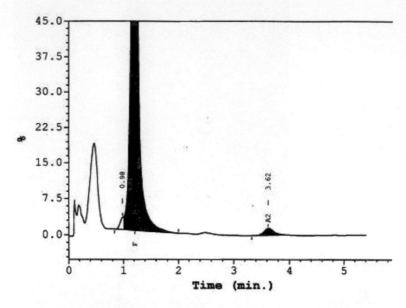

**Fig. 3.44** HPLC chromatogram from a baby of 4 months of age with β thalassaemia major (same case as in Fig. 3.42d); the haemoglobin $A_2$ was 1.4%, but otherwise the chromatogram is not distinguishable from that of a premature neonate; from left to right, peaks are post-translationally modified F, haemoglobin F and haemoglobin $A_2$.

haemoglobin $A_2$ percentage may be normal, elevated or, occasionally, reduced. A Kleihauer test shows that haemoglobin F is irregularly distributed between cells.

Biochemical tests show increased bilirubin, increased urinary urobilinogen and hyperuricaemia. Haptoglobin is decreased or absent, free haemoglobin may be detectable in the plasma and methaemalbumin may be present.

## The δβ and γδβ thalassaemias

### The δβ and ᴬγδβ thalassaemias

$δβ^0$ or $(δβ)^0$ (delta beta zero) thalassaemia (sometimes also designated $^{Gγ Aγ}(δβ)^0$ thalassaemia) results from the deletion of both δ and β genes, but with preservation of the γ genes. $^{Aγ}δβ^0$ or $(^{Aγ}δβ)^0$ thalassaemia (sometimes also designated $^{Gγ}(^{Aγ}δβ)^0$ thalassaemia) results from deletions of the $^{Aγ}$, δ and β genes. The phenotype of heterozygotes resembles that of β thalassaemia trait, but the haemoglobin $A_2$ percentage is not increased; as one δ gene has been lost, it might be expected that haemoglobin $A_2$ would be reduced, but in fact it is often normal [160]. Haemoglobin F is consistently elevated, varying from 5% to 20%. The distribution of haemoglobin F, best observed by flow cytometry, is heterocellular. The blood film features

(Fig. 3.45) are very similar to those of β thalassaemia trait. Because of the increased synthesis of haemoglobin F, homozygotes and compound heterozygotes who also have a severe $β^+$ or $β^0$ mutation may have thalassaemia intermedia rather than thalassaemia major. Homozygotes for δβ or $^{Aγ}δβ$ thalassaemia have 100% haemoglobin F. In δβ thalassaemia homozygotes, $^{Gγ}$ and $^{Aγ}$ globin chains are present in similar amounts, whereas homozygotes for $^{Aγ}δβ$ thalassaemia have only $^{Gγ}$ globin chains. Heterozygotes for either of these types of thalassaemia usually have splenomegaly and a haemoglobin concentration of 8–13 g/dl. The MCV may be reduced or low-normal and the MCH may be reduced or normal.

There are at least nine mutations giving rise to δβ thalassaemia. This type of thalassaemia is observed in many ethnic groups, including some Mediterranean populations (Italians, Greeks and Turks). There are at least 11 mutations giving rise to $^{Aγ}δβ$ thalassaemia. This type of thalassaemia also occurs in many ethnic groups, including Indians and Chinese.

An unusual molecular mechanism underlying δβ thalassaemia is a δβ fusion gene, observed in a Senegalese family, which results in a $δ^0β^+$ thalassaemia with the δ promoter controlling β chain synthesis [161]. The heterozygote described had thalassaemia trait with a normal haemoglobin $A_2$ percentage and 2.7% haemoglobin F. It is more usual for δβ fusion

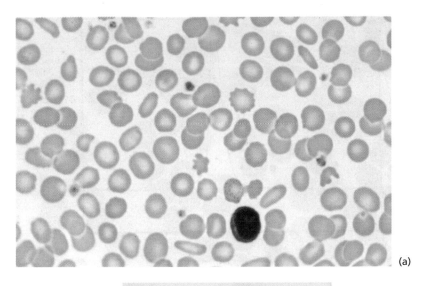

(a)

a
b
c
d
e
f
g
AFSC

(b)

**Fig. 3.45**  (a) Blood film and (b) haemoglobin electrophoresis on cellulose acetate at alkaline pH (strip b) in an adult male with δβ thalassaemia trait. The red cell indices were RBC $6.04 \times 10^{12}$/l, Hb 14 g/dl, Hct 0.42, MCV 69 fl, MCH 23.2 pg and MCHC 33.4 g/dl; AFSC, control sample containing haemoglobins A, F, S and C.

genes to lead to synthesis of haemoglobin Lepore (see below).

The Sardinian type of 'δβ thalassaemia trait' is actually a phenocopy of δβ thalassaemia trait caused by coinheritance (in *cis*) of the codon 39 nonsense mutation, which is a common cause of $\beta^0$ thalassaemia in the Mediterranean area, and a mutation of the $^A\gamma$ promoter leading to overproduction of the γ chain. There are thalassaemic indices with normal haemoglobin $A_2$ and 15–20% haemoglobin F [9]. In one described homozygote, there was microcytosis, but the haemoglobin concentration was normal and the condition was clinically silent; there was 99.8% haemoglobin F and 0.2% haemoglobin $A_2$ [162]. Another phenocopy, initially described in Corfu, was caused by coinheri-

tance of a deletion, extending downstream from the ψβ gene and encompassing the δ gene, and a point mutation in the β gene. Heterozygotes have the phenotype of δβ thalassaemia trait, while homozygotes have almost 100% haemoglobin F, traces of haemoglobin A and no haemoglobin $A_2$ [9].

Haemoglobin Lepore (see above) can be regarded as a type of $\delta\beta^+$ thalassaemia as there is a reduced rate of synthesis of both δ and β chains.

### The εγδβ thalassaemias

There are at least 12 mutations that either delete the entire β gene cluster (eight examples) or inactivate all genes of the cluster because the upstream regulatory

HPFH has also been defined in terms of the proportion of F cells, with less than 4% F cells being classified as normal, 4–8% as equivocal and more than 8% as diagnostic [166]. There are other inherited (Table 3.12) and acquired (Table 6.2) causes of an increased proportion of haemoglobin F. HPFH can result from deletions within the β globin cluster or from mutations or polymorphisms of regulatory genes, either on chromosome 11 or elsewhere. The deletional HPFHs result from relatively large deletions which include the δ and β genes. As there is no β gene on the affected chromosome, deletional HPFH behaves as if it were an allele of the β globin gene; both homozygotes for HPFH and compound heterozygotes for HPFH and a β chain variant totally lack haemoglobin A. The non-deletional HPFHs are a heterogeneous group of disorders, some of which are allelic to the β gene and some of which are not. The difference between deletional HPFH and $\delta\beta^0$ thalassaemia is one of degree. The former has 15–30% haemoglobin F and almost balanced α and non-α chain synthesis, whereas the latter has 5–15% haemoglobin F and unbalanced chain synthesis. The distribution of haemoglobin tends to be pancellular in the former and heterocellular in the latter (Table 3.13). However, there is actually a continuous spectrum of disorders

**Table 3.12** Inherited conditions associated with high haemoglobin F percentage.

**Inherited abnormalities of globin genes**
*Heterozygotes and homozygotes for hereditary persistence of fetal haemoglobin*
Deletional
Non-deletional

*β thalassaemia*
Heterozygotes for β thalassaemia (some cases, particularly those with deletions of the 5′ part of the β gene or promoter mutations)
Compound heterozygotes and homozygotes for β thalassaemia (β thalassaemia intermedia and major)
Heterozygotes and homozygotes for δβ and $^A\gamma\delta\beta$ thalassaemia
Heterozygotes and homozygotes for haemoglobin Lepore
Heterozygotes for haemoglobin Kenya

*Sickle cell trait*
Some cases, particularly Saudi/Indian haplotype

*Sickle cell anaemia and other forms of sickle cell disease*
Some cases, particularly during treatment with hydroxycarbamide, or with certain haplotypes: higher in Senegal haplotype than in Benin and Bantu haplotypes; particularly high in Saudi/Indian haplotype found in eastern province of Saudi Arabia and India

*Unstable haemoglobins*

**Inherited abnormalities other than those of globin genes**
*Haematological disorders*
Congenital aplastic anaemia (Fanconi's anaemia)
Blackfan–Diamond syndrome, particularly during corticosteroid administration
Congenital dyserythropoietic anaemia [168]
Shwachman–Diamond syndrome [169]

*Metabolic disorders*
β-ketothiolase deficiency (high levels of butyric acid) [170]
Disorders of proprionate metabolism [171]

*Other*
Osteopetrosis [172]

**Table 3.13** Distribution of haemoglobin F in various conditions associated with an increased haemoglobin F percentage.

| Heterocellular | Pancellular |
| --- | --- |
| Some types of non-deletional HPFH | Some types of non-deletional HPFH |
| $\delta\beta$ thalassaemia | Deletional HPFH |
| Haemoglobin Lepore trait | Haemoglobin Kenya trait |
| Sickle cell anaemia, sickle cell/haemoglobin C disease and sickle cell/$\beta$ thalassaemia | Sickle cell/deletional HPFH compound heterozygosity |
| $\beta$ thalassaemia heterozygosity and haemoglobin E/$\beta$ thalassaemia compound heterozygosity | $\beta$ thalassaemia homozygosity and compound heterozygosity |

HPFH, hereditary persistence of fetal haemoglobin.

rather than two distinct groups, and one condition that was previously designated type 6 HPFH [173,174] is now considered to be more correctly characterized as $^{A}\gamma\delta\beta^{0}$ thalassaemia [160]. The molecular basis of the difference is not clearly understood; juxtaposition of a downstream enhancer to the $\gamma$ genes in HPFH, but not in $\delta\beta$ thalassaemia, has been proposed as a mechanism [175].

The distribution of haemoglobin F between cells in various conditions associated with an increased percentage of haemoglobin F is best determined by flow cytometry.

## Deletional hereditary persistence of fetal haemoglobin

Deletional HPFH can result from a number of deletions of the $\beta$ globin gene cluster, which are shown diagrammatically in Fig. 3.48. The haematological features of heterozygous subjects are summarized in Table 3.14 [160,176–185]. Deletional HPFH is quite common in some ethnic groups. Its prevalence in Afro-Americans is about 1 in 1000.

The first type of deletional HPFH to be recognized was the so-called Negro type of $\delta\beta^{0}$ HPFH, described in an Afro-American child from Baltimore. An alternative terminology is $^{G}\gamma^{A}\gamma\delta\beta^{0}$ HPFH. There are now known to be at least six different deletions classified as $\delta\beta^{0}$ HPFH, two occurring in subjects of African descent, one in Indians, two in Italians and one in Vietnamese/South-East Asians [160,176,177].

In all of these, both the $\delta$ and $\beta$ genes are deleted, but the two $\gamma$ genes are intact. As homozygotes have no $\beta$ or $\delta$ genes, they cannot synthesize haemoglobin A or $A_{2}$. Haemoglobin F comprises 100% of haemoglobin. Both $^{G}\gamma$ and $^{A}\gamma$ chains are synthesized, but the proportion varies in the different subtypes. The synthesis of the $\gamma$ chain is almost sufficient to compensate for the lack of $\beta$ chain synthesis so that there is no anaemia.

Heterozygotes for $\delta\beta^{0}$ HPFH have a variable haemoglobin F percentage, depending on the precise deletion (Table 3.14). The haemoglobin $A_{2}$ percentage is either mildly reduced or normal, averaging around half of the normal mean level in most subtypes. The haemoglobin concentration is normal, but the MCV and MCH may be somewhat reduced. The mean MCH varies from $c$. 26 pg in HPFH-1 to $c$. 28 pg in HPFH-3 [160]. The MCV shows a similar variation between subtypes from a mean that is below the lower limit of normal to a mean that is clearly normal [160]. The blood film (Fig. 3.49) may be normal or show an occasional target cell. A Kleihauer test or flow cytometry shows a pancellular distribution of haemoglobin F, but there is some variation from cell to cell. The globin chain synthesis ratio ($\alpha$:non-$\alpha$) is approximately normal.

Homozygotes are not anaemic. In fact, because haemoglobin F has a higher oxygen affinity than haemoglobin A, there may be mild polycythaemia. In some homozygotes, the red cell indices resemble those of $\beta$ thalassaemia trait with an increased RBC

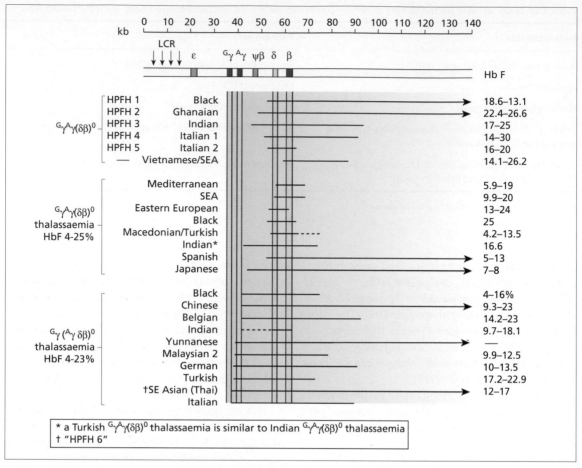

**Fig. 3.48** Deletions resulting in hereditary persistence of fetal haemoglobin or in δβ thalassaemia (modified from reference 160); $^{G}\gamma^{A}\gamma(\delta\beta)^{0}$ thalassaemia = $\delta\beta^{0}$ thalassaemia, $^{G}\gamma(^{A}\gamma\delta\beta)^{0}$ thalassaemia = $^{A}\gamma\delta\beta^{0}$ thalassaemia.

and reduced MCV and MCH. In others, the RBC is towards the top and the MCV and MCH towards the bottom of their respective normal ranges. The reticulocyte count is normal. The blood film may show anisocytosis, poikilocytosis, mild hypochromia, mild microcytosis and target cells. 'Cells resembling spherocytes' (probably irregularly contracted cells) have been described [178]. Globin chain synthesis shows an imbalance similar to that in β thalassaemia trait with an α:non-α ratio of about 1.4–3.0. A Kleihauer test shows a pancellular distribution of haemoglobin F, an inevitable feature as only haemoglobin F is present.

Heterozygosity for haemoglobin Kenya produces a variant of deletional pancellular HPFH. As one δ gene has been deleted, there is a reduced proportion of haemoglobin $A_2$. Heterozygotes may be haematologically normal or show slight anaemia and occasional target cells. Globin chain synthesis is balanced.

*Interactions with other haemoglobinopathies*

Deletional HPFH coinherited with $\beta^{S}$ leads to a very mild sickling disorder with about 30% haemoglobin F and about 70% haemoglobin S [179,186]. Haemoglobin $A_2$ may be low-normal or decreased.

Compound heterozygotes for deletional HPFH and β thalassaemia have about 70% haemoglobin F. The phenotype is variable. In the case of the two

**Table 3.14** Haematological features of heterozygosity for deletional hereditary persistence of fetal haemoglobin (HPFH) [160,176–185].

| Type of HPFH | Usual haemoglobin F (%) | Usual haemoglobin $A_2$ (%) | Usual $^G\gamma:^A\gamma$ ratio | Molecular defect | Reference |
|---|---|---|---|---|---|
| Afro-American $\delta\beta^0$ (HPFH-1) | 15–30* | 1.2–2.7 | 40:60 | Deletion including δ and β genes | [179] |
| African (Ghanaian) $\delta\beta^0$ (HPFH-2) | 20–30† | Reduced | 40:60 | Deletion including δ and β genes | |
| Indian $\delta\beta^0$ (HPFH-3) | 17–25 | 1.6–2.2 | 70:30 | Deletion including δ and β genes | [180,181] |
| Italian 1 (southern mainland Italy) $\delta\beta^0$ (HPFH-4) | 14–30 | 1.7–2.0 | 35:65 | Deletion including δ and β genes | [182] |
| Italian 2 (Sicilian) $\delta\beta^0$ (HPFH-5) | 16–20 | 2–2.1 | 15:85 | Deletion including δ and β genes | [183] |
| Vietnamese/South-East Asian | 20.7±3.8 | Increased (3.8±0.6) | 60:40 | Deletion of β gene | [160] |
| Haemoglobin Kenya | 5–15‡ | 1.4–1.8 | Mainly $^G\gamma$ | Deletion of part of the $^A\gamma$ gene, all of the δ gene and part of the β gene with $^A\gamma\beta$ fusion | |

*The percentage of haemoglobin F is very significantly reduced by coexisting iron deficiency [184].
†The percentage of haemoglobin F is very significantly reduced by coexisting iron deficiency [185].
‡Plus 5–27% (usually 7–12%) of haemoglobin Kenya ($\alpha_2{}^A\gamma\beta_2$).

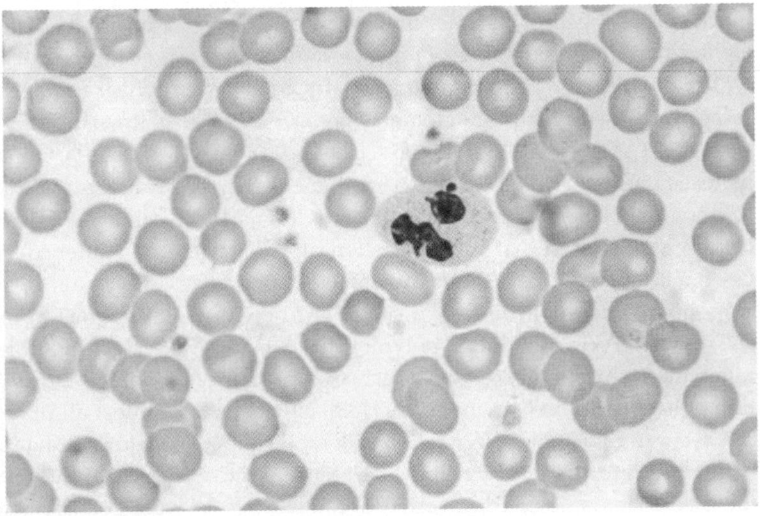

**Fig. 3.49** Blood film in an adult African woman with hereditary persistence of fetal haemoglobin. The red cell indices were RBC $4.2\times10^{12}$/l, Hb 12 g/dl, MCV 88 fl, MCH 28.6 pg and MCHC 32.4 g/dl; there was 23% haemoglobin F and 1.6% haemoglobin $A_2$.

African types, the compound heterozygous state is phenotypically very mild, whereas, in the Indian type, although the heterozygotes do not have thalassaemic features, the compound heterozygotes have the clinical picture of thalassaemia intermedia [181,186].

When coinherited with haemoglobin H disease in one family, HPFH was associated with some improvement in the haemoglobin concentration, a reduced proportion of haemoglobin H and 11% haemoglobin Bart's, suggesting that the reduced number of α chains were demonstrating a greater affinity for β chains than for γ chains [187].

## Non-deletional hereditary persistence of fetal haemoglobin

Non-deletional HPFH is a heterogeneous group of disorders. The most common form is associated with a polymorphism in regulatory sequences of the β globin gene cluster. There is a C→T change at position −158 from the $^G\gamma$ gene, which is readily detected because it creates a cleavage site for the enzyme $Xmn1$. For the sake of brevity, −158 $^G\gamma$ C→T is used here to indicate this mutation and a similar notation is used for other mutations leading to non-deletional HPFH. A further polymorphism also influences the percentage of haemoglobin F, although it is not usually categorized with the HPFHs. It is based on repeat sequences within hypersensitive site 2 (HS2) of the LCR of the β globin cluster. The sequence is designated $(AT)_xN_{12}GT(AT)_y$ where $x$ and $y$ are variable numbers of repeats of a sequence. There are at least eight different combinations of repeat sequences, of which $(AT)_9N_{12}GT(AT)_{10}$ is associated with an increased synthesis of haemoglobin F. Both C→T at −158 and $(AT)_9N_{12}GT(AT)_{10}$ are associated with an increased number of F cells (and a small increase in haemoglobin F percentage) in normal individuals. It has been suggested that the association of −158 $^G\gamma$ C→T with increased synthesis of haemoglobin F is consequent only on its linkage disequilibrium with $(AT)_9N_{12}GT(AT)_{10}$, the latter polymorphism being much more strongly linked to an increased production of haemoglobin F in one study [188]. However, this seems unlikely in view of the considerable number of other studies that have linked −158 $^G\gamma$ C→T to increased haemoglobin F in a variety of contexts.

The haemoglobin F concentration is also affected by genes encoding *trans*-acting factors. One is the determinant at Xp22 which influences F cell production and another has been mapped to 6q23 [83]. These give rise to increased synthesis of both $^G\gamma$ and $^A\gamma$ globin chains and to $^G\gamma^A\gamma$ HPFH.

Non-polymorphic non-deletional HPFH results mainly from point mutations (or occasionally a small deletion or insertion) involving the β globin gene cluster, but not the δ and β globin genes themselves. The mutations are in and around highly conserved promoter motifs 5′ to either the $^G\gamma$ or the $^A\gamma$ gene. They are at −114, −117 or −175 from the transcription initiation sites of these genes or clustered around −158 to −161 or −195 to −202. These mutations are likely to alter the binding of *trans*-acting factors to the promoter. This type of non-deletional HPFH can be further categorized according to whether there is increased synthesis of $^G\gamma$ or $^A\gamma$ chain. Increased synthesis of $^G\gamma$ chain results from mutations upstream of the $^G\gamma$ gene and increased synthesis of $^A\gamma$ chain results from mutations upstream of the $^A\gamma$ gene. Interestingly, the same mutations have often been observed in the same position 5′ to one or other of these genes.

In non-deletional HPFH, there is increased synthesis of haemoglobin F, but haemoglobins A and $A_2$ continue to be synthesized, although at a reduced rate, so that α:non-α chain synthesis is fairly balanced. Whether the distribution of haemoglobin F is pancellular or heterocellular is partly a function of the proportion of haemoglobin F present and the sensitivity of the method used for its detection.

The reported types of non-deletional HPFH for which a molecular mechanism has been defined are shown in Table 3.15 [160,166,167,176,177,186–212]. It should be noted that, although the same mutation can occur 5′ to either the $^G\gamma$ or the $^A\gamma$ genes, the percentage of haemoglobin F characteristically seen may differ considerably.

Typical of pancellular $^G\gamma$ HPFH are the two point mutations at −202 and −175 from the $^G\gamma$ gene, observed in subjects of African ancestry. They show 15–25% and 17–30%, respectively, of haemoglobin F, almost all of $^G\gamma$ type. The compound heterozygous state with haemoglobin S indicates that the β gene in *cis* of the HPFH determinant continues to be expressed, albeit at a reduced rate. The second of these

**Table 3.15** Haematological features of non-deletional hereditary persistence of fetal haemoglobin (HPFH). (Based on references [160,166,167,176,186–212].)

| Type of HPFH | Ethnic group | Molecular defect | Haemoglobin F in heterozygotes (%) | Haemoglobin F in erythropoietic stress (%) | Reference |
|---|---|---|---|---|---|
| $^{G}\gamma$ | Black | $-202\,^{G}\gamma\,C{\to}G$ | 15–25* | 19.9 and 23.5 with $\beta^S$ in *trans* | [186] |
| | Tunisian | $-200\,^{G}\gamma+C$ | 18–27 (48 and 49 in homozygotes) | | [160,195] |
| | Black/Sardinian/ British | $-175\,^{G}\gamma\,T{\to}C$ | 17–30* | 29.5 with $\beta^S$ in *trans* | [190–192] |
| | | $-161\,^{G}\gamma\,G{\to}A$ | Slight increase | More marked increase | [167] |
| | Many ethnic groups, frequency of 0.32–0.35 | $-158\,^{G}\gamma\,C{\to}T$ | 2–3 (but not always elevated if otherwise genetically normal) | More marked increase with β thalassaemia in *trans*; 10 with $\beta^S$ in *trans*; 15 with SS | [193] |
| | Black (Atlanta) | $-158\,^{G}\gamma^{G}\gamma\,C{\to}T\dagger$ | 2.3–3.8 | | [193] |
| | Australian | $-114\,^{G}\gamma\,C{\to}G$ | 8.5 | | [194] |
| | Japanese | $-114\,^{G}\gamma\,C{\to}T$ | 11–14 | | |
| | Yugoslav | $^{G}\gamma^{G}\gamma^{A}\gamma\ddagger$ | About 5 | | [196] |
| | Portuguese (one family) | $^{G}\gamma^{AG}\gamma^{AG}\gamma^{AG}\gamma^{AG}\gamma^{A}\gamma$ | 0.3–8 | | [197] |
| $^{A}\gamma$ | Black | $-202\,^{A}\gamma\,C{\to}T$ | 1.6–3.9 | 1.6–9 with S in *cis*; 25 with SS | [97] |
| | British/Australian | $-198\,^{A}\gamma\,T{\to}C$ | 3.5–10* (20 in homozygote) | | |
| | Italian/Chinese | $-196\,^{A}\gamma\,C{\to}T^{\S}$ | 12–21* | 38 and 40 with β thalassaemia in *trans*; 20 with $\beta^0$ in *cis*¶ | [198,199] |
| | Brazilian (black, white or mixed) | $-195\,^{A}\gamma\,C{\to}G$ | 4.5–8.5 | 7 with hereditary spherocytosis | [200] |
| | Black | $-175\,^{A}\gamma\,T{\to}C$ | | 38 with $\beta^C$ in *trans* and $-158\,^{G}\gamma\,C{\to}T$ in *cis* | [198] |
| | Cretan | $-158\,^{A}\gamma\,C{\to}T^{**}$ | Slight increase | | [160] |
| | Greek/Sardinian/ black | $-117\,^{A}\gamma\,G{\to}A$ | 7–20* (mean 13 in one series, 9.7 in another); 24 in two homozygotes and 37.6 in another; 13.5 in compound heterozygosity with $-158\,^{G}\gamma\,C{\to}T$ | 20–50 with β thalassaemia in *trans* | [202–208] |

*Continued on p. 126.*

**Table 3.15** *Continued.*

| Type of HPFH | Ethnic group | Molecular defect | Haemoglobin F in heterozygotes (%) | Haemoglobin F in erythropoietic stress (%) | Reference |
|---|---|---|---|---|---|
| | Black (Georgia) | $-114\,^A\gamma\,C\rightarrow T$ | 3–5 | | [209] |
| | Black | del $^A\gamma$ −114 to −102 | | 30 and 31 with sickle cell trait | [210] |
| | Chinese | del $^A\gamma$ −226 to −223 (AAGC del) | 5.4 in homozygote, 3.2 in heterozygote | | [211] |
| $^G\gamma^A\gamma$ | Many ethnic groups ('Swiss type') | Locus at Xp22.2–22.3 | 0.7–3.0 | | |
| | Indian | Locus at 6q22.3–23.1 | Interaction with $-158\,^G\gamma\,C\rightarrow T$ | | [212] |
| | British | Unknown autosomal locus other than 6q22.3–23.1 | 1–10.8 (interaction with $-158\,^G\gamma\,C\rightarrow T$) | | 166 |
| | | Locus on 8q | | | |

* Distribution of haemoglobin F is pancellular.
† Both γ genes are $^G\gamma$.
‡ However, triplication of the γ gene does not necessarily lead to increased haemoglobin F.
§ In Sardinia, occurs with a $\beta^0$ mutation in *cis* producing the phenotype of δβ thalassaemia.
¶ So-called Sardinian δβ thalassaemia — actually this mutation plus $\beta^0$ thalassaemia.
** This mutation occurs in *cis* to −158 $^G\gamma\,C\rightarrow T$.

mutations has also been observed in Sardinians and white British individuals. Other $^G\gamma$ promoter mutations, leading to either heterocellular or pancellular HPFH, have been observed in blacks, Japanese, Yugoslavians, white Australians and Japanese (Table 3.15).

Typical of pancellular $^A\gamma$ HPFH is −117 $^A\gamma$ G→A, observed initially in Greeks, but subsequently in Sardinians, Chinese and subjects of African ancestry. The percentage of haemoglobin F, of mainly $^A\gamma$ type, has generally been around 10–20%. Globin chain synthesis is balanced and there is no haematological abnormality. Two homozygotes have been described with approximately 75% haemoglobin A, 24% haemoglobin F and 0.8% haemoglobin $A_2$, indicating that the δ and β genes in *cis* to the HPFH determinant are expressed, albeit at a reduced level.

Other $^A\gamma$ promoter mutations, leading to either pancellular or heterocellular HPFH, have been described in black, white (British, Australian, Italian) and Chinese individuals and in Brazilians of various ethnic origins (Table 3.15). They generally result from point mutations, but, in one mutation, described in two individuals with sickle cell trait, there was a 13-base pair deletion involving the distal CCAAT box at −115 to −111 [211].

### Coinheritance with other abnormalities of globin chain synthesis

Coinheritance of non-deletional HPFH ameliorates sickle cell anaemia and homozygous and heterozygous β thalassaemia. For example, in both conditions, −158 $^G\gamma$ C→T and the $(AT)_9N_{12}GT(AT)_{10}$

polymorphism are associated with an increase in haemoglobin F synthesis. Homozygosity for $-158\ ^G\gamma$ C→T is also associated with an increased haemoglobin F percentage in haemoglobin E/β thalassaemia and haemoglobin E disease [213].

A child with both $-117\ ^A\gamma$ G→A non-deletional HPFH and the genotype of haemoglobin H disease has been reported [187]. The percentage of haemoglobin F was that expected for the genotype (9.5%) and haemoglobin $A_2$ was 1.3%. There was no haemoglobin H, but haemoglobin Bart's was 11%, indicating that the reduced amount of α chain was combining preferentially with β chains rather than with γ chains.

The findings in other interactions of non-deletional HPFH and other haematological abnormalities are summarized in Table 3.15.

## Other inherited abnormalities and haemoglobin F level

An increased proportion of haemoglobin F is observed in a variety of inherited conditions, related and unrelated to the β globin gene cluster (Table 3.12).

A number of haemoglobinopathies are associated, in a proportion of cases, with an increased percentage of haemoglobin F. The increase in haemoglobin F can sometimes be linked to the nature of the β globin gene mutation. Heterozygotes for non-deletional β thalassaemia and 3′ deletional β thalassaemia have been found to have a slight elevation of haemoglobin F (e.g. 1.5% in comparison with a normal of 0.7%), whereas haemoglobin Lepore heterozygotes have around 3% haemoglobin F and heterozygotes for 5′ deletional β thalassaemia have around 3.5% haemoglobin F [186]. Elevation of haemoglobin F in individuals with abnormalities of the β globin gene can also often be linked either to polymorphisms within the β globin gene cluster that affect binding of transcription factors or to other genetic factors. Heterozygotes for β thalassaemia or haemoglobin Lepore with a high haemoglobin F percentage have been found to have either the common $-158\ ^G\gamma$ C→T or $(AT)_9T_5$ instead of $(AT)_7T_7$ at $-540$ from the β gene [214]. Both of these polymorphisms were shown to exert an influence on haemoglobin F levels when found either in *cis* or in *trans* to the abnormal β or δβ

globin gene. The $(AT)_9T_5$ polymorphism was also linked to an increased percentage of haemoglobin F in β thalassaemia major [214].

The haemoglobin F level in sickle cell anaemia is determined by many factors (see p. 163), including age, sex, possibly the X chromosome F-cell determining locus, various determinants in the β globin gene cluster and the number of α genes. However, it should be noted that interpretation of the haemoglobin F percentage in sickle cell anaemia is complicated by the preferential survival of F-containing cells.

In β thalassaemia major, the haemoglobin F percentage is greatly elevated, constituting almost all of the haemoglobin in homozygotes for $β^0$ thalassaemia.

Inherited metabolic disorders can affect haemoglobin F synthesis when gene expression is altered by an abnormal metabolite. Very abnormal haemopoiesis, e.g. in congenital dyserythropoietic and congenital aplastic anaemias, can also be associated with an elevation of haemoglobin F percentage.

## Check your knowledge

One to five answers may be correct. Answers to almost all questions can be found in this chapter or can be deduced from the information given. The correct answers are given on p. 138.

3.1  An increased percentage of haemoglobin $A_2$ is expected in
(a) α thalassaemia trait
(b) β thalassaemia trait
(c) δβ thalassaemia trait
(d) γδβ thalassaemia trait
(e) silent β thalassaemia trait

3.2  Genes forming part of the β gene cluster include
(a) α
(b) β
(c) γ
(d) δ
(e) ε

3.3  Moderate to marked microcytosis is usually a feature of
(a) haemoglobin H disease
(b) $α^0$ thalassaemia trait

(c) β thalassaemia trait

(d) heterozygosity for hereditary persistence of fetal haemoglobin

(e) haemoglobin Lepore trait

3.4 Suitable methods for quantifying haemoglobin $A_2$ for the diagnosis of β thalassaemia trait include

(a) inspection of an electrophoretic strip

(b) microcolumn chromatography

(c) cellulose acetate electrophoresis followed by densitometric scanning

(d) high performance liquid chromatography

(e) cellulose acetate electrophoresis followed by elution and spectrophotometry

3.5 Haemoglobin Bart's hydrops fetalis

(a) is expected in about 50% of fetuses if both parents have $\alpha^0$ thalassaemia

(b) is a likely outcome in West Africans if both parents have α thalassaemia trait

(c) is associated with an increased incidence of pregnancy-associated hypertension

(d) can cause developmental abnormalities in limbs

(e) is associated with good oxygen delivery to tissues

3.6 A decreased percentage of haemoglobin $A_2$ may be a feature of

(a) α thalassaemia trait

(b) β thalassaemia trait

(c) haemoglobin Lepore trait

(d) iron deficiency anaemia

(e) δβ thalassaemia trait

3.7 $\alpha^0$ thalassaemia

(a) is common in Afro-Caribbeans

(b) in its homozygous form, leads to haemoglobin H disease

(c) is most often caused by deletion of both α genes on a single chromosome

(d) cannot usually be suspected from the red cell indices

(e) can be diagnosed by haemoglobin electrophoresis

3.8 Hereditary persistence of fetal haemoglobin can be caused by

(a) deletions that include the β and δ genes

(b) deletion of an α gene

(c) deletion of a γ gene

(d) mutation in a gene on chromosome 16

(e) point mutations upstream of either the $^G\gamma$ or the $^A\gamma$ globin gene

3.9 δβ thalassaemia

(a) leads to an increased percentage of haemoglobin F

(b) leads to an increased percentage of haemoglobin $A_2$

(c) usually results from deletion of the δ and β genes

(d) when homozygous, may lead to the phenotype of thalassaemia intermedia

(e) may be simulated by the coinheritance of δ and β thalassaemia

3.10 Haemoglobin Bart's hydrops fetalis

(a) usually results from homozygosity for $\alpha^+$ thalassaemia

(b) is mainly seen in those of Chinese or South-East Asian origin

(c) is characterized by worse tissue hypoxia than would be predicted from the haemoglobin concentration

(d) is characterized by low serum albumin and generalized oedema

(e) occurs occasionally in Greeks and Cypriots

3.11 The phenotype associated with β thalassaemia homozygosity or compound heterozygosity may be ameliorated by

(a) coinheritance of ααα (triple alpha)

(b) coinheritance of γ thalassaemia

(c) coinheritance of non-deletional hereditary persistence of fetal haemoglobin

(d) coinheritance of $\alpha^0$ thalassaemia heterozygosity

(e) coinheritance of $\alpha^+$ thalassaemia homozygosity

3.12 The following variant haemoglobins lead to an α or β thalassaemia phenotype

(a) haemoglobin S

(b) haemoglobin C

(c) haemoglobin E

(d)  haemoglobin Lepore

(e)  haemoglobin Constant Spring

3.13  β thalassaemia trait with a normal haemoglobin A$_2$ percentage may be caused by

(a)  coexisting δ thalassaemia

(b)  dominant β thalassaemia

(c)  a β thalassaemia mutation associated with only a minor reduction of β chain synthesis

(d)  coinherited triple α

(e)  β thalassaemia caused by deletion of the locus control region

## Further reading

Bernini LF and Harteveld CL (1998) α-thalassaemia. *Bailliere's Clin Haematol* **11**, 53–90.

Bollekens JA and Forget BG (1991) δβ thalassemia and hereditary persistence of fetal hemoglobin. *Hematol Oncol Clin North Am* **5**, 399–422.

Higgs DR (1993) α-Thalassaemia. *Bailliere's Clin Haematol* **6**, 117–150.

Steinberg MH, Forget BG, Higgs DR and Nagel RL, eds. *Disorders of Hemoglobin: Genetics, Pathophysiology, and Clinical Management*. Cambridge University Press, Cambridge, 2001.

Thein SL (1998) β-thalassaemia. *Bailliere's Clin Haematol* **11**, 91–126.

Weatherall D and Clegg JB. *The Thalassaemia Syndromes*, 4th edn. Blackwell Science, Oxford, 2001.

Weatherall DJ. The Thalassemias. In: Stamatoyannopoulos G, Nienhuis AW, Majerus PW and Varmus H, eds. *The Molecular Basis of Blood Diseases*, 3rd edn. W. B. Saunders, Philadelphia, PA, 2001, pp. 183–226.

## References

1  Cooley TB and Lee P (1925) A series of cases of splenomegaly in children with anemia and peculiar bone changes. *Trans Am Pediatr Soc* **37**, 29.

2  Whipple GH and Bradford WL (1936) Mediterranean disease-thalassemia (erythroblastic anemia of Cooley); associated pigment abnormalities simulating hemochromatosis. *J Pediatr* **9**, 279–311.

3  Rigas DA, Koler RD and Osgood EE (1955) New hemoglobin possessing a higher electrophoretic mobility than normal adult hemoglobin. *Science* **121**, 372.

4  Fessas P and Papaspyrou A (1957) New 'fast' hemoglobin associated with thalassemia. *Science* **126**, 1119.

5  Edington GM and Lehman H (1954) A new haemoglobin found in a West African. *Lancet* **267**, 173–174.

6  Ager JAM and Lehmann H (1958) Observations on some 'fast' haemoglobins: K, J, N and Bart's. *Br Med J* **i**, 929–931.

7  Higgs DR, Sharpe JA and Wood WG (1998) Understanding α globin gene expression: a step towards effective gene therapy. *Semin Hematol* **356**, 93–104.

8  Bernini LF and Harteveld CL (1998) α-thalassaemia. *Bailliere's Clin Haematol* **11**, 53–90.

9  Weatherall DJ. The Thalassemias. In: Stamatoyannopoulos G, Nienhuis AW, Majerus PW and Varmus H, eds. *The Molecular Basis of Blood Diseases*, 3rd edn. W. B. Saunders, Philadelphia, PA, 2001, pp. 183–226.

10  Morlé F, Francina A, Ducrocq R, Wajcman H, Gonnet C, Philippe N *et al.* (1995) A new α chain variant Hb Sallanches [α 2 104(G11) Cys → Tyr] associated with HbH disease in one homozygous patient. *Br J Haematol* **91**, 608–611.

11  Hill AVS (1992) Molecular epidemiology of the thalassaemias (including haemoglobin E). *Bailliere's Clin Haematol* **5**, 209–238.

12  Çürük MA, Baysal E, Gupta RB, Sharma S and Huisman THJ (1993) An IVS-I-117 (G A) acceptor splice site mutation in the α1-globin gene is a nondeletional α-thalassaemia-2 determinant in an Indian population. *Br J Haematol* **83**, 148–153.

13  Higgs DR (1993) α-Thalassaemia. *Bailliere's Clin Haematol* **6**, 117–150.

14  Hall GW, Thein SL, Newland AC, Chisholm M, Traeger-Synodinos J, Kanavakis E *et al.* (1993) A base substitution (T → G) in codon 29 of the α2-globin gene causes α thalassaemia. *Br J Haematol* **85**, 546–552.

15  Kattamis AC, Camaschella C, Sivera P, Surrey S and Fortina P (1996) Human α-thalassemia syndromes: detection of molecular defects. *Am J Hematol* **53**, 81–91.

16  Chui DHK and Waye JS (1998) Hydrops fetalis caused by α-thalassaemia: an emerging health care problem. *Blood* **91**, 2213–2222.

17  Barbour VM, Tufarelli C, Sharpe JA, Smith ZE, Ayyub H, Heinlein CA *et al.* (2000) α-Thalassemia resulting from a negative chromosomal position effect. *Blood* **96**, 800–807.

18  Higgs DR. Molecular mechanisms of α thalassemia. In: Steinberg MH, Forget BG, Higgs DR and Nagel RL, eds. *Disorders of Hemoglobin: Genetics, Pathophysiology, and Clinical Management*. Cambridge University Press, Cambridge, 2001, pp. 405–430.

19 Gibbons RJ and Higgs DR. The alpha thalassemia/mental retardation syndrome. In: Steinberg MH, Forget BG, Higgs DR and Nagel RL, eds. *Disorders of Hemoglobin: Genetics, Pathophysiology, and Clinical Management.* Cambridge University Press, Cambridge, 2001, pp. 470–488.

20 Viprakasit V, Kidd AMJ, Ayyub H, Horsley S, Hughes J and Higgs DR (2003) *De novo* deletion within the telomeric region flanking the human α globin locus as a cause of α thalassaemia. *Br J Haematol* **120**, 867–875.

21 Weatherall DJ. Genetic disorders of haemoglobin. In: Hoffbrand AV, Lewis SM and Tuddenham EGD, eds. *Postgraduate Haematology*, 5th edn. Blackwell Publishing, Oxford, 2005, pp. 85–103.

22 Flint J, Harding RM, Boyce AJ and Clegg JB (1998) The population genetics of the haemoglobinopathies. *Bailliere's Clin Haematol* **11**, 1–51.

23 Hurst D, Tittle B, Kleman KM, Embury SH and Lubin BH (1982) Anemia and hemoglobinopathies in South East Asian refugee children. *J Pediatr* **102**, 692–697.

24 Cabrera A and de Pablos JM (1984) Betathalassaemia minor in gypsies from the south of Spain. *Br J Haematol* **58**, 377.

25 Livingstone FB. *Frequencies of Hemoglobin Variants.* Oxford University Press, Oxford, 1985.

26 Yenchitsomanus PT, Summers KM, Bhatia KK, Cattani J and Board PG (1985) Extremely high frequencies of α-globin gene deletion in Madang and on Kar Kar Island, Papua New Guinea. *Am J Hum Genet* **37**, 7778–7784.

27 Petrou M, Brugiatelli M, Old J, Hurley P, Ward RHT, Wong KP *et al.* (1992) Alpha thalassaemia hydrops fetalis in the UK: the importance of screening pregnant women of Chinese, other South East Asian and Mediterranean extraction for alpha thalassaemia trait. *Br J Obstet Gynaecol* **99**, 985–989.

28 Mukherjee MB, Lu CY, Ducrocq R, Gangakhedkar RR, Colah RB, Kadam MD *et al.* (1997) Effect of α-thalassaemia on sickle cell anemia linked to the Arab–Indian haplotype in India. *Am J Hematol* **55**, 104–109.

29 Van den Broek NR, Letsky EA, White SA and Shenkin A (1998) Iron status of pregnant women: which measurements are valid? *Br J Haematol* **103**, 817–824.

30 Segbena AY, Prehu C, Wajcman H, Bardakdjian-Michau J, Messie K, Feteke L *et al.* (1998) Hemoglobins in Togolese newborns: Hb S, Hb C, Hb Bart's, and α-globin gene status. *Am J Hematol* **59**, 208–213.

31 Sirdah M, Bilto YY, El Jabour S and Najjar KH (1998) Screening secondary school students in the Gaza strip for β-thalassaemia trait. *Clin Lab Haematol* **20**, 279–283.

32 Daar S, Hussein HM, Merghoub T and Krishnamoorthy R (1998) Spectrum of β-thalassemia mutations in Oman. *Ann NY Acad Sci* **850**, 404–406.

33 Romana M, Kéclard L, Froger A, Berchel C and Mérault G (1998) Spectrum of β-thalassemia mutations in Guadeloupe (French West Indies) and interactions with other hemoglobinopathies. *Ann NY Acad Sci* **850**, 423–425.

34 Casas-Castaneda M, Hernandez-Lugo I, Torres O, Barajas H, Cibrian S, Zamudio G *et al.* (1998) Alphathalassemia in a selected population of Mexico. *Rev Invest Clin* **50**, 395–398.

35 Ruiz-Reyes G (1998) Abnormal hemoglobins and thalassemias in Mexico. *Rev Invest Clin* **50**, 163–170.

36 Ko TM, Caviles AP, Hwa HL, Liu CW, Hsu PM and Chung YP (1998) Prevalence and molecular characterization of β-thalassaemia in Filipinos. *Ann Hematol* **77**, 257–260.

37 Ko TM, Hwa HL, Liu CW, Li SF, Chu JY and Cheung YP (1999) Prevalence study and molecular characterization of α-thalassaemia in Filipinos. *Ann Hematol* **78**, 355–357.

38 Gill PS and Modell B (1999) Thalassaemia among Asians in Britain. *Lancet* **318**, 873.

39 de Silva S, Fisher CA, Premawardhena A, Lamabadusuriya SP, Peto TEA, Perera G *et al.* (2000) Thalassaemia in Sri Lanka: implications for the future health burden of Asian populations. *Lancet* **355**, 786–791.

40 Badens C, Martinez di Montmuros F, Thuret I, Michel G, Mattei J-F, Cappellini M-D and Lena-Russo D (2000) Molecular basis of haemoglobinopathies and G6PD deficiency in the Comorian population. *Hematol J* **1**, 264–268.

41 Moule R, Bodo JM, Mpele DM, Feingold J and Galacteros F (2000) β-Globin gene haplotypes and α-thalassaemia analysis in Babinga pygmies from Congo-Brazzaville. *Hum Biol* **72**, 379–383.

42 Moule R, Pambou O, Feingold J and Galacteros F (2000) α-Thalassaemia in Bantu population from Congo-Brazzaville: its interaction with sickle cell anemia. *Hum Hered* **50**, 118–125.

43 Diejomaoh FME, Haider MZ, Dalal H, Abdulaziz A, D'Souza TM and Adekile AD (2000) Influence of α-

thalassemia trait on the prevalence and severity of anemia in pregnancy in women in Kuwait. *Acta Haematol* **104**, 92–94.

44 Rund DG, Jackson N, Oron-Kami V, Filon D and Oppenheim A (2001) An unexpected high frequency of carriership for alpha-thalassemia in Ashkenazi Jews. *Hematol J* **1**, Suppl. 1, 52.

45 Loukopoulos D and Kollia P. Worldwide distribution of β thalassemia. In: Steinberg MH, Forget BG, Higgs DR and Nagel RL, eds. *Disorders of Hemoglobin: Genetics, Pathophysiology, and Clinical Management*. Cambridge University Press, Cambridge, 2001, pp. 861–877.

46 Bernini LF. Geographic distribution of α thalassemia. In: Steinberg MH, Forget BG, Higgs DR and Nagel RL, eds. *Disorders of Hemoglobin: Genetics, Pathophysiology, and Clinical Management*. Cambridge University Press, Cambridge, 2001, pp. 878–894.

47 Schrier SL, Bunyaratvej A, Khuhapinant A, Fucharoen S, Aljurf M, Snyder LM *et al.* (1997) The unusual pathobiology of hemoglobin Constant Spring in red blood cells. *Blood* **89**, 1762–1769.

48 Higgs DR and Bowden DK. Clinical and laboratory features of the α-thalassemia syndromes. In: Steinberg MH, Forget BG, Higgs DR and Nagel RL, eds. *Disorders of Hemoglobin: Genetics, Pathophysiology, and Clinical Management*. Cambridge University Press, Cambridge, 2001, pp. 431–469.

49 Pootrakul P, Winichagoon P, Fucharoen S, Pravatmuang P, Piankijagum A and Wasi P (1981) Homozygous haemoglobin Constant Spring: a need for revision of concept. *Hum Genet* **59**, 250–255.

50 Krishnamurti L and Little JA (1998) Homozygous hemoglobin Constant Spring with normal electrophoresis: a possible cause of under diagnosis. *Ann NY Acad Sci* **805**, 415–419.

51 Graham EA, Felgenhauer J, Detter JC and Labbe RF (1996) Elevated zinc protoporphyrin associated with thalassemia trait and hemoglobin E. *J Pediatr* **129**, 105–110.

52 Harthoorn-Lasthuizen EJ, Lindemans J and Langenhuijsen MMAC (1998) Combined use of erythrocyte zinc protoporphyrin and mean corpuscular volume in differentiation of thalassemia from iron deficiency anemia. *Eur J Haematol* **60**, 245–251.

53 Fucharoen S, Winichagoon P, Wisedpanichkij R, Sae-Ngow B, Sriphanich R, Oncoung W *et al.* (1998) Prenatal and postnatal diagnosis of thalassemias and hemoglobinopathies by HPLC. *Clin Chem* **44**, 740–748.

54 McFarlane AG, Barth D, Crowther MA and Lafferty JD (2003) The percentage of haemoglobin Barts as a predictor for the alpha thalassemia genotype in cord blood samples. *Blood* **102**, 33b.

55 Rees DC, Williams TN, Maitland K, Clegg JB and Weatherall DJ (1998) Alpha thalassaemia is associated with increased soluble transferrin receptor levels. *Br J Haematol* **103**, 365–369.

56 Ausavarungnirum R, Winichagoon P, Fucharoen S, Epstein N and Simkins R (1998) Detection of γ-globin chains in cord blood by ELISA (enzyme-linked immunosorbent assay): rapid screening for α-thalassemia 1 (Southeast Asian type). *Am J Hematol* **57**, 283–286.

57 Fairweather RB, Chaffee S, McBride KL, Snow K, Kubik KS, Hoyer JD *et al.* (1999) Hyperunstable Hb Dartmouth [α2-66(E15)Leu→Pro (CTG→CCG)] in association with α-thalassemia-1 (SE Asian) causes transfusion-dependent α thalassemia. *Blood* **94**, Suppl. 1, 24b.

58 Lam TH, Ghosh A, Tang MHY and Chan V (1997) The risk of α-thalassaemia in offspring of β-thalassaemia carriers in Hong Kong. *Prenatal Diagnosis* **17**, 733–736.

59 Ma SK, Chan AYY, Chan LC, Chui DHK and Waye JS (2000) Compound heterozygosity for triplicated α-globin gene and (– –$^{SEA}$) α-globin gene deletion: implication for thalassaemia screening. *Br J Haematol* **110**, 498–499.

60 Chui GHK, Fucharoen S and Chan V (2003) Hemoglobin H disease is not necessarily a benign disorder. *Blood* **101**, 791–800.

61 Lorey F, Charoenkwan P, Witkowska HE, Lafferty J, Patterson M, Eng B *et al.* (2001) Hb H hydrops foetalis syndrome: a case report and review of the literature. *Br J Haematol* **115**, 72–78.

62 Viprakasit V, Green S, Height S, Ayyub H and Higgs DR (2002) Hb H hydrops fetalis syndrome associated with the interaction of two common determinants of α thalassaemia (– –$^{MED}$/α$^{TSAUDI}$α). *Br J Haematol* **117**, 759–762.

63 Hewes LB, Alvarado CS, Holley LL, Gomez K, Dykes F, Kutlar A and Kutlar F (2001) Hemoglobin H hydrops fetalis due to compound heterozygosity for double α gene deletion and point mutation at codon 59, GGC≡GAC (Gly≡Asp), of an α$_2$ gene in an infant of Asian descent. *Blood* **98**, 22b.

64 Chen FE, Ooi C, Ha SY, Cheung BMY, Todd D, Liang R *et al.* (2000) Genetic and clinical features of hemoglobin H disease in Chinese patients. *N Engl J Med* **343**, 544–550.

65 Kanavakis E, Papassotirou I, Karagiorga M, Vrettou C, Metaxotou-Mavrommati A, Stamoulakatou A *et al.* (2000) Phenotypic and molecular diversity of haemoglobin H disease: a Greek experience. *Br J Haematol* **111**, 915–923.

66 Kurosawa K, Asoh M, Akatsuka A, Matsuo T, Ochiai Y and Maekawa K (1996) A Japanese patient with X-linked α-thalassaemia/mental retardation syndrome: an additional case report. *Jpn J Hum Genet* **41**, 329–332.

67 Kuno T, Ideguchi H, Yoshida N, Masuyama T, Ohta M, Nishimura S *et al.* (1997) A case of X-linked α-thalassaemia/mental retardation syndrome: analysis of hemoglobin by an automated glycated hemoglobin analyzer. *Acta Pediatr Jpn* **39**, 615–618.

68 Wada T, Nakamura M, Matsushita Y, Yamada M, Yamashita S, Iwamoto H *et al.* (1998) Three Japanese children with X-linked α-thalassaemia/mental retardation syndrome (ATR-X) *No To Hattatsu* **30**, 283–289.

69 O'Brien RT (1973) The effect of iron deficiency on the expression of hemoglobin H. *Blood* **41**, 853–856.

70 Saleem A, Irani DR, Bart JB and Alfrey CP (1987) Suppression of hemoglobin H in disorders of iron metabolism. *Acta Haematol* **77**, 34–37.

71 Fucharoen S, Winichagoon P, Siritanaratkul N, Chowthaworn JEW and Pootrakul P (1998) α- and β-thalassaemia in Thailand. *Ann NY Acad Sci* **850**, 412–414.

72 Ma ESK, Chan AYY, Au WY, Yeung YM and Chan LC (2001) Diagnosis of concurrent hemoglobin H disease and heterozygous β-thalassaemia. *Haematologica* **86**, 432–433.

73 Traeger-Synodinos J, Papassotiriou I, Vrettou C, Skarmoutsou C, Stamoulakatou A and Kanavakis R (2001) Erythroid marrow activity and functional anemia in patients with the rare interaction of a single functional α-globin and β-globin gene. *Haematologica* **86**, 363–367.

74 Lie-Injo LE and Jo BH (1960) A fast moving haemoglobin in hydrops foetalis. *Nature* **185**, 698.

75 Fung TY, Kin LT, Kong LC and Keung LC (1999) Homozygous alpha-thalassaemia associated with hypospadias in three survivors. *Am J Med Genet* **82**, 225–227.

76 Goulden NJ, Kyle P, Souhail K and Pamphilon DH (2002) Normal developmental outcome in a 2-year-old child born after successful salvage of haemoglobin Barts hydrops foetalis syndrome with multiple *in utero* transfusions. *Br J Haematol* **117**, Suppl. 1, 12.

77 Chan V, Chan W-Y, Tang M, Lau K, Todd D and Chan TK (1997) Molecular defects in haemoglobin H hydrops. *Br J Haematol* **96**, 224–226.

78 Hall GW, Barnetson RA and Thein SL (1992) Beta thalassaemia in the indigenous British population. *Br J Haematol* **82**, 584–588.

79 Fucharoen S, Sanchaisuriya K, Fucharoen G and Surapot S (2001) Molecular characterization of thalassemia intermedia with homozygous Hb Malay and Hb Malay/HbE in Thai patients. *Haematologica* **86**, 657–658.

80 Smith CM, Hedlund B, Cich JA, Tukey DP, Olson M, Steinberg MH and Admas JG (1983) Hemoglobin North Shore: a variant hemoglobin associated with the phenotype of β-thalassaemia. *Blood* **61**, 378–383.

81 Russell JE and Liebhaber SA (1996) The stability of human β-globin mRNA is dependent on structural determinants positioned within its 3' untranslated region. *Blood* **87**, 5314–5322.

82 Hopmeier P, Krugluger W, Gu L-H, Smetanina NS and Huisman THJ (1996) A newly discovered frameshift at codons 120–121 (+A) of the β gene is not associated with a dominant form of β-thalassaemia. *Blood* **87**, 5393–5394.

83 Thein SL (1998) β-Thalassaemia. *Bailliere's Clin Haematol* **11**, 91–126.

84 Cabeda JM, Correia C, Estevinho A, Simões C, Amorim ML, Pinho L and Justiça B (1999) Unexpected pattern of β-globin gene mutations in β-thalassaemia patients from Northern Portugal. *Br J Haematol* **105**, 68–74.

85 Ho PJ and Thein SL (2000) Gene regulation and deregulation: a β globin perspective. *Blood Rev* **14**, 78–93.

86 Rashkind WH, Niakan KK, Wolff J, Matsushita M, Vaughan T, Stamatoyannopoulos G *et al.* (1999) Mapping of a syndrome of X-linked thrombocytopenia with thalassemia to band Xp11–12: further evidence of genetic heterogeneity. *Blood* **95**, 2262–2268.

87 Weatherall D and Clegg JB. *The Thalassaemia Syndromes*, 4th edn. Blackwell Science, Oxford, 2001.

88 Yu C, Niakan KK, Martsushita M, Stamatoyannopoulos G, Orkin SH and Raskind WH (2002) X-Linked thrombocytopenia with thalassaemia from

a mutation in the amino finger of GATA-1 affecting DNA binding rather than FOG-1 interaction. *Blood* **100**, 2040–2045.

89 Castro O, Kutlar F, Kutlar A, Holley L, Hassan S and Elshowaia S (2001) Sβ⁰ Thalassemia in a 91-year-old woman with mild sickle cell disease with two thalassemia mutations on the same chromosome. *Blood* **98**, 14b–15b.

90 Murru S, Loudianos G, Porcu S, Sciarratta GV, Agosti S, Parodi MI *et al.* (1992) A β-thalassaemia phenotype not linked to the β-globin cluster in an Italian family. *Br J Haematol* **81**, 283–287.

91 Giordano PC, Harteveld CL, Haak HL, Batelaan D, van Delft P, Plug RJ *et al.* (1998) A case of non-β-globin gene linked β thalassaemia in a Dutch family with two additional α-gene defects: the common $-\alpha^{3.7}$ deletion and the rare IVS1-116 (A→G) acceptor splice site mutation. *Br J Haematol* **103**, 370–376.

92 Millard DP, Mason K, Serjeant BE and Serjeant GR (1977) Comparison of haematological features in β⁰ and β⁺ thalassaemia traits in Jamaican Negroes. *Br J Haematol* **36**, 161–170.

93 Olivieri NF and Weatherall DJ. Clinical aspects of beta thalassemia. In: Steinberg MH, Forget BG, Higgs DR and Nagel RL, eds. *Disorders of Hemoglobin: Genetics, Pathophysiology, and Clinical Management.* Cambridge University Press, Cambridge, 2001, pp. 342–355.

94 Lewis D, Stockley RJ and Chanarin I (1982) Changes in mean corpuscular red cell volume in women with β-thalassaemia trait during pregnancy. *Br J Haematol* **50**, 423–425.

95 Mentzer WC (1973) Differentiation of iron deficiency from thalassaemia trait. *Lancet* **i**, 882.

96 England JM and Fraser PM (1973) Differentiation of iron deficiency from thalassaemia trait by routine blood count. *Lancet* **i**, 449–452.

97 Mazza U, Saglio G, Cappio FC, Camaschella C, Neretto G and Gallo E (1976) Clinical and haematological data in 254 cases of beta-thalassaemia trait in Italy. *Br J Haematol* **33**, 91–99.

98 Shine I and Lal S (1977) A strategy to detect β thalassaemia trait. *Lancet* **i**, 692–694.

99 Srivastava PC (1973) Differentiation of thalassaemia minor from iron deficiency. *Lancet* **ii**, 154–155.

100 Ricerca BM, Storti S, d'Onofrio G, Mancini S, Vittori M, Campisi S *et al.* (1987) Differentiation of iron deficiency from thalassaemia trait: a new approach. *Haematologica* **72**, 409–413.

101 Green R and King RA (1989) A new red cell discriminant incorporating volume dispersion for differentiating iron deficiency anemia from thalassaemia minor. *Blood Cells* **15**, 481–485.

102 D'Onofrio G, Zini G, Ricerca BM, Mancini S and Mango G (1992) Automated measurement of red blood cell microcytosis and hypochromia in iron deficiency and β-thalassaemia trait. *Arch Pathol Lab Med* **116**, 84–89.

103 Jiminez CV, Minchinela J and Ros J (1995) New indices from the H*2 analyser improve differentiation between heterozygous β and δβ thalassaemia and iron deficiency anaemia. *Clin Lab Haematol* **17**, 151–155.

104 Eldibany MM, Totonchi KF, Joseph NJ and Rhone D (1999) Usefulness of certain red blood cell indices in diagnosing and differentiating thalassaemia trait from iron-deficiency anemia. *Am J Clin Pathol* **111**, 676–682; and Eldibany MM (1999) Correction. *Am J Clin Pathol* **112**, 428.

105 Lafferty JD, Crowther MA, Ali MA and Levine M (1996) The evaluation of various mathematical RBC indices and their efficacy in discriminating between thalassemic and non-thalassemic microcytosis. *Am J Clin Pathol* **106**, 201–205.

106 Bain BJ. *Haemoglobinopathy Diagnosis*, 1st edn. Blackwell Publishing, Oxford, 2001.

107 Rees DC, Duley DA and Marinaki AM (2003) Pyrimidine 5′ nucleotidase deficiency. *Br J Haematol* **120**, 375–383.

108 Globin Gene Disorder Working Party of the BCSH General Haematology Task Force (1994) Guidelines for the fetal diagnosis of globin gene disorders. *J Clin Pathol* **47**, 199–204.

109 Bain BJ, Amos RJ, Bareford D, Chapman C, Davies SC, Old JM and Wild BL (Working Party of the General Haematology Task Force of the British Committee for Standards in Haematology) (1998) The laboratory diagnosis of haemoglobinopathies. *Br J Haematol* **101**, 783–792.

110 Gasperini D, Cao A, Paderi L, Barella S, Paglietti E, Perseu L *et al.* (1993) Normal individuals with high Hb A₂ levels. *Br J Haematol* **84**, 166–168.

111 Nagel RL and Steinberg MH. Hemoglobins of the embryo and fetus and minor hemoglobins of adults. In: Steinberg MH, Forget BG, Higgs DR and Nagel RL, eds. *Disorders of Hemoglobin: Genetics, Pathophysiology, and Clinical Management.* Cambridge University Press, Cambridge, 2001, pp. 197–230.

112 Huisman THJ (1977) Trimodality in the percentages of β chain variants in heterozygotes: the effect of the number of active Hbα structural loci. *Hemoglobin* **1**, 349–382.

113 Tamary H, Shalev H, Luria D, Shaft D, Zoldan M, Shalmon L *et al.* (1996) Clinical features and studies of erythropoiesis in Israeli Bedouins with congenital dyserythropoietic anaemia type I. *Blood* **87**, 1763–1770.

114 Van Kirk R, Sandhaus LM and Hoyer J (2004) Diagnosis of hemoglobin (Hb) A2′ trait by high-performance liquid chromatography (HPLC). *Am J Clin Pathol* **122**, 630.

115 Rogers M, Phelan L and Bain B (1995) Screening criteria for β thalassaemia trait in pregnant women. *J Clin Pathol* **48**, 1054–1056.

116 Huisman THJ (1997) Levels of Hb A$_2$ in heterozygotes and homozygotes for beta-thalassaemia mutations: influence of mutations in the CACCC and ATAAA motifs of the beta-globin promoter. *Acta Haematol* **98**, 187–194.

117 Serjeant BE, Mason KP and Serjeant GR (1978) The development of haemoglobin A$_2$ in normal Negro infants and in sickle cell disease. *Br J Haematol* **39**, 259–263.

118 Maragoudaki E, Vrettou C, Kanavakis E, Traeger-Synodinos J, Metaxotou-Mavrommati A and Kattamis C (1998) Molecular, haematological and clinical studies of a silent β-gene C→G mutation at 6 bp 3′ to the termination codon (+1480 C→G) in twelve Greek families. *Br J Haematol* **103**, 45–51.

119 Maragoudaki E, Kanavakis E, Traeger-Synodinos J, Vrettou C, Tzetis M, Metaxotou-Mavrommati A and Kattamis C (1999) Molecular, haematological and clinical studies of the −101 C→T substitution of the β-globin gene promoter in 25 β-thalassaemia intermedia patients and 45 heterozygotes. *Br J Haematol* **107**, 699–706.

120 Athanassiado A, Papchatzopoulou A, Zoumbos N, Maniatis GM and Gibbs R (1994) A novel β-thalassaemia mutation in the 5′ untranslated region of the β-globin gene. *Br J Haematol* **88**, 307–310.

121 Ho PJ, Rochette J, Fisher CA, Wonke B, Jarvis MK, Yardumian A and Thein SL (1996) Moderate reduction of β-globin gene transcript by a novel mutation in the 5′ untranslated region: a study of its interaction with other genotypes in two families. *Blood* **87**, 1170–1178.

122 Öner C, Agarwal S, Dimovski AJ, Efremov GD, Petkov GH, Altay C *et al.* (1991) The G–A mutation at position +22 3′ to the Cap site of the beta-globin gene and a possible cause for a beta-thalassaemia. *Hemoglobin* **15**, 67–76.

123 Scerri CA, Abela W, Galdies R, Pizzuto M, Grech JL and Felice AE (1993) The β$^+$ IVS, I-NT no. 6 (T→C) thalassaemia in heterozygotes with an associated Hb Valetta or Hb S heterozygosity in homozygotes from Malta. *Br J Haematol* **83**, 669–671.

124 Old J (2003) Screening and genetic diagnosis of haemoglobin disorders. *Blood Rev* **17**, 43–54.

125 Pagano L, Desicato S, Viola A, de Rosa C and Floretti G (1995) Identification of the −92 (C→T) mutation by the amplification refractory mutation system in Southern Italy. *Hemoglobin* **19**, 307–310.

126 Wasi P, Disthasongchan P and Na-Nakorn S (1968) The effect of iron deficiency on the levels of haemoglobin A2. *J Lab Clin Med* **71**, 85–91.

127 Alperin JB, Dow PA and Petteway MB (1972) Haemoglobin A2 levels in health and various haematological disorders. *Am J Clin Pathol* **67**, 219–226.

128 Kattamis C, Lagos P, Metaxotou-Mavromati A and Matsaniotis NJ (1972) Serum iron and unsaturated iron-binding-capacity in β thalassaemia trait: their relation to the levels of haemoglobins A, A2 and F. *J Med Genet* **9**, 154–159.

129 Galanello R, Ruggeri R, Addis M, Paglietti E and Cao A (1981) Hemoglobin A$_2$ in iron-deficient β-thalassaemia heterozygotes. *Hemoglobin* **5**, 613–618.

130 Alli NA and Mendelow BV (1998) Distinguishing β-thalassaemia carriers from normal individuals — a comparison of two methods. *Br J Haematol* **102**, 179.

131 El-Agouza I, Shahla AA and Sirdah M (2002) The effect of iron deficiency anaemia on the levels of haemoglobin subtypes: possible consequences for clinical diagnosis. *Clin Lab Haematol* **24**, 285–289.

132 Guiso L, Frogheri L, Pistidda P, Angioni L, Dore F, Pardini S and Longinotti M (1996) Frequency of δ$^+$ 27-thalassaemia in Sardinians. *Clin Lab Haematol* **18**, 241–244.

133 Liang R, Liang S, Jiang NH, Wen X-J, Zhao J-B, Nechtman JF *et al.* (1994) α and β thalassaemia among Chinese children in Guangxi Province, P.R. China: molecular and haematological characterization. *Br J Haematol* **86**, 351–354.

134 Kanavakis E, Wainscoat JS, Wood WG, Weatherall DJ, Cao A, Furbetta M *et al.* (1982) The interaction of α thalassaemia with heterozygous β thalassaemia. *Br J Haematol* **52**, 465–473.

135 Gasperini D, Cao A, Paderi L, Barella S, Paglietti E, Perseu L *et al.* (1993) Normal individuals with high Hb A$_2$ levels. *Br J Haematol* **84**, 166–168.

136 Garner C, Dew TK, Sherwood R, Rees D and Thein SL (2003) Heterocellular hereditary persistence of fetal haemoglobin affects the haematological parameters of β-thalassaemia trait. *Br J Haematol* **123**, 353–358.

137 Dacie JV. *The Haemolytic Anaemias*, Volume 2, *The Hereditary Haemolytic Anaemias*. Churchill Livingstone, Edinburgh, 1988.

138 Maehara T, Tsuukamoto N, Nijima Y, Karasawa M, Murakami H, Hattori Y and Ideguchi H (2002) Enhanced haemolysis with β-thalassaemia trait due to unstable β chain variant, Hb Gunma, accompanied by hereditary elliptocytosis due to protein 4.1 deficiency in a Japanese family. *Br J Haematol* **117**,193–197.

139 Thein SL (1999) Is it dominantly inherited β thalassaemia or just a β-chain variant that is highly unstable? *Br J Haematol* **107**, 12–21.

140 Ho PJ, Wickramasinghe S, Rees DC, Lee MJ, Eden A and Thein SL (1997) Erythroblastic inclusions in dominantly inherited β thalassaemia trait. *Blood* **89**, 322–328.

141 Faustino P, Osçrio-Almeida L, Romao L, Barbot J, Fernandes B, Justica B and Lavinha J (1998) Dominantly transmitted β-thalassaemia arising from the production of several aberrant mRNA species and one abnormal peptide. *Blood* **91**, 685–690.

142 Thein SL, Hesketh C, Taylor P, Temperley IJ, Hutchinson RM, Old JM *et al.* (1990) Molecular basis of dominantly inherited inclusion body β-thalassemia. *Proc Natl Acad Sci USA* **87** 3924–3928.

143 Thein SL (1992) Dominant β thalassaemia: molecular basis and pathophysiology. *Br J Haematol* **80**, 273–277.

144 Galanello R and Cao A (1998) Relationship between genotype and phenotype: thalassemia intermedia. *Ann NY Acad Sci* **850**, 325–333.

145 Vetter B, Neu-Yilik G, Kohne E, Arnold R, Sinha P, Gaedicke G *et al.* (2000) Dominant β thalassaemia; a highly unstable haemoglobin is caused by a novel 6 bp deletion of the β-globin gene. *Br J Haematol* **108**, 176–181.

146 Waye JS, Eng B, Patterson M, Barr RD and Chui DHK (1997) De novo mutation of the β-globin gene initiation codon (ATG→AAG) in a Northern European boy. *Am J Hematol* **56**, 179–182.

147 Ropero P, Gonzalez FA, Sanchez J, Anguita E, Asenjo S, Del Arco A *et al.* (1999) Identification of the Hb Lepore phenotype by HPLC. *Haematologica* **84**, 1081–1084.

148 Ma SK and Au WY (1999) Images in haematology: hepatic haemopoiesis in β-thalassaemia trait. *Br J Haematol* **107**, 1.

149 Aessopos A, Farmakis D, Karagiorga M, Voskaridou E, Loutradi A, Hatziliami A *et al* (2001) Cardiac involvement in thalassaemia intermedia: a multicenter study. *Blood* **97**, 3411–3416.

150 Vassilopoulos G, Papassotiriou I, Voskaridou E, Stamoulakatou A, Premetis E, Kister J *et al.* (1995) Hb Arta [β45 (CD4) Phe→Cys]: a new unstable haemoglobin with reduced oxygen affinity in trans with β-thalassaemia. *Br J Haematol* **91**, 595–601.

151 Huisman THJ (1997) Combinations of β chain abnormal hemoglobins with each other and with β-thalassaemia determinants with known mutations: influence on phenotype. *Clin Chem* **43**, 1850–1856.

152 Papassotiriou I, Traeger-Synodinos J, Prom D, Kister J, Premetis E, Stamoulakatou A *et al.* (1998) Hb Acharnes or β53(D4) Ala→Thr: an unstable electrophoretically silent haemoglobin variant in association with β-thalassaemia. *Br J Haematol* **102**, 178.

153 Rund D, Oron-Karni V, Filon D, Goldfarb A, Rachmilewitz E and Oppenheim A (1997) Genetic analysis of β-thalassaemia intermedia in Israel: diversity of mechanisms and unpredictability of phenotype. *Am J Hematol* **54**, 16–22.

154 Ho PJ, Hall GW, Luo LY, Weatherall DJ and Thein SL (1998) Beta-thalassaemia intermedia: is it possible consistently to predict phenotype from genotype? *Br J Haematol* **100**, 70–78.

155 Mohamed N and Jackson N (1998) Severe thalassaemia intermedia: clinical problems in the absence of hypertransfusion. *Blood Rev* **12**, 163–170.

156 Badens C, Mattei MG, Imbert AM, Lapouméroulie C, Martini N, Michel G and Lena-Russo D (2002) A novel mechanism for thalassaemia intermedia. *Lancet* **359**, 132–133.

157 Chang Y-PC, Littera R, Garau R, Smith KD, Dover GJ, Iannelli S *et al.* (2001) The role of heterocellular hereditary persistence of fetal haemoglobin in β$^0$-thalassaemia intermedia. *Br J Haematol* **114**, 899–906.

158 Saxon BR, Rees D and Olivieri NF (1998) Regression of extramedullary haemopoiesis and augmentation of fetal haemoglobin concentration during hydroxyurea therapy in β thalassaemia. *Br J Haematol* **101**, 416–419.

159 Fisher CA, Premawardhena A, de Silva S, Perera G, Rajapaksa S, Olivieri NA *et al.* and the Sri Lanka Thalassaemia Study Group. (2003) The molecular basis of the thalassaemias in Sri Lanka. *Br J Haematol* **121**, 662–671.

160 Wood WG. Hereditary persistence of fetal hemoglobin and δβ thalassemia. In: Steinberg MH, Forget BG, Higgs DR and Nagel RL, eds. *Disorders of Hemoglobin: Genetics, Pathophysiology, and Clinical Management.* Cambridge University Press, Cambridge, 2001, pp. 356–388.

161 Zertal-Zidani S, Ducrocq R, Weil-Oliver C, Elion J and Krishnamoorthy R (2001) A novel δβ fusion gene expresses hemoglobin A (HbA) not Hb Lepore: Senegalese $\delta^0\beta^+$ thalassaemia. *Blood* **98**, 1261–1263.

162 Galanello R, Barella S, Satta S, Maccioni L, Pintor C and Cao A (2002) Homozygosity for non-deletional $\delta$-$\beta^0$ thalassaemia resulting in a silent clinical phenotype. *Blood* **100**, 1913–1914.

163 Harteveld CL, Osborne CS, Peters M, van der Werf S, Plug R, Fraser P and Giordano PC (2003) Novel 112 kb (εGγAγ) δβ-thalassaemia deletion in a Dutch family. *Br J Haematol* **122**, 855–858.

164 Game L, Bergounioux J, Close JP, Marzouka BE and Thein SL (2003) A novel deletion causing $(\epsilon\gamma\delta\beta)^0$ thalassaemia in a Chilean family. *Br J Haematol* **123**, 154–159.

165 Huisman THJ (1997) Gamma chain abnormal human fetal hemoglobin variants. *Am J Hematol* **55**, 159–163.

166 Craig JE, Rochette J, Sampietro M, Wilkie AOM, Barnetson R, Hatton CSR *et al.* (1997) Genetic heterogeneity in heterocellular hereditary persistence of fetal hemoglobin. *Blood* **90**, 428–434.

167 Gilman JG, Mishima N, Wen XJ, Kutlar F and Huisman THJ (1988) Upstream promoter mutation associated with a modest elevation of fetal hemoglobin expression in human adults. *Blood* **72**, 78–81.

168 Wickramasinghe SN (1998) Congenital dyserythropoietic anaemias: clinical features, haematological morphology and new biochemical data. *Blood Rev* **12**, 178–200.

169 Dror Y and Freedman MH (2002) Shwachman–Diamond syndrome. *Br J Haematol* **118**, 701–713.

170 Peters F, Rohloff D, Kohlmann T, Renner F, Jantschek G, Kerner W and Fehm HL (1998) Fetal hemoglobin in starvation ketosis in young women. *Blood* **91**, 691–694.

171 Little JA, Dempsey NJ, Tuchman M and Ginder GD (1995) Metabolic persistence of fetal hemoglobin. *Blood* **85**, 1712–1718.

172 Schilirò G, Musumeci S, Pizzarelli G, Russo A, Marinucci M, Tentori L and Russo G (1978) Fetal haemoglobin in early malignant osteopetrosis. *Br J Haematol* **38**, 339–344.

173 Kosteas T, Palena A and Anagno NP (1997) Molecular cloning of the breakpoints of the hereditary persistence of fetal hemoglobin type 6 (HPFH-6) deletion and sequence analysis of the novel juxtaposed region from the 3′ end of the β-globin gene cluster. *Hum Genet* **100**, 441–445.

174 Fucharoen S, Fucharoen G, Sanchaisuriya K and Surapot S (2002) Molecular characterization of thalassaemia intermedia associated with HPFH-6/β-thalassaemia and HPTH-6/Hb E in Thai patients. *Acta Haematol* **108**, 157–161.

175 Forget BG (1998) Molecular basis of hereditary persistence of fetal hemoglobin. *Ann NY Acad Sci* **850**, 38–44.

176 Bollekens JA and Forget BG (1991) δβ Thalassemia and hereditary persistence of fetal hemoglobin. *Hematol Oncol Clin North Am* **5**, 399–422.

177 Stamatoyannopoulos G and Nienhuis AW. Hemoglobin switching In: Stamatoyannopoulos G, Nienhuis AW, Majerus PW and Varmus H, eds. *The Molecular Basis of Blood Diseases*, 2nd edn. W.B. Saunders, Philadelphia, PA, 1994, pp. 107–156.

178 Jane SM and Cunningham JM (1998) Understanding fetal globin gene expression: a step towards effective Hb F reactivation in haemoglobinopathies. *Br J Haematol* **102**, 415–422.

179 Conley CL, Weatherall DL, Richardson SN, Shepard MK and Charache S (1963) Hereditary persistence of fetal hemoglobin. A study of 79 affected persons in 15 Negro families in Baltimore. *Blood* **21**, 261–281.

180 Schroeder WH, Huisman THJ and Sukumaran PK (1973) A second type of hereditary persistence of foetal haemoglobin. *Br J Haematol* **25**, 131–135.

181 Wainscoat JS, Old JM, Wood WG, Trent RJ and Weatherall DJ (1984) Characterization of an Indian $(\delta\beta)^0$ thalassaemia. *Br J Haematol* **58**, 353–360.

182 Saglio G, Camaschella C, Serra A, Bertero T, Rege Cambrin G, Guerrasiqo A *et al.* (1986) Italian type of deletional hereditary persistence of fetal hemoglobin. *Blood* **68**, 646–651.

183 Camaschella C, Serra A, Gottardi E, Alfarano A, Revello D, Mazza U and Saglio G (1990) A new

hereditary persistence of fetal hemoglobin deletional has the breakpoint within the 3′ β-globin gene enhancer. *Blood* **75**, 1000–1005.

184 Adams JG, Coleman MB, Hayes J, Morrison WT and Steinberg MH (1985) Modulation of fetal hemoglobin synthesis by iron deficiency. *N Engl J Med* **313**, 1402–1405.

185 Landman H and Huisman TH (1998) Persistent iron and folate deficiency in a patient with deletional hereditary persistence of fetal hemoglobin: the effect of the relative levels of Hb F and $^G\gamma$ chains and the corresponding mRNAs. *Hemoglobin* **22**, 53–63.

186 Wood WG (1993) Increased Hb F in adult life. *Bailliere's Clin Haematol* **6**, 177–213.

187 Chui DHK, Patterson M, Dowling CE, Kazazian HH and Kendall AG (1990) Hemoglobin Bart's disease in an Italian boy: interaction between α-thalassaemia and hereditary persistence of fetal hemoglobin. *N Engl J Med* **323**, 179–182.

188 Merghoub T, Perichon B, Maier-Redelsperger M, Dibenedetto SP, Samperi P, Ducrocq R *et al.* (1997) Dissection of the association status of two polymorphisms in the β-globin gene cluster with variations in F-cell number in non-anemic invididuals. *Am J Hematol* **56**, 239–243.

189 Collins FS, Stoeckert CJ, Serjeant GR, Forget BG and Weissman SM (1984) $^G\gamma\beta$+ hereditary persistence of fetal hemoglobin: cosmid cloning and identification of a specific mutation 5′ to the $^G\gamma$ gene. *Proc Natl Acad Sci USA* **81**, 4894–4898.

190 Surrey S, Delgrosso K, Malladi P and Schwartz E (1988) A single base change at position −175 in the 5′-flanking region of the $^G\gamma$-globin gene from a black with $^G\gamma\beta$+HPFH. *Blood* **71**, 807–810.

191 Ottolenghi S, Nicolis S, Taramelli R, Malgaretti N, Mantovani R, Comi P *et al.* (1988) Sardinian $^G\gamma$-HPFH: a T→C substitution in a conserved 'octomer' sequence in the Gγ-globin promoter. *Blood* **71**, 815–817.

192 Craig JE, Sheerin SM, Barnetson R and Thein SL (1993) The molecular basis of HPFH in a British family identified by heteroduplex formation. *Br J Haematol* **84**, 106–110.

193 Gilman JG and Huisman THJ (1985) DNA sequence variation associated with elevated fetal Gγ globin production. *Blood* **66**, 783–787.

194 Motum PL, Deng Z-M, Huong L and Trent RJ (1994) The Australian type of nondeletional $^G\gamma$-HPFH has a C→G substitution at nucleotide −114 of the Gγ gene. *Br J Haematol* **86**, 219–221.

195 Pissard S, M'rad A, Beuzard Y and Roméo P-H (1996) A new type of hereditary persistence of fetal haemoglobin (HPFH): HPFH Tunisia β+ (+C-200)$^G\gamma$. *Br J Haematol* **95**, 67–72.

196 Efremov GD, Filipce V, Gjorgovski I, Juricic D, Stojanoski N, Harano T *et al.* (1986) $^G\gamma^A\gamma(\delta\beta)^0$-Thalassaemia and a new form of γ globin gene triplication identified in the Yugoslavian population. *Br J Haematol* **63**, 17–29.

197 Gonçalves I, Lavinha J, Ducrocq R and Osório-Almeida L (2002) A novel rearrangement of the human fetal globin genes leading to a six γ-globin gene haplotype. *Br J Haematol* **116**, 454–457.

198 Giglioni B, Casini C, Mantovani R, Merli S, Comi P, Ottolenghi S *et al.* (1984) A molecular study of a family with Greek hereditary persistence of fetal hemoglobin and β-thalassemia. *EMBO J* **3**, 2641–2645.

199 Ottolenghi S, Camaschella C, Comi P, Giglioni B, Longinotti M, Oggiani L *et al.* (1988) A frequent $^A\gamma$-hereditary persistence of fetal hemoglobin in northern Sardinia: its molecular basis and hematologic phenotype in heterozygotes and compound heterozygotes with β-thalassaemia. *Hum Genet* **79**, 13–17.

200 Bordin S, Martins JT, Gonçalves MS, Melo MB, Saad STO and Costa FF (1998) Haplotype analysis and Aγ gene polymorphism associated with Brazilian type of hereditary persistence of fetal hemoglobin. *Am J Hematol* **58**, 49–54.

201 Stoming TA, Stoming GS, Lanclos KD, Fei YJ, Altay F, Kutlar F and Huisman THJ (1989) An $^A\gamma$ type of nondeletional hereditary persistence of fetal hemoglobin with a T→C mutation at position −175 to the cap site of the $^A\gamma$ globin gene. *Blood* **73**, 329–333.

202 Fessas P and Stamatoyannopoulos G (1964) Hereditary persistence of fetal hemoglobin in Greece: a study and a comparison. *Blood* **24**, 223–240.

203 Sofroniadou K, Wood WG, Nute PE and Stamatoyannopoulos G (1975) Globin gene synthesis in the Greek type ($^A\gamma$) of hereditary persistence of fetal haemoglobin. *Br J Haematol* **29**, 137–147.

204 Collins FS, Metherall JE, Yamakawa M, Pan J, Weissman SM and Forget BG (1985) A point mutation in the $^A\gamma$-globin gene promoter in Greek hereditary persistence of fetal haemoglobin. *Nature* **313**, 325–326.

205 Gelinas R, Endlich B, Pfeiffer C, Yagi M and Stamatoyannopoulos G (1985) G to A substitution in the distal CCAAT box of the $^A\gamma$-globin gene in Greek

hereditary persistence of fetal haemoglobin. *Nature* **313**, 323–324.

206 Camaschella C, Oggiano L, Sampietro M, Gottardi E, Alfarano A, Pistidda P *et al.* (1989) The homozygous state of G to A –117 [A]γ hereditary persistence of fetal hemoglobin. *Blood* **73**, 1999–2002.

207 Dedoussis GV, Sinopoulou K, Gyparaki M and Loutradis A (1999) Fetal hemoglobin expression in the compound heterozygote state for –117(G→A) Aγ HPFH and IVSII-745 (C→G) β+ thalassemia: a case study. *Am J Hematol* **61**, 139–143.

208 Papadakis NM, Patrinos GP, Tsaftaridis P and Loutradi-Anagnostou A (2000) Foetal hemoglobin expression in compound heterozygotes for the Greek type of nondeletional HPFH and beta-thalassemia. *Hematol J* **1**, Suppl. 1, 36.

209 Öner R, Kutlar F, Gu L-H and Huisman THJ (1991) The Georgia type of nondeletional hereditary persistence of fetal hemoglobin has a C→T mutation at nucleotide –114 of the [A]γ globin gene. *Blood* **77**, 1124.

210 Gilman JG, Mishima N, Wen XJ, Stoming TA, Lobel J and Huisman THJ (1988) Distal CCAAT box deletion in the Aγ globin gene of two black adolescents with elevated fetal Aγ globin. *Nucleic Acids Res* **16**, 10 635–10 642.

211 Huang X-D, Yang XO, Huang R-B, Zhang H-Y, Zhao H-L, Zhao Y-J *et al.* (2000) A novel four base-pair deletion within the Aγ-globin gene promoter associated with slight increase of Aγ expression in adult. *Am J Hematol* **63**, 16–19.

212 Craig JE, Rochette J, Fisher CA, Weatherall DJ, Marc S, Lathrop GM *et al.* (1996) Dissecting the loci controlling fetal hemoglobin production on chromosome 11p and 6q by the regressive approach. *Nat Genet* **12**, 58–64.

213 Winichagoon P, Thonglairoam V, Fucharoen S, Wilairat P, Fukumaki Y and Wasi P (1993) Severity differences in β-thalassaemia/haemoglobin E syndromes: implication of genetic factors. *Br J Haematol* **83**, 633–639.

214 Gonçalves I, Ducrocq R, Lavinha J, Nogueira PJ, Peres MJ, Picanco I *et al.* (1998) Combined effect of two different polymorphic sequences within the β globin gene cluster on the level of Hb F. *Am J Hematol* **57**, 269–276.

## Answers to questions

| 3.1 | | | 3.4 | | | 3.7 | | | 3.10 | | | 3.13 | | |
|-----|-----|---|-----|-----|---|-----|-----|---|------|-----|---|------|-----|---|
| | (a) | F | | (a) | F | | (a) | F | | (a) | F | | (a) | T |
| | (b) | T | | (b) | T | | (b) | F | | (b) | T | | (b) | F |
| | (c) | F | | (c) | F | | (c) | T | | (c) | T | | (c) | T |
| | (d) | F | | (d) | T | | (d) | F | | (d) | T | | (d) | F |
| | (e) | F | | (e) | T | | (e) | F | | (e) | T | | (e) | T |

| 3.2 | | | 3.5 | | | 3.8 | | | 3.11 | | |
|-----|-----|---|-----|-----|---|-----|-----|---|------|-----|---|
| | (a) | F | | (a) | F | | (a) | T | | (a) | F |
| | (b) | T | | (b) | F | | (b) | F | | (b) | F |
| | (c) | T | | (c) | T | | (c) | F | | (c) | T |
| | (d) | T | | (d) | T | | (d) | F | | (d) | T |
| | (e) | T | | (e) | F | | (e) | T | | (e) | T |

| 3.3 | | | 3.6 | | | 3.9 | | | 3.12 | | |
|-----|-----|---|-----|-----|---|-----|-----|---|------|-----|---|
| | (a) | T | | (a) | T | | (a) | T | | (a) | F |
| | (b) | T | | (b) | F | | (b) | F | | (b) | F |
| | (c) | T | | (c) | T | | (c) | T | | (c) | T |
| | (d) | F | | (d) | T | | (d) | T | | (d) | T |
| | (e) | T | | (e) | T | | (e) | T | | (e) | T |

# 4 Sickle cell haemoglobin and its interactions with other variant haemoglobins and with thalassaemias

Sickle cell anaemia was first described in 1910 when a patient with severe anaemia was noted to have 'peculiar elongated and sickle shaped red blood corpuscles' [1]. Many years later, Linus Pauling and colleagues found that the sickling phenomenon was caused by haemoglobin with unusual characteristics [2] and, subsequently, Vernon Ingram and colleagues identified the causative amino acid in the β chain of haemoglobin [3]. Sickle cell haemoglobin, haemoglobin S, has a valine for glutamic acid substitution at position 6 of the β chain. The haemoglobin can be designated $\alpha_2\beta_2^{6Glu\rightarrow Val}$. Sickle cell haemoglobin can produce deleterious effects because, on deoxygenation, its solubility is reduced and polymerization occurs (Fig. 4.1). Both partially and fully deoxygenated haemoglobin S can be incorporated into a polymer. Long polymers distort the red cell into a holly-leaf or into a crescent or sickle shape that hinders blood flow through capillaries, because of both reduced deformability and increased adhesion to endothelial cells resulting from secondary changes in the red cell membrane. When fully oxygenated, haemoglobin S is as soluble as haemoglobin A. The presence of haemoglobin A in a red cell slows polymerization, although haemoglobin A can copolymerize with haemoglobin F. Haemoglobin F and haemoglobin $A_2$ are even more effective at retarding sickling whereas, in comparison with haemoglobin A, sickling is facilitated by the presence of haemoglobin C, haemoglobin D-Punjab or haemoglobin O-Arab. Haemoglobin F and haemoglobin $A_2$ cannot copolymerize with haemoglobin S and the hybrid tetramer, $\alpha_2\beta^S\gamma$, is similarly unable to polymerize. Because acidosis and a rise in temperature shift the oxygen dissociation curve to the right, they favour sickling. However, in clinical practice, exposure to cold can also provoke sickling because of slowed circulation through capillaries.

The sickle cell mutation appears to have arisen spontaneously at least five times in the history of mankind (Fig. 4.2). Such independent mutations can be recognized by their association with different β globin gene haplotypes, demonstrated by the analysis of restriction fragment length polymorphisms (RFLPs). There are three foci of haemoglobin S in Africa, associated with different haplotypes, the haplotypes being defined by RFLP analysis. They are in Senegal (Senegal type), the Central African Republic and southern Africa (Bantu or Central African Republic type) and Benin, Central, West and North Africa (Benin type) [4]. The Benin type has also spread to Spain, Portugal, Sicily (perhaps from Greece, perhaps from Sudanese soldiers in Arab armies) and southern mainland Italy, Greece (particularly Macedonia), Albania, Turkey, north-western Saudi Arabia and Oman. The Bantu type has spread to Kenya, Zambia and the Sudan. In addition to the three major foci, there may have been a further independent mutation amongst the Eton people in southern Cameroon. A fifth mutation is associated with further foci in eastern Saudi Arabia and in extensive areas of central and southern India, particularly amongst the scheduled tribes (a group living outside the caste system). It may have arisen initially in the Indus valley. The prevalence of the haemoglobin S gene is up to 25% in eastern Saudi Arabia and as high as 30% in some tribal populations in central India. The Indian/Saudi Arabian haplotype has also been found in Afghanistan, Oman, Kuwait, Bahrain and Iran and amongst Bedouin Arabs in Israel.

Migration from Africa has led to the sickle cell gene occurring also in Central and South America, in Afro-Americans and in Afro-Caribbeans in Canada, the UK and other European countries. There is a high prevalence in some populations in Mexico, Colombia, Venezuela, Guyana, Surinam, French Guyana, Brazil and Peru. All three major African haplotypes

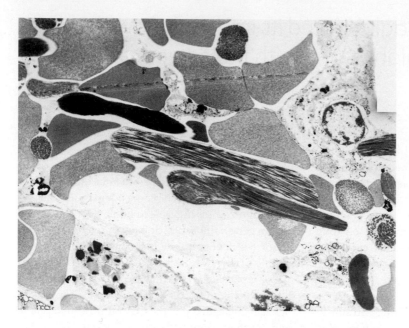

**Fig. 4.1** Transmission electron micrograph showing polymerization of haemoglobin S in a patient with compound heterozygosity for haemoglobin S and haemoglobin D-Punjab. (With thanks to Mr S. Ladva, St Mary's Hospital.)

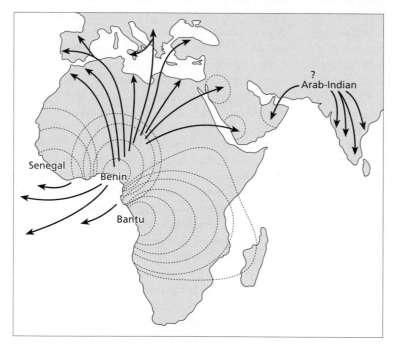

**Fig. 4.2** Multifocal origin and spread of the β^S gene.

are represented in the USA, the Caribbean and the UK. The sickle cell gene is also found in Madagascar, Mauritius (both Bantu and Arab–Indian haplotypes), Abu Dhabi, United Arab Emirates, Lebanon, Iraq, the southern part of the former USSR and amongst North African Arabs.

The wide geographical spread of this potentially deleterious gene has been attributed to the protection of heterozygotes from premature death from falciparum malaria. In areas in which malaria is endemic, the $\beta^S$ and $\beta^A$ genes may exist as a balanced polymorphism, i.e. death or serious disability from sickle cell anaemia before the age of reproduction is balanced by a decreased death rate from malaria amongst heterozygotes. The prevalence of haemoglobin S in various populations is shown in Table 4.1 [5–18].

A second mutation has occasionally occurred in a $\beta^S$ gene leading to the synthesis of a variant haemoglobin with two amino acid substitutions. Such variant haemoglobins retain their ability to sickle, but may have a different electrophoretic mobility from haemoglobin S. In heterozygous, homozygous and compound heterozygous states, these mutations have a similar, although not necessarily identical, significance to haemoglobin S. At least 10 such double mutations are known (Table 4.2) [19–22]. The most common, haemoglobin C-Harlem (initially described under the name of haemoglobin C-Georgetown), $\alpha_2\beta_2^{6Glu\rightarrow Val,73Asp\rightarrow Asn}$, is less prone to polymerization than haemoglobin S itself. The rare double substitution haemoglobin, haemoglobin S-Antilles, is even more prone to sickle than haemoglobin S itself, as is haemoglobin Jamaica Plain.

There are other haemoglobins unrelated to haemoglobin S that can polymerize *in vitro*, e.g. haemoglobin I ($\alpha$16 Lys$\rightarrow$Glu) and haemoglobin Setif ($\alpha$22 Asp$\rightarrow$Tyr). Although they are not associated with any relevant clinical abnormality, haemoglobin Setif can cause a false positive sickle solubility test [23].

Homozygosity for haemoglobin S ($\beta^S\beta^S$) causes a serious condition referred to as 'sickle cell anaemia'. Heterozygosity for haemoglobin S ($\beta\beta^S$), referred to as sickle cell trait, is usually asymptomatic. The $\beta^S$ gene may also be coinherited with another $\beta$ chain variant. When there is deleterious interaction between the sickle cell haemoglobin and the second variant haemoglobins, as is the case, for example, with haemoglobin C and haemoglobin D-Punjab, a clinically significant sickling disorder occurs. Subjects who are heterozygous for $\beta$ thalassaemia and haemoglobin S likewise suffer from the clinicopathological effects of sickle cell formation and consequent vascular occlusion. The term 'sickle cell disease' is often used as a generic term to include sickle cell anaemia and other conditions in which a clinically significant disorder results from sickle cell formation and the associated pathological processes. Some such conditions are shown in Table 4.3 [21,24–27].

## Sickle cell trait

The term 'sickle cell trait' indicates heterozygosity for the sickle cell gene ($\beta\beta^S$). Sickle cell trait is asymptomatic in the great majority of individuals, but is of genetic importance. It gives partial protection against death from *Plasmodium falciparum* malaria.

If a patient with symptoms suggestive of sickle cell disease appears to have sickle cell trait on haemoglobin electrophoresis or high performance liquid chromatography (HPLC), further detailed investigation is indicated, as this may be the result of a second mutation in a $\beta^S$ gene, e.g. haemoglobin Jamaica Plain (see below), or a second mutation in a $\beta^C$ gene, e.g. haemoglobin Arlington Park (see below). The second mutation alters the characteristics of the variant haemoglobin so that it can be confused with haemoglobin A.

## Clinical features

Subjects with sickle cell trait are usually asymptomatic. However, sickle cell formation leading to vascular occlusion can occur during high fever and under conditions of significant hypoxia, such as during travel by air (particularly but not only in unpressurized aircraft), mountain climbing, vigorous exercise and anaesthetic misadventures. Vascular occlusion in such circumstances can lead to splenic, pulmonary, pituitary, cerebral, retinal, renal and bone infarcts and also to priapism (persistent erection caused by sickling within blood vessels of the penis). Bone infarcts can lead to avascular necrosis. There is a low risk of sudden death associated with vigorous exercise, particularly exercise at a high altitude and exercise complicated by dehydration and acidosis [28]. Such circumstances can also lead to exertional rhabdomyolysis, disseminated intravascular coagulation and renal failure [29]. In a study of USA Air Force personnel, the rate of non-traumatic deaths in airmen was very low, but was 25-fold higher in those with sickle cell trait than in those without sickle cell trait [30]. Similar observations have been made in USA Army recruits. In sickle cell trait, spontaneous sickle cell formation can occur in renal papillae where oxygen tension is normally low, leading to renal papillary necrosis, episodes of haematuria and impairment of renal concentrating ability. Loss of

**Table 4.1** Prevalence (%) of haemoglobins S and C in different populations. (From references [5–18] and other sources.)

| Country or people | Haemoglobin S | Haemoglobin C |
|---|---|---|
| *West Africa* | | |
| Senegal | 3–15 | <1–6 |
| Gambia | 6–28 | <1–2 |
| Guinea Bissau | <1–25 | <1–1.5 |
| Guinea | 13–33 | |
| Sierra Leone | 22–30 | |
| Liberia | <1–29 | 1–3 |
| Ivory Coast | 2–26 | <1–50 |
| Mali | 5–17 | |
| Burkina Faso (previously Upper Volta) | 2–34 | 15–40 |
| Ghana | 3–25 | 8–40 |
| Togo | 6–28 | 7–17 |
| Benin | 5–31 | 7–27 |
| Niger | 5–23 | 1–8 |
| Nigeria | 10–41 | <1–9 |
| | | |
| *Central Africa* | | |
| Gabon | 8–32 | |
| Cameroon | <1–31 | <1 |
| Central African Republic | 2–24 | |
| The Republic of the Congo | 7–32 | |
| Democratic Republic of the Congo (previously Zaire) | 1–46 | |
| | | |
| *East Africa* | | |
| Kenya | <1–34 | |
| Uganda | 1–39 | |
| Tanzania | 1–38 | |
| Rwanda | | |
|   Tutsi | <1–5 | |
|   Hutu | 5–15 | |
| Burundi | 1.5–26 | |
| | | |
| *Southern Africa* | | |
| Angola | 8–40 | |
| Zambia | <1–30 | |
| Zimbabwe | <1–11 | |
| Malawi | 3–18 | |
| Mozambique | <1–40 | |
| Madagascar | <1–23 | |
| Botswana | <1 | |
| Namibia | 0–15 | |
| South Africa | | |
|   Bantu | <1–4 | |
|   Indian | 2–10 | |
|   Cape Coloured | <1 | <1 |
| | | |
| *North Africa* | | |
| Morocco | <1–7 | <1–6 |
| Algeria | <1–15 | <1–13 |
| Tunisia | <1–2 | |
| Libya | <1–70 | |
| Egypt | <1* | |
| Sudan | <1–17 | |

**Table 4.1** *Continued.*

| Country or people | Haemoglobin S | Haemoglobin C |
|---|---|---|
| *Horn of Africa* | | |
| Ethiopia | 0–1 | |
| Djibouti | ≈0 | |
| Somalia | ≈0 | |
| *Afro-Americans* | 6–15 | 1–3.5 |
| *Afro-Caribbeans* | | |
| Jamaica | 3.5–12 | 2–4 |
| Bahamas | 14 | 3 |
| Barbados | 4 | 3–5 |
| Cuba | 0–23 | 0–2.5 |
| Haiti | 7–17 | 1–3 |
| Dominican Republic | 6–12 | 3 |
| Puerto Rica | <1–8 | <1–2 |
| Lesser Antilles | 1–14 | 1–4.5 |
| Guadeloupe | 4.4 | |
| *Central America* | | |
| Mexico | <1–9 | <1 |
| Guatemala | <1–17 | |
| Belize | 0–25 | |
| El Salvador | <1–2 | |
| Honduras | <1–16 | |
| Nicaragua | ≈0 | |
| Costa Rica | <1–8 | |
| Panama | 0–21 | 0–2.5 |
| *South America* | | |
| Colombia | 0–15 | 0–6 |
| Venezuela | 0–9 | 0–3 |
| Guyana | <1 | |
| Surinam | 0–22 | 0–6 |
| French Guyana | 0–18 | 0–7 |
| Ecuador | ≈0 | ≈0 |
| Peru | <1 | ≈0 |
| Bolivia | ≈0 | ≈0 |
| Brazil | 0–16 | 0–4 |
| Paraguay | ≈0 | |
| Argentina | <1 | |
| Uruguay | ≈0 | |
| Chile | <1 | <1 |
| *Europe* | | |
| Greece | 0–32 | |
| Turkey | <1–34 | 0.5–1 |
| Cyprus | <1 | |
| Italy | | |
|   Sicily | <1–13 | |
|   Sardinia | ≈0 | |
|   Mainland southern Italy | 0.5–1 | |
| Portugal | <1–5 | |
| Spain | | 0.12 (southern Spain) |

*Continued on p. 144.*

**Table 4.1** *Continued.*

| Country or people | Haemoglobin S | Haemoglobin C |
|---|---|---|
| *Middle East* | | |
| Turkey | <1–34 | |
| Syria | <5–25 | |
| Lebanon | <1 | |
| Jordan | 4–6 | |
| Israel | | |
|    Arabs | 1–38 | |
|    Jews | ≈0 | |
| Iraq | 0–25 | |
| Iran | ≈0 | |
| Saudi Arabia | <1–36 | |
| Kuwait | 2 | |
| Bahrain | 2.5 | |
| Oman | 5 | Rare |
| Yemen | 1–2† | |
| Abu Dhabi | 2 | |
| United Arab Emirates | 2 | |
| *Asia* | | |
| India | 0–35‡ | |
| Pakistan | 0.5–1 | |
| Sri Lanka | Rare | |
| Thailand | | Rare |

*5–22% in various oases.
†23% in Western province.
‡5–35% in various tribal populations [17]; 15% in Orissa, Madhya Pradesh and Maharashtra states [18].

**Table 4.2** Variant haemoglobins in which the mutation of haemoglobin S is one of two mutations. (Derived from references [9,19–22].)

| Variant haemoglobin | Second substitution | Mobility on cellulose acetate at alkaline pH |
|---|---|---|
| C-Harlem | β73 Asp→Asn | C |
| C-Ziguinchor | β58 Pro→Arg | C |
| S-Travis | β142 Ala→Val | S |
| S-Antilles | β23 Val→Ile | S |
| S-Providence | β82 Lys→Asn | A |
| S-Oman | β121 Glu→Lys | Slower than C |
| S-Wake | β139 Asp→Ser | |
| Cameroon | β90 Glu→Lys | |
| Jamaica Plain | β68 Leu→Phe | S [21] |
| South End | β132 Lys→Asn | [22] |

renal concentrating ability is less if thalassaemia trait coexists [31]. If the kidney is excluded, spontaneous episodes of vascular occlusion, i.e. episodes occurring in the absence of fever, dehydration, hypoxia or acidosis, are very rare but do occur. Splenic seques-tration has likewise been described, but very rarely, in sickle cell trait [32]. During pregnancy, women with sickle cell trait may have an increased incidence of bacteriuria and pyelonephritis [33] and pregnancy-associated hypertension [34]. There is also an unexpected but quite strong association between medullary carcinoma of the kidney and sickle cell trait [35].

Despite this list of potential complications, the great majority of patients with sickle cell trait are asymptomatic, and the main reason for seeking to identify the heterozygous state is the genetic implications. If both parents have sickle cell trait, there is a 25% probability of sickle cell anaemia in a child.

**Table 4.3** Causes of sickle cell disease.

**Sickle cell anaemia (homozygosity for haemoglobin S)**

**Compound heterozygous states**
Sickle cell/haemoglobin C disease
Sickle cell/β thalassaemia
Sickle cell/haemoglobin D-Punjab
Sickle cell/haemoglobin C-Harlem
Sickle cell/haemoglobin S-Antilles
Sickle cell/haemoglobin O-Arab
Sickle cell/haemoglobin Quebec-Chori [24]
Sickle cell/haemoglobin S-Oman
Sickle cell/haemoglobin O-Tibesti
Haemoglobin S-Antilles/haemoglobin C
Sickle cell/haemoglobin Lepore
Haemoglobin C/haemoglobin C-Harlem [25]

**Mutations leading to sickle cell disease in βˢ heterozygotes**
Haemoglobin S-Antilles [19]
Haemoglobin S trait plus haemoglobin Conakry trait (an α chain variant) [26]
Haemoglobin S-Oman [27]
Haemoglobin Jamaica Plain [21]

## Laboratory features

### Blood count

The haemoglobin concentration is normal, except in those with coexisting α thalassaemia trait who may be slightly anaemic [36]. Similarly, the mean cell volume (MCV) and mean cell haemoglobin (MCH) are reduced in those with coexisting α thalassaemia trait (Table 4.4) [9,36–40], but otherwise are normal. α thalassaemia trait is somewhat more prevalent in Africans and Afro-Americans with sickle cell trait than in those with normal β globin genes [41], so that it is not rare for subjects with sickle cell trait to have borderline anaemia or reduction of the MCV and MCH.

### Blood film

The blood film may be completely normal or may show microcytosis or target cells (Fig. 4.3). If a subject with sickle cell trait develops iron deficiency, target cells are often prominent. Although classical sickle cells are not seen, small numbers of plump cells that are pointed at both ends have been reported [42]; such cells were described in about 96% of individuals with sickle cell trait in comparison with 4% of normal subjects.

During *P. falciparum* malaria, subjects with sickle cell trait have a blood film showing a lower percentage of parasitized cells than is seen in subjects without a haemoglobinopathy [43].

**Table 4.4** Mean cell volume (MCV) and percentage of haemoglobin S reported in sickle cell trait with and without deletion of α globin genes.

| | αα/αα | –α/αα | –α/–α | Reference |
|---|---|---|---|---|
| Haemoglobin S (%) | >38 | 31–38 | <31 | [37] |
| | 35–39 | 29–34 | 24–27 | [38] |
| | 35–45* | 30–35* | 25–30* | [36] |
| | 34–38 | 28–34 | 20–28 | [9] |
| | 31–43 | 29–35 | 22–29 | [39] |
| MCV (fl) (range and mean ± standard deviation) | 80–90 | 75–85 | 70–75 | [36] |
| | 84.9 ± 8.26 | 79.1 ± 5.8 | 67.8 ± 5.81 | [39] |

*These values are averages derived from published series in which the α chain deletion was –α$^{3.7}$; the deletion –α$^{4.2}$ leads to a greater reduction in haemoglobin S percentage [40].

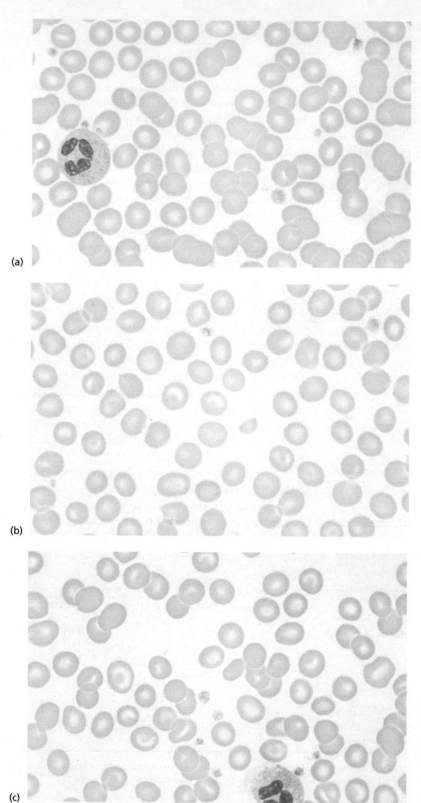

(a)

(b)

(c)

**Fig. 4.3** Blood films from three patients with sickle cell trait showing the range of features observed: (a) normal film; (b) minimal anisocytosis and poikilocytosis with occasional target cells; (c) hypochromia with occasional target cells and other poikilocytes.

*Other investigations*

It might be expected that heterozygotes for haemoglobin S ($\beta\beta^S$) would have equal amounts of haemoglobin S and haemoglobin A. In fact, haemoglobin A is somewhat more than 50% and haemoglobin S is somewhat less, usually around 40%; this is because normal $\beta$ chain has a greater affinity for $\beta^S$ than for $\alpha$ chains. Haemoglobin S is readily detected by haemoglobin electrophoresis and other techniques. Haemoglobin electrophoresis at alkaline or acid pH shows a variant haemoglobin with characteristic mobility (Fig. 4.4). Haemoglobins D and G have the same electrophoretic mobility at alkaline pH, but can be distinguished by electrophoresis at acid pH, which usually shows mobility which is the same as or very similar to that of haemoglobin A. Haemoglobin S can also be distinguished from haemoglobins A, D and G by isoelectric focusing and HPLC (Fig. 4.5; see also Fig. 2.16). A sickle solubility test (see Fig. 2.19) should always be performed when the presence of a significant proportion of haemoglobin S is suspected. It will be positive, except in the early neonatal period when the percentage may be below the detection limit. It follows that a negative sickle solubility test in a neonate with a variant haemoglobin

consistent with haemoglobin S does not exclude a diagnosis of sickle cell trait. Reagents suitable for a sickle solubility test are commercially available in kit form [44].

Haemoglobin S can also be distinguished from haemoglobin A and haemoglobin C by immunologi-

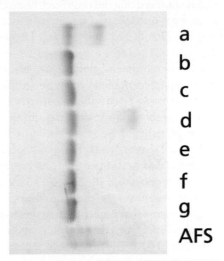

**Fig. 4.4** Haemoglobin electrophoresis on cellulose acetate at alkaline pH showing haemoglobins A and S in a patient with sickle cell trait (lane a); AFS, control sample containing haemoglobins A, F and S.

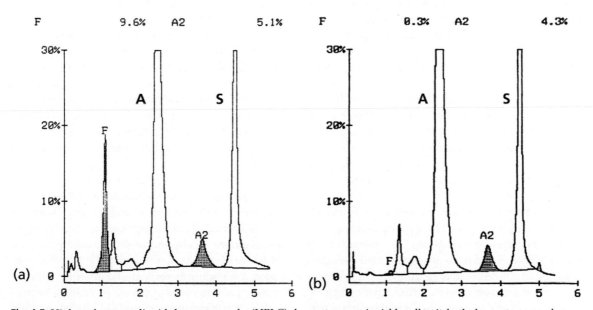

**Fig. 4.5** High performance liquid chromatography (HPLC) chromatograms in sickle cell trait; both chromatograms show haemoglobins A, $A_2$ and S and chromatogram (a) shows, in addition, increased haemoglobin F; haemoglobin A that has undergone post-translational modification appears as two peaks to the left of haemoglobin A.

cal techniques based on monoclonal antibodies to sequences including the amino acids which are substituted in haemoglobin S and haemoglobin C. It is thus possible to distinguish sickle cell trait from sickle cell anaemia and sickle cell/haemoglobin C disease. However, sickle cell/$\beta^+$ thalassaemia may not be distinguished from sickle cell trait. Such monoclonal antibodies were previously commercially available in kit form as HemoCard A plus S and HemoCard C [44].

The proportion of haemoglobin S can be quantified by scanning densitometry of an electrophoretic strip, elution from an electrophoretic strip or HPLC. The percentage shows a trimodal distribution, depending on whether there is coexisting $\alpha$ thalassaemia trait (Table 4.4). If there is coexisting haemoglobin H disease, the percentage of haemoglobin S is even lower, around 10–25% [40]. Conversely, if there are five $\alpha$ genes ($\alpha\alpha\alpha/\alpha\alpha$), the haemoglobin S percentage is somewhat higher than in those with a normal complement of $\alpha$ genes [45], about 45% rather than about 40%. The percentage of haemoglobin S correlates with the MCV and MCH as all of these variables are influenced by coexisting $\alpha$ thalassaemia trait. A rare cause of a low haemoglobin S percentage in sickle cell trait is coinheritance of a $\beta$ thalassaemia determinant in *cis*, i.e. on the same chromosome [46] (see p. 149). Haemoglobin S may then be as low as 10%. The proportion of haemoglobin S is also reduced if there is coexisting iron deficiency [47]. It has been observed to fall markedly in megaloblastic anaemia [48] and may be low in lead poisoning [49].

The percentage of haemoglobin $A_2$ may be slightly elevated in sickle cell trait. However, this is not a particularly useful investigation to perform. Adult levels of haemoglobin F are reached by 2 years of age [50]. It is not clear whether, thereafter, the frequency of an elevated haemoglobin F percentage differs from normal [9].

In the neonatal period, haemoglobin F will be present in large amounts. There will be more haemoglobin A than haemoglobin S. However, if haemoglobins S and A are present in small amounts, precise quantification may be difficult. Unless there is clearly more haemoglobin A than haemoglobin S, sickle cell/$\beta^+$ thalassaemia is a possible alternative

diagnosis. If necessary, the test should be repeated when the infant is a few months old.

Electrophoretic features suggestive of sickle cell trait despite clinical features of sickle cell disease should lead to investigation for an electrophoretically silent variant haemoglobin that may be interacting with haemoglobin S [24].

## Diagnosis

The diagnosis rests on the demonstration of the presence of haemoglobin S and haemoglobin A, with the percentage of haemoglobin S being less than the percentage of haemoglobin A. The haemoglobin S identification must be supported by two independent tests.

## Interactions of haemoglobin S heterozygosity with thalassaemias and haemoglobinopathies

The interaction of sickle cell trait and $\alpha$ thalassaemia trait has been discussed above. The coexistence of sickle cell trait and the genotype of haemoglobin H disease leads to a modification of the phenotype of haemoglobin H disease. There is a hypochromic microcytic anaemia with splenomegaly and erythroid hyperplasia, but with a normal reticulocyte count [51]. Haemoglobin S is lower than is usual in sickle cell trait with coexisting $\alpha$ thalassaemia [25,51]. Haemoglobin Bart's may be present in infancy, but haemoglobin H is not detected and only occasional inclusion-containing cells are found on a haemoglobin H preparation. Inclusions have been reported in bone marrow erythroblasts. It could be speculated that these represent $\beta^S$ precipitates, $\beta^A$ having combined preferentially with the reduced numbers of $\alpha$ chains.

The coinheritance of $\beta^S$ and various $\beta$ chain variants, $\beta$ and $\delta\beta$ thalassaemias is discussed below. The interaction of sickle cell trait and $\alpha$ chain variants is generally clinically silent, but leads to extra bands on haemoglobin electrophoresis. For example, coinheritance of sickle cell trait and $\alpha^{G\text{-Philadelphia}}$ is associated, on electrophoresis at alkaline pH, with the presence of three bands with the mobility of haemoglobins A, S (representing S and G-Philadelphia) and

C (representing an S–G hybrid) (Fig. 4.6). On agarose gel at acid pH, there are two bands, a band with the mobility of haemoglobin A (representing A plus G-Philadelphia) and a band with the mobility of haemoglobin S (representing S and S–G hybrid). On HPLC, there are four fractions distinguished by their retention times (Fig. 4.7).

A β thalassaemia mutation occurring in *cis* to a $\beta^S$ mutation differs considerably from sickle cell trait. Two individuals with this combination had haemoglobin S of 10–11%, haemoglobin $A_2$ of 6–7%, haemoglobin F of around 3% and a mild microcytic anaemia with a reticulocyte count of around 3% [46,52].

## Interactions of haemoglobin S heterozygosity with other haematological conditions

The coexistence of sickle cell trait and hereditary spherocytosis has been reported in 19 instances. Four of these individuals suffered either splenic sequestration or splenic infarction [53]. It is likely that the increased haemoglobin concentration within red cells as a result of the hereditary spherocytosis favours sickling within the spleen.

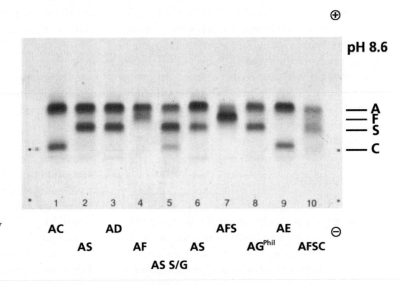

**Fig. 4.6** Haemoglobin electrophoresis on agarose gel at pH 8.6 showing three bands with the mobilities of haemoglobins A, S and C in a patient with sickle cell trait and heterozygosity for haemoglobin G-Philadelphia (lane 5); AFSC, control sample containing haemoglobins A, F, S and C.

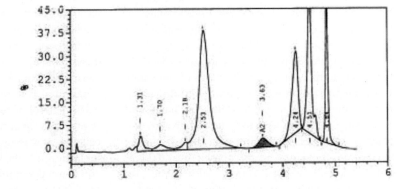

**Fig. 4.7** HPLC chromatogram in a patient with heterozygosity for both haemoglobin S and haemoglobin G-Philadelphia; from left to right, the peaks are post-translationally modified haemoglobin A (two peaks) and haemoglobins A, $A_2$, S, G-Philadelphia and hybrid ($\alpha\alpha^G\beta\beta^S$).

## Sickle cell anaemia

Sickle cell anaemia is the disease resulting from homozygosity for haemoglobin S. Individuals with sickle cell anaemia have haemoglobin S as the major haemoglobin component with a small proportion of haemoglobin $A_2$ and a variable proportion of haemoglobin F. As there is no synthesis of normal β chain, there is a total absence of haemoglobin A. Red cells sickle due to polymerization of haemoglobin S under conditions of low oxygen tension, but initially this process is reversible as the cells pass through the lungs. This process is cyclical, but eventually membrane damage leads to the red cell becoming irreversibly sickled. The irreversibly sickled cell has an increased calcium content, which triggers calcium-dependent potassium transport and loss of potassium and water. Potassium/chloride ($K^+/Cl^-$) cotransport is also increased. The dehydrated cell becomes even more rigid. The red cell membrane is damaged by oxidation and the effects of repeated polymerization with clustering of band 3 protein, binding of immunoglobulin G and phagocytosis by macrophages. Sickle cells also show increased interaction with endothelium, particularly when adhesion molecules are upregulated.

## Clinical features

The clinicopathological features of sickle cell anaemia result directly or indirectly from vascular obstruction by sickled red cells, with consequent tissue infarction. In addition to the shape change, erythrocytes show increased adhesion to endothelium, which contributes to vascular occlusion. Neonates are asymptomatic as a major part of the total haemoglobin is haemoglobin F. As the synthesis of haemoglobin F decreases and that of haemoglobin S increases, symptoms start to appear, usually from 6 months of age. In infants, bony infarction leads to avascular necrosis of the small bones of the hands and feet which presents clinically as painful swelling of the fingers and toes (dactylitis or 'hand–foot syndrome'). This can lead to failure of growth of a phalanx and later shortening of a digit (Fig. 4.8). In children, there may be splenomegaly and, occasionally, hypersplenism. Young children can also suffer from splenic sequestration in which pooling of red cells in a rapidly enlarging spleen leads to acute anaemia. Hepatic sequestration also occurs, but is less common. Cerebral haemorrhage and infarction are particular features of children with sickle cell disease, as a result of prior endothelial damage.

In older children and adults, there continues to be infarction of bones, such as the ribs, vertebrae and long bones; osteonecrosis can be detected radiologically (Fig. 4.9a). In addition, there is infarction of internal organs, including the lungs (Fig. 4.9b), abdominal organs and brain. Pulmonary infarction can be associated with pulmonary sequestration of red cells and platelets and, if recurrent, leads to pulmonary hypertension in a significant minority of patients; inactivation of nitric oxide by reactive oxygen species and by free haemoglobin in the plasma may contribute to pulmonary hypertension [54]. Bone marrow infarction may be extensive and may be complicated by embolism of necrotic bone marrow to the lungs. Infarction of bones may also be complicated by osteomyelitis, usually caused by salmonella or staphylococcus. Recurrent infarction of the spleen leads to hyposplenism, which, in turn, causes increased severity of various infections, including malaria and pneumococcal septicaemia. Splenic phagocytic function is lost first and then splenic filtering function [55]. Infarction of the skin can result in ulceration of the legs. The increased breakdown of red cells means that patients are intermittently jaundiced (Fig. 4.10). There is a high incidence of pigment gallstones (Fig. 4.11) consequent on this chronic haemolysis. Increased erythropoiesis occurs as a response to haemolytic anaemia, leading to overexpansion of the bone marrow cavity. In some patients, this causes frontal bossing of the skull and malpositioned teeth. On skull radiology, there may be thickening of the cranial bones (Fig. 4.12) and a 'hair-on-end' appearance. Patients with sickle cell anaemia may suffer rapid worsening of anaemia during infection by parvovirus B19. The mechanism is pure red cell aplasia, which is transient but, because of the shortened red cell life span, rapidly leads to anaemia. In some countries, patients with sickle cell anaemia show an increased incidence of megaloblastic anaemia, which has been attributed to inadequate intake of folic acid in the face of an increased need for this vitamin.

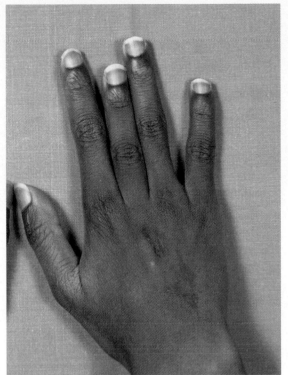

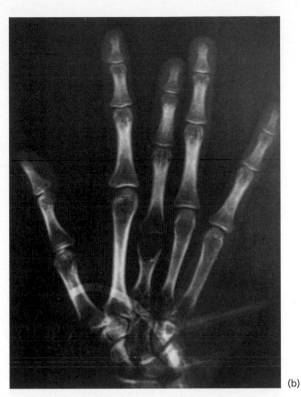

(a)

(b)

**Fig. 4.8** Long-term result of 'dactylitis' in sickle cell anaemia: (a) the hand of an 18-year-old Nigerian man; (b) X-ray of the hand. (Reproduced from Hoffbrand AV and Pettit JE. *Essential Haematology*, 3rd edn. Blackwell Scientific Publications, Oxford, 1993, by kind permission of Professor A. V. Hoffbrand.)

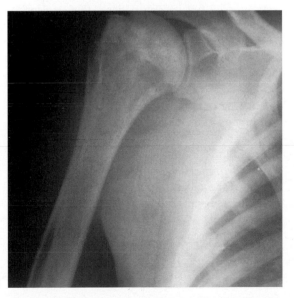

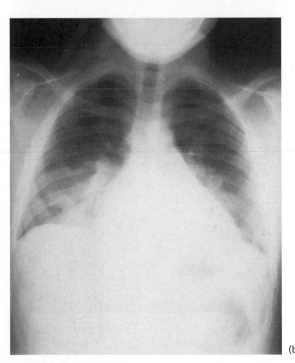

(a)

(b)

**Fig. 4.9** (a) Radiograph of the head of the humerus showing areas of reduced radiodensity consequent on previous infarction. (By courtesy of Professor I. Roberts.) (b) Chest radiograph showing opacities in the lower half of both lung fields representing pulmonary infarction as a result of sickle cell formation and vascular occlusion. (By courtesy of Professor I. Roberts.)

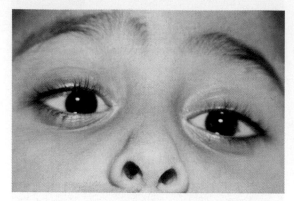

**Fig. 4.10** Face of a child with sickle cell anaemia showing pallor and jaundice. (By courtesy of Professor I. Roberts.)

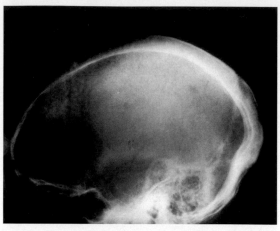

**Fig. 4.12** Skull radiograph in sickle cell anaemia showing expansion of the bony cavity resulting from hyperplastic erythropoiesis.

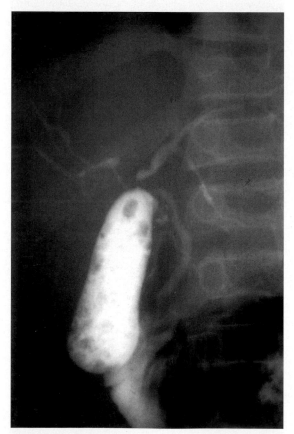

**Fig. 4.11** Cholecystogram showing gallstones (negative images) caused by increased bilirubin production resulting from haemolysis. (By courtesy of Professor I. Roberts.)

Patients who require regular or intermittent blood transfusions often develop red cell alloantibodies. If a delayed transfusion reaction occurs, the haemoglobin concentration may fall rapidly to levels below the pre-transfusion level. This is due mainly to the destruction of transfused red cells while haemopoiesis is suppressed, but, in some patients, there is also 'bystander' destruction of the patient's own red cells [56]. In addition, transfusion may be followed by hyperhaemolysis without any evidence of red cell incompatibility [57].

The causes of anaemia in homozygotes for haemoglobin S are summarized in Table 4.5.

Death in sickle cell anaemia is most often attributable to infection, cerebrovascular accidents or respiratory failure, the latter consequent on extensive sickling within pulmonary blood vessels. In the absence of parental education and vigilance, death of infants can result from splenic sequestration. In African countries, it is likely that many deaths in infants and children with sickle cell anaemia are attributable to malaria and some to severe anaemia. Patients with sickle cell anaemia who survive childhood and adolescence may die from end-organ failure consequent on recurrent tissue infarction, e.g. from renal or hepatic failure.

The survival of individuals with sickle cell anaemia has improved greatly in recent decades. In one study in the USA, the median life expectancy was

**Table 4.5**  Causes of anaemia in sickle cell anaemia.

**Causes of steady state anaemia**
Haemolysis
Reduced oxygen affinity leading to reduced erythropoietic drive

**Causes of worsening of anaemia**
Splenic, hepatic or pulmonary sequestration
Hypersplenism (usually only in infants and children)
Parvovirus B19 infection
Suppression of erythropoiesis in other infections
Megaloblastic anaemia resulting from folic acid deficiency
Bone marrow infarction
Hyperhaemolysis following blood transfusion
Renal failure

**Table 4.6**  Factors ameliorating sickle cell anaemia or some features of the disease.

Coinheritance of hereditary persistence of fetal haemoglobin, or other factors either linked or unlinked to the β globin locus, leading to a high percentage of haemoglobin F; the haemoglobin F level is highest in the Arab–Indian and Senegal haplotypes, lowest in the Central African Republic haplotype and intermediate in the Benin haplotype

Coinheritance of certain α chain variant haemoglobins, e.g. haemoglobin Memphis or haemoglobin Hopkins II

Coinheritance of α thalassaemia trait — ameliorates haemolysis [61], ameliorates soft tissue end-organ damage [4], reduces leg ulcers [64], reduces the frequency of stroke [60,64] and is associated with longer preservation of splenic function [55]; however, does not ameliorate painful crises [61] and possibly increases their frequency [60], increases the frequency of retinopathy [64] and aggravates osteonecrosis [4,64]; does not improve survival [58]

Iron deficiency (ameliorates haemolysis) [62]

42 years for men and 48 years for women [58], and in another in Jamaica it was 58 years for men and 66 years for women [59]. Despite the severity of the disease in many patients, there are a significant minority who are asymptomatic for prolonged periods. For example, in one French study of 299 patients, 9% were asymptomatic for 3 years or more [60].

## Ameliorating factors and interaction with α thalassaemia trait

The clinical course of sickle cell anaemia is very variable. This is largely unexplained, although some factors have been identified that appear to ameliorate the condition and lead to later presentation, milder symptoms and a better life expectancy. Some of these are shown in Table 4.6 [4,55,58,60–64]. Elevation of haemoglobin F to more than 20% is usually sufficient to render sickle cell anaemia largely asymptomatic. Coexisting α thalassaemia trait is common in sickle cell disease. For example, 30% of Afro-Americans with homozygosity for haemoglobin S have a single α gene deletion and 5% have two α genes deleted [63]. The effect of coexisting α thalassaemia trait is complex, with some features being ameliorated and others being worsened. In a study of sickle cell anaemia associated with the Arab–Indian haplotype, a tribal Indian group with a very high incidence of α thalassaemia trait had significantly fewer painful crises, infections and episodes of hospitalization than a non-tribal group with a much lower incidence

of α thalassaemia trait [65]. In another study, deletion of two α genes was associated with an increased prevalence of avascular necrosis, retinopathy and splenomegaly and a decreased prevalence of leg ulcers and cerebrovascular accidents [64]. For the effects demonstrated in other studies, see Table 4.6. The complex effects of the presence of α thalassaemia in patients with sickle cell anaemia may be the result of two conflicting factors: (i) reduced polymerization, leading to less membrane damage, fewer dehydrated and irreversibly sickled cells and improved red cell survival; and (ii) higher haemoglobin concentration, leading to increased blood viscosity. In a large study of sickle cell anaemia in a population with the $β^S$ gene associated with a variety of haplotypes, overall life expectancy was not altered by coexisting α thalassaemia [58]; presumably, therefore, the beneficial and adverse effects of coexisting thalassaemia trait balance out.

## Laboratory features

### Blood count

The blood count is normal at birth. During the first year, as haemoglobin F is replaced by haemoglobin S, there is a fall in haemoglobin concentration and a rise in the reticulocyte count. Mean values differ from controls by 1–2 months of age [66,67]. Anaemia and reticulocytosis continue throughout childhood, adolescence and adult life. The haemoglobin concentration reported in adults is most often between 6 and 10 g/dl, but can range from 5 to 12 g/dl or even higher. In a personally observed series of 29 mainly Afro-Caribbean patients, the haemoglobin concentration ranged from 7.6 to 13.8 g/dl, with a mean of 9 g/dl. In males, there is a significant post-pubertal rise in the haemoglobin concentration, averaging between 1 and 2 g/dl [9]. Patients with a higher percentage of haemoglobin F tend to have a higher haemoglobin concentration [9]. The haemoglobin concentration is of some prognostic significance [58]. During complications such as splenic sequestration, parvovirus infection or megaloblastic anaemia, the haemoglobin concentration may fall to as low as 1.5–3 g/dl. Bacterial infection is also associated with some worsening of the anaemia. In older patients with sickle cell anaemia, a slow fall in the haemoglobin concentra-

tion without any alteration in the red cell indices may be found to be consequent on the onset of renal failure. Although the reticulocyte count is elevated in sickle cell anaemia, usually to 5–20%, it is not increased in proportion to the reduction in haemoglobin concentration. This is because haemoglobin S has a lower oxygen affinity than haemoglobin A and the drive to erythropoiesis is therefore less than would be anticipated from the haemoglobin concentration. For the same reason, the serum erythropoietin concentration is lower than would be expected for the degree of anaemia [68]. In patients with no associated α thalassaemia, the red cell indices are normal [38, 69]. However, the MCV and MCH are not elevated in keeping with the reticulocyte count, suggesting a relative microcytosis. The MCV tends to be higher in those with a higher haemoglobin F percentage [9]. The mean cell haemoglobin concentration (MCHC) may be slightly increased and the proportion of cells with a high haemoglobin concentration is increased (Fig. 4.13). The red cell distribution width (RDW) is generally markedly increased and correlates with

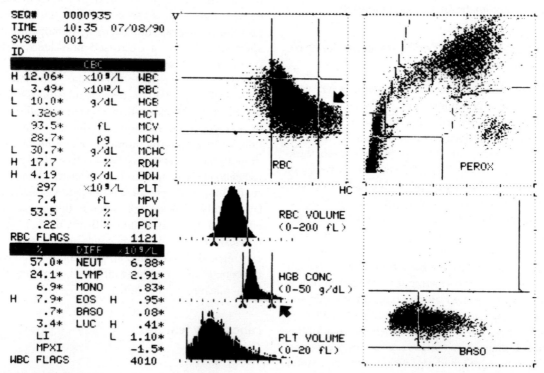

**Fig. 4.13** Red cell cytogram and histograms showing an increase in hyperchromic cells (arrows), representing irreversibly sickled cells, and increased hypochromic macrocytes, representing reticulocytes.

disease severity [70]. The total nucleated cell count may be increased as a consequence of significant numbers of circulating erythroblasts. The neutrophil count may be increased between as well as during crises. The baseline white blood cell count (WBC) has been found to correlate with the frequency of acute chest syndrome [71] and to be predictive of earlier death from sickle cell disease [58]. The monocyte count and the lymphocyte count are also increased [72], the latter possibly as a feature of hyposplenism. The platelet count is increased and there is an increased proportion of large platelets. Both of these features are attributable to hyposplenism.

Patients with sickle cell disease who also have α thalassaemia trait have a lower MCV, MCH and MCHC than those with four α genes [38]. The haemoglobin concentration is, on average, 1–2 g/dl higher and the reticulocyte count is lower [40,73]. The percentage of hyperdense cells is reduced. Patients with sickle cell anaemia with a high haemoglobin F percentage tend to have a higher haemoglobin concentration and MCV and a lower percentage of hyperdense cells. Those with the highest haemoglobin F levels, e.g. patients with the Saudi/Indian haplotype, also have a lower reticulocyte count.

Coexisting iron deficiency leads to a lower haemoglobin concentration, MCV, MCH and MCHC. There is an associated amelioration of haemolysis [62]. Patients who are maintained on folic acid have an MCV, on average, 4 fl lower than patients not so maintained [74].

Changes occur in the blood count quite early in sickle cell crisis. There is a fall in the haemoglobin concentration, a rise in the reticulocyte percentage and a rise in the MCHC, RDW, haemoglobin distribution width (HDW) and percentage of hyperdense cells [75]. The HDW is a measurement of the variation in haemoglobin concentration between individual red cells; its increase is a reflection of the increased number of hyperdense cells. Later in a crisis, there is a return of the RDW, HDW and percentage of hyperdense cells towards baseline values; the percentage of hyperdense cells may fall below baseline values, probably because the densest, least deformable cells are being preferentially trapped in the spleen and destroyed. The WBC and the neutrophil count increase during painful crises and the platelet count may also increase. When a sickle cell crisis is complicated by an acute chest syndrome caused by pulmonary fat embolism, there is leucocytosis and usually a marked fall in haemoglobin concentration and platelet count [76]. Irregularly contracted cells may appear in quite significant numbers.

Patients whose sickle cell anaemia is treated with hydroxycarbamide, with a consequent increase in the haemoglobin F percentage, show characteristic changes in the haemoglobin concentration and red cell indices. The haemoglobin concentration and the MCV rise, while the MCHC, percentage of dense cells and reticulocyte count fall. The WBC, neutrophil count and platelet count may fall as a consequence of the cytotoxic effect of hydroxycarbamide.

### Blood film

The blood film is usually normal at birth and in the early neonatal period as the haemoglobin S percentage is relatively low, but this is not necessarily so (Fig. 4.14). Abnormalities are usually detectable around 6 months of age (Fig. 4.15) when occasional sickle cells, target cells and Howell–Jolly bodies start to appear [66]. The majority of infants have features of hyposplenism by 1 year of age [66] and circulating erythroblasts, sickle cells and Howell–Jolly bodies are much more common thereafter. In an adult with sickle cell disease, the blood film shows a variable number of crescent or sickle-shaped sickle cells (Fig. 4.16a). These represent irreversibly sickled cells, which have not corrected their shape on exposure to atmospheric oxygen. The number of sickle cells is very variable, ranging from only occasional cells to 30–40%. They are less numerous in those with a lower MCHC [9]. In addition to classical sickle cells, there are elongated cells pointed at one or both ends (Fig. 4.16b) [77]; these have been referred to as boat-shaped or oat-shaped cells or as plump sickle cells. There is polychromasia and, in some patients, microcytosis and hypochromia. Small numbers of irregularly contracted cells may be seen (Fig. 4.16c) and sometimes there are cells in which the haemoglobin appears to have retracted into one half of the cell ('hemi-ghosts' or 'blister cells'); both of these features are particularly common in patients with widespread pulmonary infarction and hypoxia; these abnormal red cells have increased density; their formation has been attributed to oxidant damage

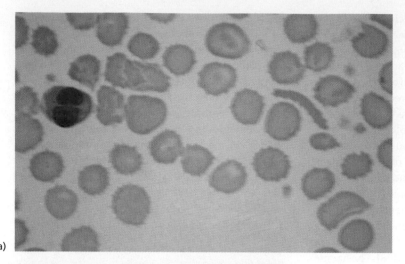

(a)

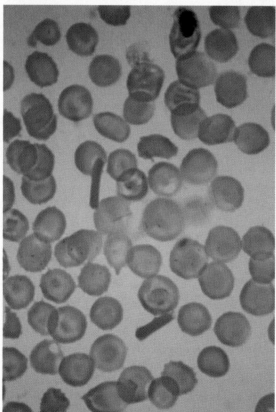

(b)

**Fig. 4.14** Blood film of a neonate with sickle cell anaemia showing one sickle cell (a) and other poikilocytes consistent with reversibly sickled cells (b).

leading to transcellular bonding of damaged regions of the red cell membrane with trapping of haemoglobin within pseudovacuoles [78]. Linear red cell fragments may be present; these were first described in a patient with cold agglutinins and a positive antiglobulin test [79], but in fact they are not rare if specifically looked for. There are features of hyposplenism (Fig. 4.16d), specifically Howell–Jolly bodies, target cells, Pappenheimer bodies, an increased platelet count, increased platelet anisocyto-

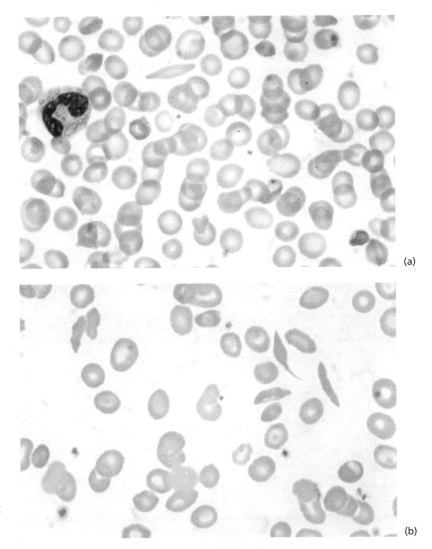

(a)

(b)

**Fig. 4.15** Blood films of a child with sickle cell anaemia: (a) at the age of 5 months showing mild anisopoikilocytosis and one sickle cell; (b) at the age of 13 years showing more marked anisocytosis and sickle cell formation.

sis and sometimes an increased lymphocyte count. Acanthocytes, which are usually present in small numbers in hyposplenic individuals, are not usually a feature of hyposplenism in sickle cell disease. There are variable numbers of nucleated red cells. The neutrophil count may be increased. Phagocytosis of erythrocytes by monocytes or neutrophils may be observed, but is quite uncommon.

In patients with sickle cell anaemia with a high haemoglobin F, the abnormalities in the blood film are much less (Fig. 4.17). Sickle cells are less frequent and polychromasia and anaemia are less. The onset

of features of hyposplenism is delayed. Coexisting α thalassaemia trait has also been observed to protect against the loss of splenic function [55,80], although, surprisingly, hyposplenism was not found to be related to age or haemoglobin F concentration [80]. Coexisting α thalassaemia trait (particularly homozygous $\alpha^+$ thalassaemia trait) is associated with a blood film showing more target cells but fewer sickle cells [9].

Therapy with hydroxycarbamide leads to macrocytosis, a reduction in the number of sickle cells and boat-shaped cells and lessening of polychromasia.

Various other complications of sickle cell anaemia may be apparent from the full blood count (FBC) and the blood film. Parvovirus B19 infection may be suspected when there is worsening anaemia with a lack of polychromasia. The platelet count is also often reduced. When recovery occurs, there is initially the appearance of numerous nucleated red cells in the peripheral blood, followed by reticulocytosis and thrombocytosis. In splenic sequestration, there is an acute fall in the haemoglobin concentration with reticulocytosis and increasing numbers of nucleated red blood cells. The platelet count may also be reduced. In chronic hypersplenism, there is worsening anaemia, thrombocytopenia and reticulocytosis. When there is complicating megaloblastic anaemia, there may be macrocytes, oval macrocytes and hypersegmented neutrophils; polychromasia is less than would otherwise be expected in a patient with sickle cell anaemia. Patients with coexisting sickle cell anaemia and homozygosity for $\alpha^+$ thalassaemia who develop megaloblastic anaemia may show an increase in the MCV and MCH, but with both values remaining within the normal range rather than exceeding it. Because of the shortened red cell life span, megaloblastic anaemia may also have an acute onset with pancytopenia and a rapidly falling haemoglobin concentration without macrocytosis. In patients with a delayed transfusion reaction, some spherocytes are seen, but it can be difficult to recognize the morphological features of a transfusion reaction in a patient with sickle cell anaemia. The direct antiglobulin test is positive. Patients with sickle cell disease may develop hyperhaemolysis following blood transfusion with both homologous and autologous cells being destroyed. During intercurrent infections, the patient with sickle cell anaemia is likely to show neutrophilia, left shift, toxic granulation and sometimes an increase in the platelet count; rarely organisms, e.g. pneumococci, are found within neutrophils.

*Other investigations*

In the adult, haemoglobin electrophoresis and HPLC show haemoglobins S, F and $A_2$ (Fig. 4.18). Haemoglobin S is the major haemoglobin present, usually comprising 90–95% of total haemoglobin. Haemoglobin A is totally absent. Haemoglobin $A_2$ may be

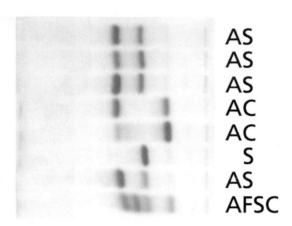

**Fig. 4.18** Haemoglobin electrophoresis on cellulose acetate at alkaline pH showing a patient with sickle cell anaemia (third lane from bottom) with almost all the haemoglobin being haemoglobin S; AFSC, control sample containing haemoglobins A, F, S and C; AS, sickle cell trait; AC, haemoglobin C trait.

present in normal amounts or may be slightly elevated (usually 2–4%) [9,38]. Higher percentages are seen in those who also have $\alpha$ thalassaemia trait, although there is considerable variation in the mean levels reported in different series of patients (Table 4.7) [9,50,63,83,84]. Haemoglobin F is usually only slightly elevated (see below). Inevitably, the percentage of haemoglobin S correlates inversely with the percentage of haemoglobin F. The percentage of haemoglobin S also varies with the number of $\alpha$ genes and with the MCV and MCH. Looked at in another way, the coexistence of $\alpha$ thalassaemia trait with sickle cell anaemia leads to a reduction in the MCV and MCH and a slight reduction in the haemoglobin S percentage.

Neonates with sickle cell anaemia usually have predominantly haemoglobin F with haemoglobin S comprising only a low percentage of total haemoglobin (Fig. 4.19). Sometimes only haemoglobin F is present and repeat testing when the baby is a few months of age is then necessary for diagnosis. In the neonatal period, diagnostic confusion can occur not only with sickle cell/$\beta^0$ thalassaemia, but also with sickle cell/$\beta^+$ thalassaemia [85] (see below). The postnatal fall in haemoglobin F is slower in babies with sickle cell anaemia than in normal babies, with mean levels of about 20% at 1 year of age [66].

**Table 4.7** Haematological characteristics and percentages of various haemoglobins in adults with sickle cell anaemia and other conditions with haemoglobins S, F and $A_2$ only. (Derived from references [9,50,63,83,84] and other sources.)

| Genotype | Usual Hb (g/dl) | Usual MCV (fl) | Usual reticulocyte count (%) | Usual haemoglobin F (%) | Usual haemoglobin $A_2$ (%) |
|---|---|---|---|---|---|
| SS | 6–10 | 70–100 | 5–20 | Usually 5–10 but up to 40* | 1.6–3.6† (occasionally up to 5)‡ |
| S$\beta^0$ | 7–11 | 60–80 | 8–9 | 5–15 | 4–5.6† |
| S/$\delta\beta^0$ | 10–12 | 76–83 | 2–4 | 15–25 | 1.9–2.3 |
| S/HPFH | >12 | 68–88§ | Normal | 20–30 | 1.1–2.2 in the majority |

Hb, haemoglobin concentration; HPFH, hereditary persistence of fetal haemoglobin; MCV, mean cell volume.

* Influenced by coinheritance of non-deletional HPFH as well as by the haplotype associated with the $\beta^S$ gene [83,84]: Arab–Indian haplotype, 10–25% haemoglobin F; Senegal haplotype, 7–10% haemoglobin F; Benin or Bantu haplotype, 6–7% haemoglobin F; Cameroon haplotype, 5–6% haemoglobin F. Mean ± standard deviation of 6.06 ± 4.23% for 120 SS adults in the UK [50].

† Some overlap occurs, particularly when coexisting homozygous $\alpha^+$ thalassaemia raises the $A_2$ percentage in cases of SS [9]; in one series, the reported mean haemoglobin $A_2$ levels were 2.8% with four $\alpha$ genes, 3.3% with three $\alpha$ genes and 3.8% with two $\alpha$ genes [83]; in another series, the reported levels were higher—3.5%, 3.7% and 4.9%, respectively [63].

‡ High levels are characteristically seen in the Arab–Indian mutation.

§ Normal if there is no coexisting $\alpha$ thalassaemia trait.

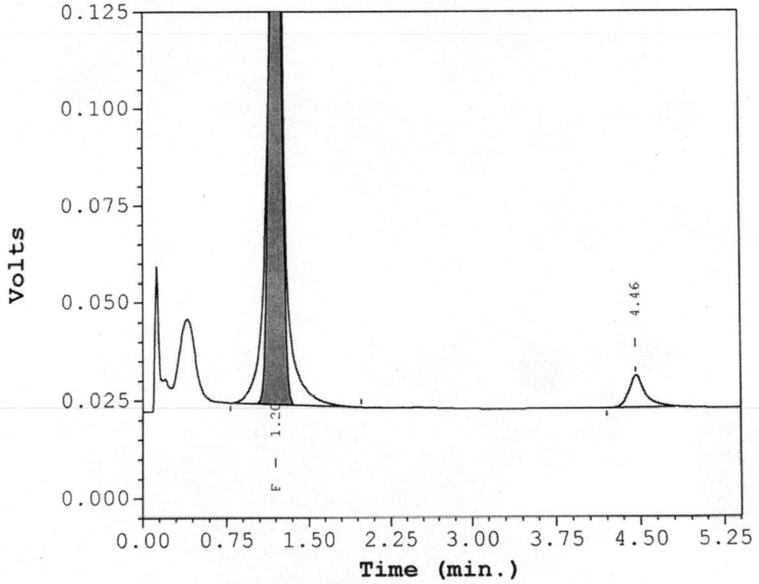

**Fig. 4.19** HPLC chromatogram in a neonate with sickle cell anaemia showing mainly haemoglobin F, total absence of haemoglobin A and presence of haemoglobin S; haemoglobin S was 5.5% and the retention time was 4.46 min; the peaks on the left of the chromatogram represent altered F.

The sickle solubility test is positive and immunoassays [86] demonstrate the presence of haemoglobin S with no haemoglobin A.

The oxygen dissociation curve shows reduced oxygen affinity, i.e. a right-shifted curve and an increased $P_{50}$ (the $P_{O_2}$ at which haemoglobin is 50% saturated) [87]. The right shift is less in those with a high haemoglobin F percentage, either as a feature of the disease or as a consequence of hydroxycarbamide therapy. Resting arterial oxygen saturation when not in crisis is usually greater than 95%, but in patients with significant pulmonary damage may be reduced, e.g. to 80–95%.

Studies of globin chain synthesis show balanced synthesis of α and β$^S$ globin chains unless there is coexisting α thalassaemia trait.

The bilirubin concentration is increased, the bilirubin being mainly unconjugated. Lactate dehydrogenase (LDH) is increased approximately two-fold. Hyperuricaemia is common. Serum haptoglobin is usually absent and Schumm's test for methaemalbumin may be positive. Red cell survival studies show a half-life of about 7–14 days, less if there is splenomegaly. Heterozygous α$^+$ thalassaemia is as-sociated with longer red cell survival. Coexisting iron deficiency leads to a considerable improvement in red cell survival, associated with a fall in bilirubin concentration and LDH [62]. Hydroxycarbamide therapy also leads to improved red cell survival and reduced biochemical evidence of haemolysis [88].

A bone marrow aspirate shows erythroid hyperplasia and the presence of sickle cells (Fig. 4.20). Macrophages are increased and may contain sickled cells (Fig. 4.21). Foamy macrophages and sea-blue histiocytes may be increased. A trephine biopsy like-

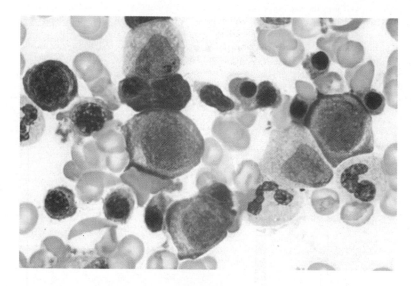

**Fig. 4.20** Bone marrow aspirate in sickle cell anaemia showing erythroid hyperplasia and two sickle cells.

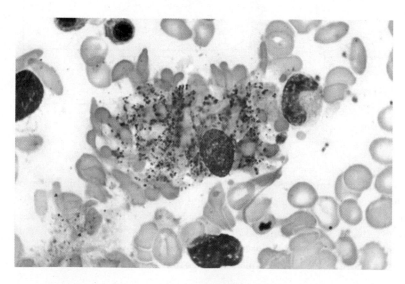

**Fig. 4.21** Bone marrow aspirate in sickle cell anaemia showing a sea-blue histiocyte packed with sickle cells.

wise shows erythroid hyperplasia and sickle cells inside macrophages and within blood vessels (Fig. 4.22).

## Haemoglobin F percentage

In sickle cell anaemia, haemoglobin F is usually around 5–10% but may be higher, sometimes comprising up to 40% of total haemoglobin (Table 4.7). The level is higher in infancy and tends to be higher in women than in men [70]. The switch from $\gamma$ to $\beta^S$ synthesis is delayed compared with the $\gamma$ to $\beta$ switch in normal subjects. The percentage of haemoglobin F falls most rapidly in the first 3 years of life and then more slowly until the age of 10 years; by this time, levels approximate those in adult life, although there may be a continued slow fall up to the age of 20 years. The percentage of haemoglobin F in an individual is determined by factors related and unrelated to the $\beta$ globin gene cluster. There is a clear relationship to the haplotype of the chromosome carrying $\beta^S$. The Arab–Indian haplotype is usually associated with a haemoglobin F level of 10–25% [84]. The Senegal haplotype is also associated with a relatively high haemoglobin F level, e.g. 7–10% in adults, whereas the Bantu and Benin haplotypes have lower levels, in adults averaging around 6–7%, but with a wide range [83,84]. The Cameroon haplotype tends to be associated with the lowest haemoglobin F level,

averaging 5–6% [83]. The relationship of haplotype to haemoglobin F percentage appears to result from an association between haplotype and determinants of non-deletional hereditary persistence of fetal haemoglobin. Both the Arab–Indian haplotype and the Senegal haplotype are linked with the common $-158\ ^{G}\gamma\ C{\rightarrow}T$ polymorphism [89], whereas the Benin haplotype, which has a low percentage of haemoglobin F, is not linked with $-158\ ^{G}\gamma\ C{\rightarrow}T$. A polymorphism at $^{A}\gamma$ IVS2 has also been linked to the high haemoglobin F level observed when the $\beta^S$ gene is associated with the Senegal and Arab–Indian haplotypes [90]. In addition, the Arab–Indian haplotype is associated with a polymorphism at $-530$ base pairs (bp), where there is $(AT)_9 T_5$ rather than $(AT)_7 T_7$, causing increased affinity for BP-1 (a negative *trans*-acting factor) and repression of $\beta^S$ synthesis. The higher haemoglobin F in sickle cell anaemia associated with the Arab–Indian haplotype, in comparison with that in the Senegal haplotype, may be related to the combined effect of the $(AT)_x(T)_y$ polymorphism and the $-158\ ^{G}\gamma\ C{\rightarrow}T$ and $^{A}\gamma$ IVS2 polymorphisms. The $^{G}\gamma{:}^{A}\gamma$ ratio is increased in individuals with a high haemoglobin F in association with the Saudi Arabian or Senegal haplotype [81]. The $^{G}\gamma$ promoter associated with the Bantu haplotype has been shown to be associated with low $^{G}\gamma$ synthesis [91].

The percentage of F cells (i.e. cells containing haemoglobin F) is increased in sickle cell anaemia. In

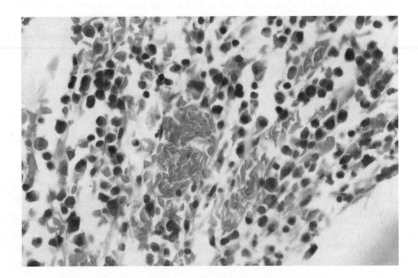

**Fig. 4.22** Trephine biopsy in sickle cell anaemia showing erythroid hyperplasia and two vessels packed with sickle cells.

one study, the mean count was 55% (range 17–94%), the normal level being 0.5–7% [92]. The logarithm of the haemoglobin F concentration correlated with the percentage of F cells. In one study, the X-linked F-cell production locus was found to be the major determinant of haemoglobin F percentage in patients with sickle cell anaemia in association with the three major African haplotypes [93]. Factors linked to the $\beta$ gene haplotype were next most important. The effect of the X-linked F-cell locus may be the reason why women with sickle cell anaemia, like haematologically normal women, tend to have a higher haemoglobin F level than men.

Individuals with coexisting $\alpha$ thalassaemia trait have been observed to have a significantly higher proportion of haemoglobin F in the first decade of life [73], but thereafter have a somewhat lower proportion, than those with four $\alpha$ genes [38,94].

The haemoglobin F percentage in sickle cell anaemia is of prognostic significance [58], the prognosis being more favourable when the percentage is high. The haemoglobin F percentage is increased 2–16-fold by hydroxycarbamide therapy [88].

## Diagnosis

The diagnosis rests on the demonstration of haemoglobins S, F and $A_2$ only, with the presence of haemoglobin S as the sole variant haemoglobin being confirmed by at least two independent techniques. It is important not to misdiagnose compound heterozygous states for haemoglobin S and haemoglobins D, G, Korle Bu or Lepore as sickle cell anaemia. Recognizing the presence of haemoglobins D, G, Korle Bu or Lepore in compound heterozygous states with haemoglobin S is more complex than recognizing the simple heterozygous state, as all of these have a single band on cellulose acetate electrophoresis and a positive sickle solubility test (whereas the simple heterozygous state for any of these variant haemoglobins may simulate sickle cell trait on cellulose acetate electrophoresis at alkaline pH, but is easily distinguished as the sickle solubility test is negative). In patients with microcytosis or with a significant increase in haemoglobin F, the possibility of compound heterozygosity for haemoglobin S and $\beta^0$ or $\delta\beta^0$ thalassaemia or haemoglobin S and deletional hereditary persistence of fetal haemo-

globin, respectively, must also be considered before a diagnosis of sickle cell anaemia is made.

## Interactions of haemoglobin S homozygosity with other thalassaemias, haemoglobinopathies and other inherited erythrocyte abnormalities

The modification of sickle cell anaemia by coinheritance of $\alpha$ thalassaemia trait or non-deletional hereditary persistence of fetal haemoglobin has been discussed above.

The coinheritance of certain $\alpha$ chain variants, including haemoglobin Korle Bu, haemoglobin Memphis and haemoglobin Hopkins II, ameliorates sickle cell anaemia.

The coinheritance of other $\alpha$ chain variants, e.g. haemoglobin G-Philadelphia and haemoglobin Stanleyville II, has no significant effect on the clinical or haematological features of sickle cell anaemia [95,96]. The results of haemoglobin electrophoresis may be complex. With sickle cell anaemia and haemoglobin G-Philadelphia, there are two bands, an S band and a G-Philadelphia–S hybrid band (which has the same mobility at alkaline pH as haemoglobin C). The proportion of haemoglobin S is greater than the proportion of the hybrid band [95]. At acid pH, there is a single band with the mobility of haemoglobin S as, at this pH, the hybrid has the same mobility as S. Coinheritance with the $\alpha$ chain variant, haemoglobin Montgomery, also produces a hybrid band which has characteristics resembling those of haemoglobin C on both cellulose acetate electrophoresis and HPLC [97].

Glucose-6-phosphate dehydrogenase deficiency is common in many of the ethnic groups who carry the $\beta^S$ gene. However, it has no effect on the clinical or haematological features of sickle cell anaemia [81].

## Sickle cell/haemoglobin C disease

Sickle cell/haemoglobin C disease is consequent on the coinheritance of the $\beta^S$ and $\beta^C$ genes. There is no normal $\beta$ gene and therefore no haemoglobin A. This compound heterozygous state leads to a sickling disorder that is similar to sickle cell anaemia but, on average, is somewhat less severe. The degree of haemolysis is less, with red cells surviving around

27 days, in comparison with around 17 days in sickle cell anaemia. The life expectancy is considerably better than that of sickle cell anaemia. In the USA, the average survival is 60 years for men and 68 years for women [58].

Sickle cell/haemoglobin C disease is characterized by an increased density of red cells, which is attributable to increased $K^+/Cl^-$ cotransport with the loss of intracellular potassium and resultant cellular dehydration [98]. This, in turn, increases the likelihood of polymerization of haemoglobin S and, together with the higher haemoglobin S percentage (averaging 50% rather than 40%), helps to explain why the compound heterozygous state generally causes significant disease, whereas sickle cell trait does not [98].

Variant haemoglobins in which there is a second mutation in the $\beta^C$ gene are likely to interact with haemoglobin S in a similar manner to haemoglobin C itself. One such haemoglobin is haemoglobin Arlington Park ($\beta^{6Glu \to Lys}$, $\beta^{95Lys \to Glu}$), which will be missed on cellulose acetate electrophoresis at alkaline pH as there is no net charge change in comparison with haemoglobin A [99,100].

## Clinical features

Sickle cell/haemoglobin C disease leads to a chronic haemolytic anaemia and to intermittent sickle cell crises, similar to those of sickle cell anaemia but less frequent. Dactylitis is quite uncommon [101]. The haemoglobin concentration is higher than in sickle cell anaemia and the degree of haemolysis is less; the higher haemoglobin concentration is mainly due to a smaller reduction in the oxygen affinity rather than to less severe haemolysis. Aseptic necrosis (Fig. 4.23) and probably also bone marrow infarction with embolism of necrotic bone marrow to the lungs are more common than in sickle cell anaemia. In one series of patients, 15% suffered osteonecrosis of the femoral or humoral heads or vertebral bodies and two of 284 patients died of bone marrow embolism (two of 25 deaths) [101]. Retinal disease (retinitis proliferans and vitreous haemorrhage) is more frequent and more severe; in one series of patients, it was seen in 21% and in another in 23% [101]. Splenomegaly persists for longer, so that splenic infarction and splenic sequestration can occur in adults as well as in children, while the onset of hyposplenism, consequent

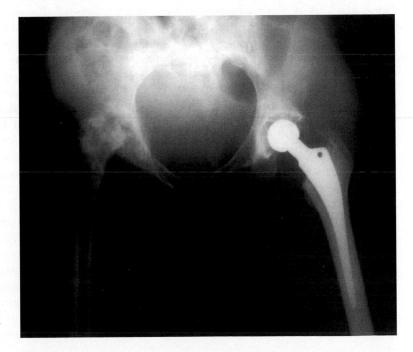

**Fig. 4.23** Radiograph of the hips and pelvis in a patient with sickle cell/haemoglobin C compound heterozygosity showing osteonecrosis of one hip resulting from vascular occlusion by sickle cells; the other hip had already been replaced because of the same process. (By courtesy of Professor I. Roberts.)

on recurrent splenic infarction, is delayed. In contrast with patients with sickle cell anaemia, in whom the spleen is atrophic as a result of infarction, patients with sickle cell/haemoglobin C disease occasionally suffer splenic infarction during aeroplane flights [102]. As a consequence of the delay in the development of hyposplenism, life-threatening infections are less common than in sickle cell anaemia. Splenomegaly can lead to hypersplenism with chronic thrombocytopenia [103]. Because the red cell life span is considerably longer than in sickle cell anaemia, clinically apparent parvovirus-induced aplastic crises are uncommon and gallstones are less common.

## Laboratory features

### Blood count

The haemoglobin concentration is higher than in sickle cell anaemia, ranging from about 8 g/dl up to the top of the normal range [104]. In a personally observed series of 29 patients, the range was 8.9 to 15.6 g/dl with a mean of 12.2 g/dl. A concentration of 10 g/dl gives a fairly good separation between sickle cell anaemia and sickle cell/haemoglobin C disease. In one large study of adult patients originating in North Africa, West Africa and the Caribbean area, there were no individuals with sickle cell/haemoglobin C disease with a haemoglobin concentration of less than 11 g/dl [105]. In children, splenomegaly has been associated with a lower haemoglobin concentration and platelet count [103]. The MCV is lower than in sickle cell anaemia with a mean level around the lower limit of the normal range [104,106]. The MCH is similar, whereas the MCHC is more often elevated and the percentage of hyperdense cells is higher. The RDW is increased, but generally less than in sickle cell anaemia [70,107]. The HDW is increased [107]. The reticulocyte count is less markedly elevated than in sickle cell anaemia, with a mean level around 3–6%. The accuracy of measurement of red cell indices in sickle cell/haemoglobin C disease is dependent on the automated instrument used; cells in this disease are less deformable than normal, leading to a false elevation of the MCV and reduction of the MCHC on impedance counters and on some earlier light-scattering instruments [107].

Splenic sequestration is associated not only with a fall in the haemoglobin concentration, but also with a fall in the platelet count [103].

Individuals of African descent with sickle cell/haemoglobin C disease show a similar prevalence of α thalassaemia trait to those without this condition. The prevalence has varied between 20% and 35% in different series of patients [101]. Coexisting α thalassaemia trait leads to a higher red cell count and a lower MCV and MCH in comparison with other patients with sickle cell/haemoglobin C disease. In contrast with sickle cell anaemia, concomitant α thalassaemia trait does not alter the haemoglobin concentration [40,101,105,108], but a lower reticulocyte count and lower LDH indicate that there is less haemolysis [105].

The WBC, neutrophil count and monocyte count are elevated in sickle cell/haemoglobin C disease, but less so than in sickle cell anaemia [72].

When sickle cell/haemoglobin C disease is treated with hydroxycarbamide, there is an increase in the MCV and a fall in the MCHC and the proportion of hyperdense cells. The reticulocyte count falls.

### Blood film

The peripheral blood features of sickle cell/haemoglobin C disease are compared with those of sickle cell anaemia and haemoglobin C disease in Table 4.8 [77]. In contrast with sickle cell anaemia, the blood film does not often show classical sickle cells. Boat-shaped cells are more common than classical sickle cells, but they are less common than in sickle cell anaemia. Occasional cells may contain straight-edged six-sided haemoglobin C crystals. Around one-half of patients with sickle cell/haemoglobin C disease show characteristic poikilocytes (Fig. 4.24), which are not seen in either sickle cell anaemia or haemoglobin C disease [72,109]. These misshapen cells have complex forms. Some have crystals of varying shape and size jutting out at various angles. Others are curved, thus resembling sickle cells, but also appear to contain crystals with straight edges or with blunt-angled rather than pointed ends. Haemoglobin C will copolymerize with haemoglobin S (as occurs in the rare sickle cells and in the more common boat-shaped cells in the compound heterozygous state) [110]. Haemoglobin S will cocrystallize with

**Table 4.8** Blood film features of sickle cell anaemia, sickle cell/haemoglobin C disease and haemoglobin C disease or Cβ⁰ thalassaemia. (From reference [77].)

| Genotype | SS | SC | CC or Cβ⁰ thalassaemia |
|---|---|---|---|
| Number of cases | 29 | 29 | 10 |
| Sickle cells | 24 | 6 | 0 |
| Boat-shaped cells | 24 | 16 | 1 |
| Haemoglobin C crystals | 0 | 4 | 5 |
| SC poikilocytes | 0 | 16 | 0 |
| Irregularly contracted cells | 5 | 25 | 9 |
| Howell–Jolly bodies | 29 | 5 | 0 |
| Pappenheimer bodies | 25 | 7 | 1 |
| Target cells | 27 | 29 | 9 |
| Spherocytes | 10 | 3 | 1 |
| Polychromasia | 24 | 9 | 3 |
| Nucleated red blood cells | 26 | 15 | 7 |

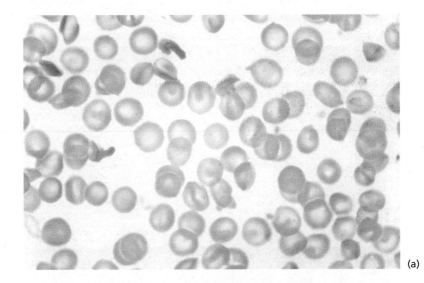

(a)

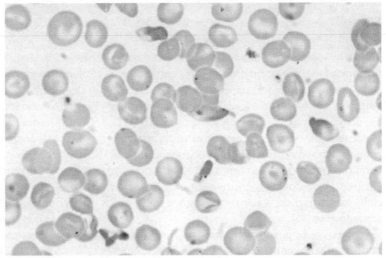

**Fig. 4.24** Blood films in four patients with sickle cell/haemoglobin C compound heterozygosity showing the range of abnormalities observed: (a) target cells and SC poikilocytes; (b) SC poikilocytes and a boat-shaped cell. (*Continued on p. 168.*)

(b)

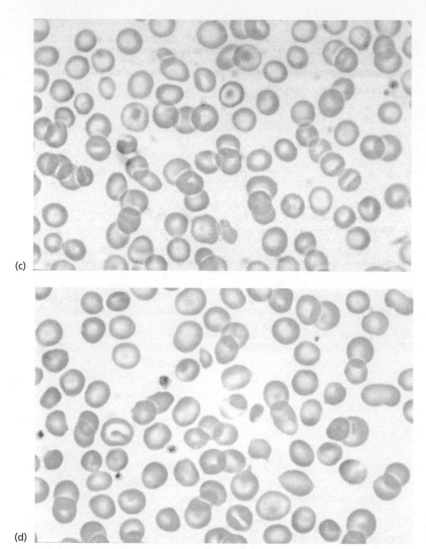

(c)

(d)

**Fig. 4.24** *Continued.* (c) hypochromia and target cells; (d) irregularly contracted cells, a 'hemi-ghost', a target cell and a stomatocyte.

haemoglobin C (as occurs in the less common cells containing haemoglobin C crystals) [111]. Deoxygenation favours S-like polymerization, whereas oxygenation favours C-like crystallization [110,112]. It seems likely that the formation of SC poikilocytes is consequent on both processes occurring simultaneously in the one cell. On scanning electron microscopy, the forms seen include folded cells (compared to a taco), triconcave cells and stomatocytes [98].

Features of hyposplenism, such as Howell–Jolly bodies and Pappenheimer bodies, are less common than in sickle cell anaemia. Polychromasia and nucleated red blood cells are likewise less common, whereas target cells (Fig. 4.24c) show a similarly high frequency and irregularly contracted cells (Fig. 4.24d) are much more common. 'Hemi-ghosts' may be present (Fig. 4.24d). An assessment of the blood count and film usually permits the distinction between sickle cell/haemoglobin C disease and sickle cell anaemia. However, those cases that lack sickle cells, boat-shaped cells and SC poikilocytes (Fig. 4.24d) can be difficult to distinguish from haemoglobin C disease.

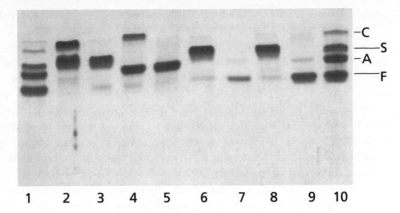

**Fig. 4.25** Haemoglobin electrophoresis on agarose gel at pH 6.2 showing a patient with sickle cell/haemoglobin C disease (lane 2); lanes 1 and 10, control sample containing haemoglobins F, A, S and C.

## Other investigations

Haemoglobins S and C are present in similar proportions (Fig. 4.25). The haemoglobin F percentage ranges from normal to slightly elevated, with mean values of 1.1–3.3% having been reported in different studies. The haemoglobin F percentage is significantly higher in females than in males [105]. As in sickle cell anaemia, the haemoglobin F percentage is affected by the β gene haplotype, averaging 3.2% with the Senegal haplotype and 1.5% and 1.4% with the Benin and Bantu haplotypes, respectively [105]. In 98 UK subjects, the mean haemoglobin F was 1.46% (standard deviation 1.81%), with adult levels being reached by 9 years of age [50]. The percentage of F cells is increased; in one study, the mean level was 27% (range 5–73%), in comparison with normal levels of 0.5–7% [92]. Little information is available on the haemoglobin $A_2$ percentage in sickle cell/haemoglobin C disease as, on cellulose acetate electrophoresis, haemoglobin $A_2$ comigrates with haemoglobin C.

The sickle solubility test is positive and immunoassays demonstrate the presence of haemoglobins S and C with no haemoglobin A.

Bilirubin is normal or mildly elevated. LDH is elevated in comparison with control subjects, but is less elevated than in sickle cell anaemia. The red cell life span ranges from moderately shortened to slightly less than normal. The oxygen dissociation curve shows reduced oxygen affinity, i.e. a right-shifted curve and a higher $P_{50}$. The reduction in oxygen affinity is less than that seen in sickle cell anaemia [87].

## Diagnosis

The diagnosis rests on the demonstration of the presence of haemoglobin S and haemoglobin C with haemoglobin A being absent. The identity of the two variant haemoglobins must be confirmed by at least two independent techniques. It is important not to confuse compound heterozygous states for haemoglobin S and haemoglobin C-Harlem, O-Arab or E (see pp. 175, 176 and 178) with sickle cell/haemoglobin C disease, as all have two bands in the same positions on cellulose acetate electrophoresis at alkaline pH. In compound heterozygosity for haemoglobins S and E, the band in the C position constitutes a lower percentage than the S band. Homozygous haemoglobin S with coexisting haemoglobin G-Philadelphia will also have bands in the positions of S and C, but the band in the C position, which represents the hybrid $\alpha^{\text{G-Philadelphia}}\beta^S$ haemoglobin, constitutes an appreciably lower percentage than the band representing S plus G-Philadelphia.

## Interactions with other haemoglobinopathies and other haematological diseases

There is conflicting evidence as to the effect of coexisting α thalassaemia trait. In one series of patients, α thalassaemia trait was associated with a lower risk of osteonecrosis and retinopathy, but an earlier series did not show this [101].

Individuals with sickle cell/haemoglobin C disease who are also heterozygous for the α chain variant, haemoglobin G-Philadelphia, have disease of variable severity. One reported case was more severe than is usual in sickle cell/haemoglobin C disease [113], while another had a mild clinical course with abundant crystals in circulating cells and numerous folded cells [114]. The latter is considered to be the more typical clinical picture, attributable to the presence of the G-Philadelphia $\alpha$ chain both increasing the likelihood of crystallization of haemoglobin C and decreasing the likelihood of polymerization of haemoglobin S [98]. Haemoglobin electrophoresis is complex. At alkaline pH, there are bands with the mobility of haemoglobins S (about 35%), C (about 47%) and a slow G–C hybrid (about 15%) [113]. The 'S' band represents haemoglobins S and G-Philadelphia. The 'C' band represents haemoglobin C and the S–G hybrid. At acid pH, there are two bands with the mobility of haemoglobins S and C.

A severe phenotype has been observed with coincidental hereditary spherocytosis [81].

## Sickle cell/β thalassaemia

Sickle cell/β thalassaemia is a compound heterozygous state for $\beta^S$ and either $\beta^+$ thalassaemia or $\beta^0$ thalassaemia [115,116]. In sickle cell/$\beta^0$ thalassaemia, there is no haemoglobin A, whereas, in sickle cell/$\beta^+$ thalassaemia, a variable amount of haemoglobin A is present. The reduced concentration of haemoglobin S within red cells, together with the greater or lesser increase in the percentages of haemoglobins $A_2$ and F, lessens the likelihood of sickling and lessens the haemolysis (in comparison with sickle cell anaemia); however, this is counterbalanced by the higher haemoglobin concentration and increased blood viscosity.

## Clinical features

Patients with sickle cell/$\beta^0$ thalassaemia have less evidence of haemolysis than patients with sickle cell anaemia but, despite this, the frequency of painful crises is, if anything, greater [61]. The explanation may lie in the higher haemoglobin concentration. Patients with sickle cell/$\beta^+$ thalassaemia may have both less haemolysis and a reduced incidence of painful crises in comparison with individuals with sickle cell anaemia. The amelioration of the disease is proportional to the percentage of haemoglobin A present. They may, however, have a higher incidence of proliferative retinopathy, as a consequence of the higher haemoglobin concentration [81]. Splenomegaly persists longer than in sickle cell anaemia, particularly in those with sickle cell/$\beta^+$ thalassaemia. Patients with sickle cell/$\beta^+$ thalassaemia and persisting splenomegaly remain susceptible to splenic infarction during aeroplane flights, whereas those with sickle cell/$\beta^0$ thalassaemia resemble patients with sickle cell anaemia as they are likely to have suffered recurrent splenic infarction and consequent atrophy and therefore do not remain susceptible [102]. Sometimes massive splenomegaly leads to hypersplenism. Overexpansion of the bone marrow cavity in the skull may cause frontal bossing. Sickle cell/β thalassaemia is generally more severe in Mediterranean populations than in those of African descent because of the greater prevalence of $\beta^0$ thalassaemia in the former group.

## Laboratory features

### Blood count

Anaemia is milder than in sickle cell anaemia, the haemoglobin concentration varying from about 5 g/dl to within the normal range. The distribution of haemoglobin concentration is bimodal, being higher in those with sickle cell/$\beta^+$ thalassaemia than in those with sickle cell/$\beta^0$ thalassaemia; mean values in one study were 10.7 and 8.1 g/dl, respectively [9]. The MCV, MCH and MCHC are reduced, again showing a bimodal distribution. Mean values observed were 72 and 69.8 fl for MCV, 22.6 and 20.1 pg for MCH and 31.5 and 28.8 g/dl for MCHC [116]. For both groups, sickle cell/$\beta^0$ thalassaemia and sickle cell/$\beta^+$ thalassaemia, the mean values for MCV, MCH and MCHC are lower than those in sickle cell anaemia, but overlap occurs. The RDW is markedly increased in sickle cell/$\beta^0$ thalassaemia and moderately increased in sickle cell/$\beta^+$ thalassaemia [70]. It should be noted that, in patients with sickle cell/β thalassaemia who develop megaloblastic anaemia, the MCV and MCH, although elevated in comparison with baseline values, may be within the normal range.

The reticulocyte count is elevated, in sickle cell/$\beta^0$ thalassaemia to around 8–9% on average and in sickle cell/$\beta^+$ thalassaemia to around 3% on average [104]. During complicating bacterial or parvovirus infection or megaloblastic anaemia, the usual elevation of the reticulocyte count is lacking.

Coexisting $\alpha$ thalassaemia increases the haemoglobin concentration, MCV and MCH and reduces the reticulocyte count [9].

*Blood film*

The blood film abnormalities are more severe in sickle cell/$\beta^0$ thalassaemia (Fig. 4.26) than in sickle cell/$\beta^1$ thalassaemia (Fig. 4.27). Classical sickle cells are quite uncommon, particularly in sickle cell/$\beta^+$ thalassaemia. There are some boat-shaped cells. There is hypochromia and microcytosis, and circulating nucleated red blood cells show defective haemoglobinization. Target cells are prominent and basophilic stippling may be apparent. Features of hyposplenism may be present, particularly in sickle cell/$\beta^0$ thalassaemia. In patients with hyposplenism, Pappenheimer bodies are often very prominent. Polychromasia is present unless there is associated erythropoietic failure caused by infection or megaloblastosis.

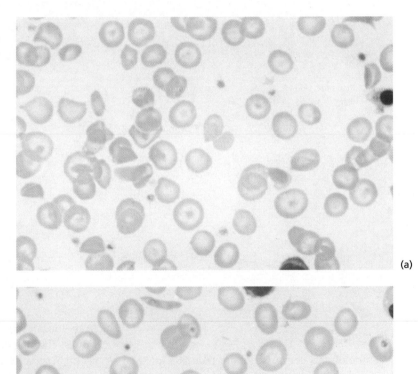

(a)

(b)

**Fig. 4.26** Blood films in two patients with sickle cell/$\beta^0$ thalassaemia showing: (a) target cells, a nucleated red blood cell and a number of partly sickled cells; (b) hypochromia, microcytosis, target cells and a number of partly sickled cells.

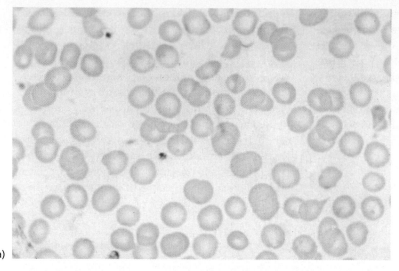

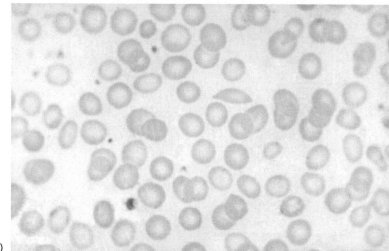

(a)

(b)

**Fig. 4.27** Blood films in two patients with sickle cell/$\beta^+$ thalassaemia showing: (a) hypochromia, poikilocytosis and a probable sickle cell; (b) hypochromia, microcytosis and one partly sickled cell. The first patient had 70% haemoglobin S, 24% haemoglobin A, 6% haemoglobin $A_2$, red blood cell count (RBC) $5.07 \times 10^{12}/l$, haemoglobin concentration (Hb) 10.6 g/dl, mean cell volume (MCV) 64 fl, mean cell haemoglobin (MCH) 21 pg and mean cell haemoglobin concentration (MCHC) 32.9 g/dl. The second patient had 59% haemoglobin S, 25% haemoglobin A and $A_2$, 13% haemoglobin F, RBC $4.71 \times 10^{12}/l$, Hb 10.6 g/dl, haematocrit (Hct) 0.32, MCV 68 fl, MCH 22.5 pg and MCHC 33 g/dl.

### Other investigations

Haemoglobin S comprises more than 50% of total haemoglobin, in contrast with sickle cell trait when it is less than 50%. In patients with sickle cell/$\beta^0$ thalassaemia, there is no haemoglobin A, whereas, in those with sickle cell/$\beta^+$ thalassaemia (Fig. 4.28), the amount of haemoglobin A varies from almost undetectable to, rarely, as high as 45% (Table 4.9) [117–120]. Haemoglobin F is usually 5–15% and the percentage of F cells is considerably increased. As for sickle cell anaemia, the haemoglobin F concentration is influenced by the $\beta$ gene haplotype associated with the $\beta^S$ mutation, being higher with the Senegal and Arab–Indian haplotypes. Because of the overlap in values, the haemoglobin F percentage is not very useful in separating sickle cell/$\beta^0$ thalassaemia from sickle cell anaemia; in one series of Jamaican patients, the F percentage tended to be higher in compound heterozygotes, but the difference was not significant [116]. Haemoglobin $A_2$ tends to be somewhat elevated, usually 3.5–5.5%, with the level being higher when the $\beta$ thalassaemia gene is $\beta^0$ rather than $\beta^+$ [121]. Higher levels of haemoglobins F and $A_2$ (and a milder clinical course) have been observed when the $\beta$ thalassaemia mutation is a large (290-bp) deletion [122]. The higher level of haemoglobin $A_2$ in sickle cell/$\beta^0$ thalassaemia can be useful in helping to make a distinction between the compound heterozygous state and sickle cell anaemia with microcytosis consequent on coexisting α thalassaemia trait, in which haemoglobin $A_2$ is usually in the range of 2–4%. Although there is some overlap in haemoglobin $A_2$ percentages, this is the most useful variable for making the distinction; the haemoglobin concentration, reticulocyte count and haemoglobin F percentage show more overlap (Table 4.7).

The red cell life span is reduced, particularly in sickle cell/$\beta^0$ thalassaemia, but not to the same extent as in sickle cell anaemia. The α:β chain synthesis ratio in peripheral blood reticulocytes is increased in sickle cell/β thalassaemia, whereas it is normal in sickle cell anaemia.

In the neonatal period, the diagnosis of sickle cell/$\beta^+$ thalassaemia can be difficult [85]. Confusion with sickle cell trait can occur if almost all the haemoglobin present is haemoglobin F and the proportions

of haemoglobins S and A are so low that it is not clear which is present in the greater amount. Neonates with sickle cell/$\beta^+$ thalassaemia may also have only haemoglobins S and F, so that confusion with sickle cell anaemia and sickle cell/$\beta^0$ thalassaemia is possible. Only a provisional diagnosis can be made in this circumstance. Family studies and follow-up are needed for a definitive diagnosis.

The bone marrow aspirate (Fig. 4.29) shows erythroid hyperplasia, sickle cells and a variable degree of iron overload.

## Diagnosis

The diagnosis of compound heterozygosity for haemoglobin S and $\beta^+$ thalassaemia is straightforward, merely requiring the demonstration of both haemoglobin A and haemoglobin S by two independent techniques and the confirmation that haemoglobin S is present as a larger proportion than haemoglobin A. The diagnosis of compound heterozygosity for haemoglobin S and $\beta^0$ thalassaemia is more difficult as a distinction must be made from sickle cell anaemia with microcytosis (e.g. due to coexisting α thalassaemia) (see above). When a precise diagnosis is important, e.g. for genetic counselling, and is not clear from family studies and from a consideration of the proportions of various haemoglobins, DNA analysis should be carried out. A distinction also needs to be made from compound heterozygosity for haemoglobin S and deletional hereditary persistence of fetal haemoglobin, particularly with coexisting α thalassaemia trait; in this instance, clinical features, haemoglobin concentration, MCV and haemoglobin F percentage are useful (Table 4.7).

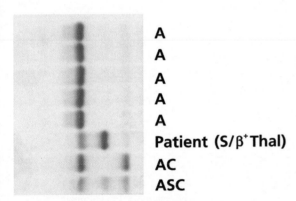

**Fig. 4.28** Haemoglobin electrophoresis on cellulose acetate at alkaline pH in a patient with sickle cell/$\beta^+$ thalassaemia compound heterozygosity; ASC, control sample containing haemoglobins A, S and C.

| **Mutation and ethnic group** | **Haemoglobin A (%)** |
|---|---|
| C→G at IVS2, position 745 (Greek/Turkish) | 3–5 |
| G→C at IVS1, position 5 (Indian) | 3–5 |
| G→A at IVS1, position 110 (Greek/Turkish) | 8–14 |
| C→T at –88 (black) | 18–25 |
| A→G at –29 (black) | 18–25 |
| G→T at IVS1, position 5 (Greek/Turkish) | 18–25 |

**Table 4.9** Percentage of haemoglobin A in compound heterozygosity for haemoglobin S and $\beta^+$ thalassaemia. (Derived from references [115–120].)

Labels on figure: A, A, A, A, A, Patient (S/β⁺Thal), AC, ASC

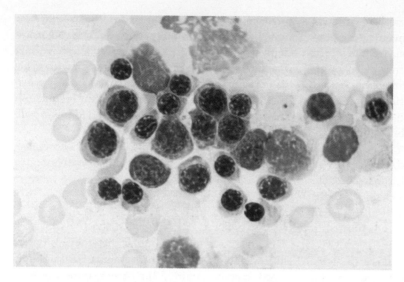

**Fig. 4.29** Bone marrow aspirate in sickle cell/$\beta^0$ thalassaemia compound heterozygosity showing erythroid hyperplasia and one sickle cell.

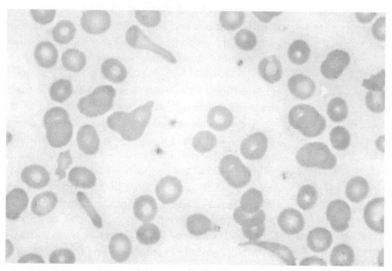

**Fig. 4.30** Blood film in sickle cell/haemoglobin D-Punjab compound heterozygosity.

## Other causes of sickle cell disease

### Sickle cell/haemoglobin D-Punjab/D-Los Angeles disease

Compound heterozygosity for sickle cell haemoglobin and haemoglobin D-Punjab (D-Los Angeles) leads to sickle cell disease which is, on average, slightly milder than sickle cell anaemia [9,96,123–127]. This compound heterozygous state has been observed in Afro-Americans, Afro-Caribbeans, Central and South Americans (Mexicans and Venezuelans) and Turks and, in addition, in a number of individuals of mixed ancestry (Northern European/American Indian, English/African, English/Afro-Caribbean) including several individuals who appeared to have only Mediterranean or Northern European ancestry. The clinical features are a mild or moderate haemolytic anaemia with sickling crises. Persisting splenomegaly is more common than in sickle cell anaemia. The haemoglobin concentration is usually between 5 and 10 g/dl and the reticulocyte count between 5% and 20% (occasionally higher). The MCV is very variable, but macrocytosis is quite common with some individuals having an MCV of 110–120 fl. The blood film (Fig. 4.30) shows anisocytosis, poikilocytosis, target cells, sickle cells, boat-shaped cells, nucleated red cells and sometimes macrocytes. The bone marrow shows erythroid hyperplasia and sickle cells (Fig. 4.31). On cellulose acetate electrophoresis at alkaline pH, haemoglobins S and D-Punjab show the same electrophoretic mobility, but HPLC and electrophoresis at acid pH separate these two haemoglobins from each other. Haemoglobin D forms a somewhat higher proportion of total haemoglobin than does haemoglobin S [127]. In a few cases, haemoglobin F is significantly elevated, e.g. 13–20% [126], but usually is present in only small amounts. Haemoglobin $A_2$ may be slightly elevated [127].

It should be noted that coinheritance of haemoglobin S and haemoglobin D variants other than haemoglobin D-Punjab/haemoglobin D-Los Angeles does not have the same adverse effects as sickle cell/haemoglobin D-Punjab compound heterozygosity. For example, two Nigerians with haemoglobin S/haemoglobin D-Ibadan were asymptomatic [125]. Similarly, haemoglobin D-Iran does not interact adversely with haemoglobin S.

## Sickle cell/haemoglobin O-Arab disease

Compound heterozygosity for sickle cell haemoglobin and haemoglobin O-Arab ($\alpha_2\beta_2^{121Glu \to Lys}$) leads to sickle cell disease that is generally severe

[9,96,128–130]. Sickle cell/haemoglobin O-Arab has been observed in Arabs, Africans (Sudanese and Kenyans), Afro-Caribbeans, Afro-Americans and Americans who appeared to be of Caucasian ancestry. The haemoglobin concentration in adults varies between 6.1 and 9.9 g/dl. The reticulocyte count is usually between 8% and 10% (1–15% reported). The reported MCVs have been quite variable, from normal to moderately macrocytic levels (82–110 fl in adults). The blood film (Fig. 4.32) is similar to that in sickle cell anaemia. The oxygen affinity is reduced, comparable to that seen in sickle cell anaemia. On electrophoresis on cellulose acetate at alkaline pH, haemoglobin O-Arab has a similar mobility to haemoglobin C (Fig. 4.33), but, at acid pH, the mobility depends on the electrophoresis medium. On agarose gel, it is slightly slower than haemoglobin S (Fig. 4.34). On HPLC, there are two abnormal peaks, one in the position of haemoglobin S and the other between haemoglobins S and C (Fig. 4.35). Haemoglobin O-Arab and haemoglobin C-Harlem can easily be confused with each other when present in the compound heterozygous state with haemoglobin S. The difference in mobility on citrate agar at acid pH is most useful in making the distinction (Table 4.10). Haemoglobin S forms a somewhat higher proportion of total haemoglobin than does haemoglobin O-Arab [127].

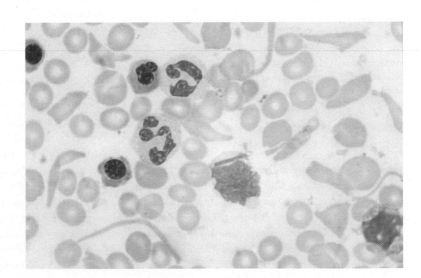

**Fig. 4.31** Bone marrow aspirate in sickle cell/haemoglobin D-Punjab compound heterozygosity showing prominent sickle cell formation.

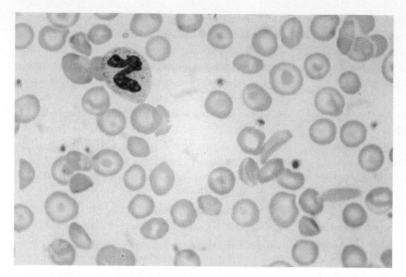

**Fig. 4.32** Blood film in sickle cell/haemoglobin O-Arab compound heterozygosity showing hypochromia, target cells and partially sickled cells. (Note: O-Arab in this patient was misidentified as C-Harlem in the previous edition of this book; the correct identity has been confirmed by family studies, citrate agar electrophoresis and mass spectrometry.)

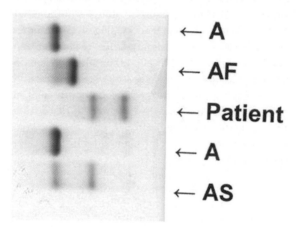

**Fig. 4.33** Haemoglobin electrophoresis on cellulose acetate at alkaline pH in sickle cell/haemoglobin O-Arab compound heterozygosity (Patient). By this technique, the pattern cannot be distinguished from that of sickle cell/haemoglobin C compound heterozygosity; other samples contain the haemoglobins indicated.

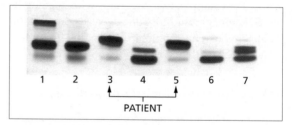

**Fig. 4.34** Haemoglobin electrophoresis on agarose gel at acid pH in sickle cell/haemoglobin O-Arab compound heterozygosity (lanes 3 and 5) showing a faint F band and broadening of the S band in the direction of C by the presence of O-Arab. From left to right, lanes are: (1) F, A and C; (2) F and A; (3) S plus O-Arab; (4) F and A; (5) S plus O-Arab; (6) F; (7) F, A and S. The mobility of O-Arab on this medium is more readily apparent in the absence of haemoglobin S (see Fig. 5.24).

## Sickle cell/haemoglobin C-Harlem compound heterozygosity

This condition is slightly milder than sickle cell anaemia. The blood film shows similar features. Haemoglobin electrophoresis at alkaline pH resembles that of sickle cell/haemoglobin C disease, whereas, at acid pH on citrate agar (but not agarose gel), there is a single band with the mobility of haemoglobin S (Table 4.10).

## Sickle cell/haemoglobin Lepore

Compound heterozygosity for sickle cell haemoglobin and haemoglobin Lepore-Boston [131,132] has been reported in Mediterranean (Greek and Italian), Afro-Caribbean and Afro-American populations. Sickle cell/haemoglobin Lepore leads to sickle cell disease of variable severity, but resembling sickle cell/β thalassaemia more closely than sickle cell anaemia. Of the 10 cases reported up to 1997, three were severe and seven were mild [132].

The haematological variables reported in adults [9,96,132] have included a haemoglobin concentra-

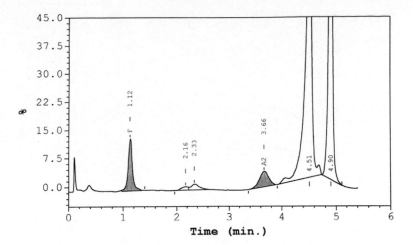

**Fig. 4.35**  HPLC chromatogram in a patient with haemoglobin S/O-Arab compound heterozygosity; the haemoglobin O-Arab in this and another patient had retention times on a Bio-Rad Variant II of 4.89 and 4.90 min respectively; from left to right, the peaks are altered F, haemoglobin F, altered S and haemoglobins $A_2$, S and O-Arab.

**Table 4.10**  Making a distinction between haemoglobin O-Arab and haemoglobin C-Harlem.

|  | Haemoglobin O-Arab | Haemoglobin C-Harlem |
| --- | --- | --- |
| Frequency | Uncommon | Rare |
| Clinical severity of compound heterozygous state with haemoglobin S | As severe as sickle cell anaemia | Somewhat milder than sickle cell anaemia |
| Sickle solubility test | Negative | Positive |
| Mobility on cellulose acetate electrophoresis at alkaline pH | Mobility of C | Mobility of C |
| Mobility on agarose gel electrophoresis at acid pH | Slightly slower than S (i.e. slightly towards C) | With S |
| Mobility on citrate agar electrophoresis at acid pH | Somewhat faster than S (i.e. slightly on the A side of S) | With S |
| High performance liquid chromatography | Between S and C | Between S and C |
| Isoelectric focusing | With E | With E |

tion of 8–13.3 g/dl, MCV of 66.5–83 fl, MCH of 24.3–27.6 pg and reticulocyte count of 3–13% (33% in one case). The blood film shows anisocytosis, hypochromia, microcytosis and some sickle cells.

As haemoglobin Lepore has the same mobility as haemoglobin S on electrophoresis at alkaline pH, the only bands apparently present are haemoglobins F, S and $A_2$, and diagnostic confusion with sickle cell anaemia and sickle cell/$\beta^0$ thalassaemia can therefore occur. However, other techniques, such as HPLC, show that haemoglobin Lepore is usually around 10–12% of total haemoglobin (20% in one

case), while haemoglobin S is 63–90% and haemoglobin F is 5–25%. Electrophoresis at acid pH shows two bands, one with the mobility of haemoglobin A, which represents haemoglobin Lepore. The proportion of haemoglobin $A_2$ is variable, having been reported to be reduced, normal or slightly elevated in different cases (0.9–4%) [9,132].

## Sickle cell/$\delta\beta^0$ thalassaemia

Sickle cell/$\delta\beta^0$ thalassaemia has been observed in Mediterranean populations (Greek, Sicilian, other

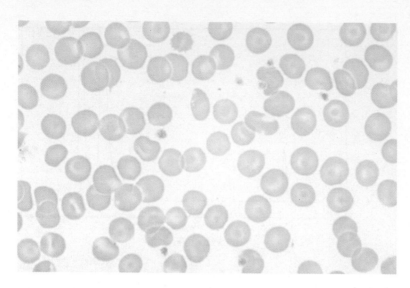

**Fig. 4.36** Blood film in sickle cell/hereditary persistence of fetal haemoglobin compound heterozygosity showing mild poikilocytosis and target cell formation.

Italian), Arabs and Afro-Americans [9,96]. This compound heterozygous state is generally much milder than sickle cell anaemia because the high percentage of haemoglobin F protects against sickling. There is mild anaemia and splenomegaly.

The blood count shows a haemoglobin concentration of around 10–12 g/dl and the MCV is slightly reduced (76–83 fl). The reticulocyte count is slightly elevated, usually 2–4%. The blood film shows anisocytosis, poikilocytosis and hypochromia. Haemoglobin S is the major haemoglobin component, with haemoglobin F being 15–37% of total haemoglobin. The proportion of haemoglobin $A_2$ is normal or low (1.5–3.1%). Sickle cell/$\delta\beta^0$ thalassaemia differs from microcytic cases of sickle cell anaemia, having a higher haemoglobin concentration, lower reticulocyte count and lower haemoglobin $A_2$ percentage (Table 4.7). However, definitive diagnosis requires DNA analysis.

### Sickle cell/hereditary persistence of fetal haemoglobin

Compound heterozygosity for haemoglobin S and deletional or pancellular hereditary persistence of fetal haemoglobin (HPFH) is either asymptomatic or produces quite mild sickle cell disease [96]. Haemoglobin S/HPFH has been reported in Africans, Afro-Caribbeans and Afro-Americans. There may be mild

haemolytic anaemia and splenomegaly or minor clinical features consequent on sickling. The haemoglobin and reticulocyte count are usually normal, but microcytosis is common and occasionally there is mild anaemia and reticulocytosis of 2–4%. The blood film (Fig. 4.36) may show anisocytosis, microcytosis and target cells. Haemoglobin electrophoresis or HPLC shows haemoglobin F of 15–35% (usually 20–30%), low-normal or slightly reduced haemoglobin $A_2$ and haemoglobin S comprising around 60–80% of total haemoglobin. Virtually all cells are F cells [92]. Haemoglobin A is absent. The proportions of various haemoglobins in haemoglobin S/HPFH are similar to those in haemoglobin S/$\beta^0$ thalassaemia. Distinction between the two is aided by the usual lack of symptoms and by the fact that the haemoglobin concentration and reticulocyte count are often normal in haemoglobin S/HPFH (Table 4.7). Definitive diagnosis requires family studies or DNA analysis.

### Sickle cell/haemoglobin E compound heterozygosity

Compound heterozygosity for haemoglobin S and haemoglobin E produces a condition that is either asymptomatic or clinically mild [9,96,133–136]. Sickle cell/haemoglobin E has been observed in Turks, Afro-Americans, Afro-Caribbeans, Saudi Arabians

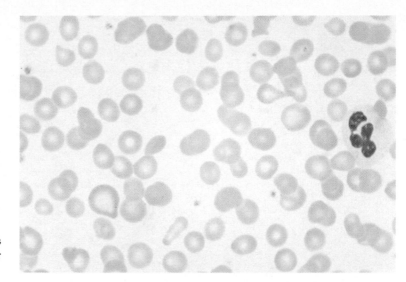

**Fig. 4.37** Blood film in sickle cell/haemoglobin E compound heterozygosity showing microcytosis and poikilocytosis. (By courtesy of Dr R. Gupta.)

and a Pakistani. There are sometimes minor symptoms that are probably related to sickling. There may be mild haemolysis, often compensated, and splenomegaly. Recurrent splenic infarction during aeroplane flights has been reported [134]. The haemoglobin concentration may be normal or reduced (8–14.6 g/dl) with sometimes a slight increase in the reticulocyte count (1.5–4%). The MCV may be normal or reduced (71–97 fl in adults). The blood film (Fig. 4.37) may show target cells which are sometimes numerous. Sickle cells have been observed [133], but this is not usual. Haemoglobin S is a larger proportion of total haemoglobin than haemoglobin E, e.g. around 60% [127,134,136] (Fig. 4.38). The haemoglobin E percentage tends to be higher than in individuals with haemoglobin E trait [127]. Haemoglobin F may be normal or slightly elevated [127,135].

## Sickle cell/$\delta^0\beta^+$ thalassaemia

Sickle cell/$\delta^0\beta^+$ thalassaemia, as the result of the formation of a $\delta\beta$ fusion gene, has been reported in four brothers in a Senegalese family. The haemoglobin concentration varied from 10.9 to 13.4 g/dl, MCV from 76 to 85 fl, haemoglobin S from 58% to 70%, haemoglobin A from 12% to 16% and haemoglobin F from 12% to 30% [137]. The propositus was asymptomatic.

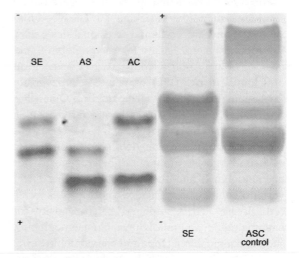

**Fig. 4.38** Haemoglobin electrophoresis at acid and alkaline pH in sickle cell/haemoglobin E compound heterozygosity; the first three lanes from the left are cellulose acetate electrophoresis at alkaline pH; the two lanes on the right are agarose gel electrophoresis at acid pH; ASC, control sample containing haemoglobins A, S and C. (By courtesy of Dr R. Gupta, Mr M. Jarvis and Dr A. Yardumian.)

## Other rare compound heterozygous states

Compound heterozygosity for haemoglobin C and haemoglobin C-Harlem appears to produce a much milder disease than sickle cell/haemoglobin C disease. One reported patient who presented with

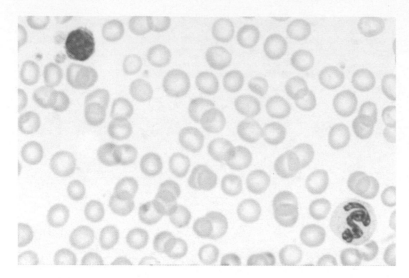

**Fig. 4.39** Blood film from a 1-year-old child with haemoglobin S/haemoglobin Siriraj compound heterozygosity showing anisocytosis and hypochromia. The red cell indices were RBC $4.87 \times 10^{12}$/l, Hb 11.2 g/dl, MCV 67 fl, MCH 23.3 pg and MCHC 34.4 g/dl.

haematuria had anaemia and splenomegaly, but no symptoms suggestive of sickling [7]. The blood film showed many target cells and occasional sickle cells. Compound heterozygosity for haemoglobin S and haemoglobin S-Antilles produces a very severe form of sickle cell disease [19]. Compound heterozygosity for haemoglobin S and haemoglobin S-Oman has been described, presenting at the age of 1 year [138]; it is likely that the phenotype will be severe as this double substitution haemoglobin can cause disease in heterozygotes. Compound heterozygosity for haemoglobin S and the electrophoretically silent variant, haemoglobin Quebec-Chori, causes sickle cell disease [24]. Compound heterozygosity for haemoglobin S and mildly unstable haemoglobins, such as haemoglobin Hope and haemoglobin Siriraj (Fig. 4.39), can cause mild haemolysis [96]. A compound heterozygote for haemoglobin S and haemoglobin Hofu (a fast-moving haemoglobin) had significant anaemia (haemoglobin concentration 9.6 g/dl), 73% haemoglobin S and apparently clinical features of sickling [127]. Compound heterozygosity for haemoglobin S and the $\gamma\beta$ fusion haemoglobin, haemoglobin Kenya, has an interestingly mild phenotype, given that haemoglobin S is 60–70% of total haemoglobin [139]. Haemoglobin Kenya is about 18% and haemoglobin F about 8%; haemoglobins F and $A_2$ will inhibit sickling and one might be tempted to postulate that this could also be true of haemoglo-

bin Kenya. Compound heterozygosity for haemoglobin S and various other variant haemoglobins can cause haematological abnormalities as a result of the characteristics of the second variant, rather than as a result of any interaction between the two variant haemoglobins; this appears to be true of haemoglobins I-Toulouse (unstable), San Diego (high oxygen affinity), Shelby (mildly unstable), Hope (unstable and low oxygen affinity) and North Shore ('thalassaemic') [52]. Compound heterozygosity for haemoglobin S and haemoglobin Monroe leads to a clinical syndrome resembling haemoglobin $S/\beta^0$ thalassaemia, as haemoglobin Monroe is unstable and constitutes only about 2% of total haemoglobin [140].

There are many $\beta$ chain variants that do not interact with haemoglobin S, so that compound heterozygotes have clinical and haematological features resembling those of sickle cell trait. These include haemoglobins Camden, Caribbean, D-Ouled Rabah, D-Ibadan, Detroit, G-Galveston, G-San Jose, G-Szuhu, J-Amiens, J-Baltimore, J-Bangkok, K-Ibadan, K-Matupo, Korle Bu, K-Woolwich, Mobile, N-Baltimore, Ocho-Rios, Osu-Christiansborg, Pyrgos and Richmond [54,69].

## Sickle cell disease in heterozygotes

Three variant haemoglobins in which the $\beta^{6Glu \rightarrow Val}$ substitution is one of two substitutions are capable of

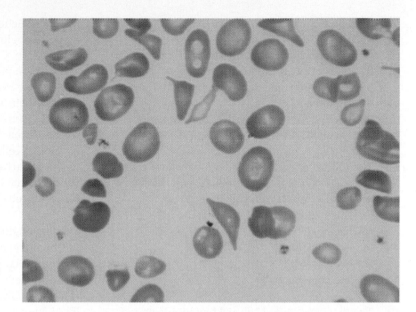

**Fig. 4.40** Blood film from a patient with compound heterozygosity for haemoglobin S and haemoglobin S-Oman showing the 'Napoleon hat' red cells that are characteristic of haemoglobin S-Oman. (With thanks to Dr Samir Al Azzawi, Muscat, Sultanate of Oman.)

producing sickle cell disease in heterozygotes. They are haemoglobin S-Antilles, haemoglobin S-Oman and haemoglobin Jamaica Plain (Table 4.2). In the case of haemoglobin S-Oman, severe disease occurs in heterozygotes with coinheritance of $-\alpha/\alpha\alpha$, who have 20–27% of the variant haemoglobin, whereas those with coinheritance of $-\alpha/-\alpha$, who have 13–15% of haemoglobin S-Oman, have no significant clinical disease. The morphology of sickle cells in patients who are simple or compound heterozygotes for haemoglobin S-Oman differs from the morphology of classical sickle cells. There are cells that are pointed at both ends but fat in the middle; they have been compared to a yarn/knitting needle or to 'Napoleon hats' [138] (Fig. 4.40). Affected heterozygotes also differ clinically from individuals with sickle cell anaemia in that splenomegaly can persist into adult life.

Sickle cell disease can also occur in heterozygotes if there is coinheritance of another condition leading to a high concentration of 2,3-diphosphoglycerate (2,3-DPG) and reduced oxygen affinity. For example, a patient who had coinherited a severe pyruvate kinase deficiency had a two-fold increase in 2,3-DPG leading to reduced oxygen affinity and symptomatic sickling crises [26].

## Check your knowledge

One to five answers may be correct. Answers to almost all questions can be found in this chapter or can be deduced from the information given. The correct answers are given on p. 189.

4.1 The coinheritance of haemoglobin S and the following haemoglobins usually produces a clinically significant sickling disorder
  (a) haemoglobin C
  (b) haemoglobin G-Philadelphia
  (c) haemoglobin D-Punjab
  (d) haemoglobin Lepore
  (e) haemoglobin A

4.2 Haemoglobin S occurs in a significant proportion of individuals from the following ethnic groups
  (a) Australian aboriginals
  (b) Greeks
  (c) southern Italians and Sicilians
  (d) Saudi Arabs
  (e) Nigerians

4.3 Recognized features of sickle cell trait include
(a) a defect in urine concentrating ability
(b) an increased incidence of gallstones
(c) an increased reticulocyte count
(d) leg ulcers
(e) susceptibility to clinically significant sickling in conditions of severe hypoxia

4.4 The following variant haemoglobins have the same mobility as haemoglobin S on cellulose acetate electrophoresis at alkaline pH
(a) haemoglobin C
(b) haemoglobin D
(c) haemoglobin E
(d) haemoglobin F
(e) haemoglobin G

4.5 The likelihood of red cell sickling occurring is increased by
(a) acidosis
(b) a lower partial pressure of oxygen
(c) an increased percentage of haemoglobin F
(d) reduced blood flow through tissues
(e) a lower mean cell haemoglobin concentration

4.6 In comparison with individuals with sickle cell anaemia, patients with compound heterozygosity for haemoglobin S and haemoglobin C usually have
(a) a higher percentage of haemoglobin A
(b) more severe anaemia
(c) a higher incidence of proliferative retinopathy
(d) a higher incidence of ischaemic necrosis of the femoral head
(e) earlier onset of blood film features of hyposplenism

4.7 Significant disease would be predicted in 25% of offspring if the partner of a pregnant woman with sickle cell trait had
(a) α thalassaemia trait
(b) β thalassaemia trait
(c) δ thalassaemia trait
(d) δβ thalassaemia trait

(e) non-deletional hereditary persistence of fetal haemoglobin

4.8 The disease phenotype is usually appreciably less severe than that of homozygosity for haemoglobin S in
(a) sickle cell/haemoglobin C disease
(b) sickle cell/$\beta^+$ thalassaemia
(c) sickle cell/deletional hereditary persistence of fetal haemoglobin
(d) sickle cell/$\delta\beta^0$ thalassaemia
(e) sickle cell/haemoglobin E

4.9 On haemoglobin electrophoresis at alkaline pH, homozygosity for haemoglobin S cannot be distinguished from
(a) sickle cell/haemoglobin C disease
(b) sickle cell/$\beta^0$ thalassaemia
(c) sickle cell/haemoglobin D-Punjab
(d) sickle cell/haemoglobin Lepore
(e) heterozygosity for both haemoglobin S and haemoglobin G-Philadelphia

4.10 A higher mortality rate in sickle cell anaemia correlates with
(a) a higher white cell count
(b) coexisting α thalassaemia trait
(c) a lower percentage of haemoglobin F
(d) male gender
(e) previous cerebrovascular accident

4.11 The blood count in sickle cell/haemoglobin C disease is characterized by
(a) generally mild anaemia
(b) reticulocytosis
(c) increased mean cell volume
(d) increased mean cell haemoglobin concentration
(e) increased red cell distribution width and haemoglobin distribution width

4.12 The haemoglobin F percentage in sickle cell anaemia is affected by
(a) age
(b) gender
(c) haplotype of the β globin gene cluster
(d) the F-cell locus on the X chromosome
(e) hydroxycarbamide (hydroxyurea) therapy

# Further reading

Bunn HF. Sickle hemoglobin and other hemoglobin mutants. In: Stamatoyannopoulos G, Nienhuis AW, Majerus PW and Varmus H, eds. *The Molecular Basis of Blood Diseases*, 2nd edn. W. B. Saunders, Philadelphia, PA, 1994, pp. 207–256.

Dacie J. *The Haemolytic Anaemias*, Volume 2, *The Hereditary Haemolytic Anaemias*, Part 2, 3rd edn. Churchill Livingstone, Edinburgh, 1988.

Lehmann H and Huntsman RG. *Man's Haemoglobins including the Haemoglobinopathies and their Investigation*. North Holland Publishing Company, Amsterdam, 1974.

Serjeant GR and Sergeant BE. *Sickle Cell Disease*, 3rd edn. Oxford University Press, Oxford, 2001.

Steinberg MH, Forget BG, Higgs DR and Nagel RL, eds. *Disorders of Hemoglobin: Genetics, Pathophysiology, and Clinical Management*. Cambridge University Press, Cambridge, 2001.

# References

1 Herrick JB (1910) Peculiar elongated and sickle shaped red blood corpuscles in a case of severe anemia. *Ann Intern Med* **6**, 517–521.

2 Pauling L, Itano HA, Singer SJ and Wells IC (1949) Sickle cell anaemia, a molecular disease. *Science* **110**, 543–548.

3 Ingram VM (1956) A specific chemical difference between the globins of normal human and sickle cell anaemia haemoglobin. *Nature* **178**, 792–794.

4 Powars DR (1991) $\beta^S$-gene-cluster in sickle cell anemia: clinical and hematologic features. *Hematol Oncol Clin North Am* **5**, 475–493.

5 White JM (1983) The approximate gene frequency of sickle haemoglobins in the Arabian peninsula. *Br J Haematol* **55**, 563–564.

6 Livingstone FB. *Frequencies of Hemoglobin Variants*. Oxford University Press, Oxford, 1985.

7 de Pablos JM (1985) Incidence of Hb C trait in an area of southern Spain. *Br J Haematol* **60**, 584–585.

8 Nagel RL and Fleming AF (1992) Genetic epidemiology of the $\beta^S$ gene. *Bailliere's Clin Haematol* **5**, 331–365.

9 Serjeant GR. *Sickle Cell Disease*, 2nd edn. Oxford University Press, Oxford, 1992.

10 Talafih K, Hunaiti AA, Gharaibeh N, Gharaibeh M and Jaradat S (1996) The prevalence of hemoglobin S and glucose-6-phosphate dehydrogenase deficiency in Jordanian newborn. *J Obstet Gynaecol Res* **22**, 417–420.

11 Wurie AT, Wurie JM, Gevao SM and Robbin-Coker DJ (1996) The prevalence of sickle cell trait in Sierra Leone: a laboratory profile. *West Afr J Med* **15**, 201–203.

12 Flint J, Harding RM, Boyce AJ and Clegg JB (1998) The population genetics of the haemoglobinopathies. *Bailliere's Clin Haematol* **11**, 1–51.

13 Segbena AY, Prehu C, Wajcman H, Bardakdjian-Michau J, Messie K, Feteke L *et al.* (1998) Hemoglobins in Togolese newborns: Hb S, Hb C, Hb Bart's, and $\alpha$-globin gene status. *Am J Hematol* **59**, 208–213.

14 St John MA and Lungu FN (1999) Haemoglobin electrophoresis patterns in Barbados. *West Indian Med J* **48**, 221–222.

15 de Silva S, Fisher CA, Premawardhena A, Lamabadusuriya SP, Peto TEA, Perera G *et al.* (2000) Thalassaemia in Sri Lanka: implications for the future health burden of Asian populations. *Lancet* **355**, 786–791.

16 Serjeant GR (2001) Historical review: the emerging understanding of sickle cell disease. *Br J Haematol* **112**, 3–18.

17 Kaur M, Das GP and Verma IC (1997) Sickle cell trait and disease among tribal communities in Orissa, Madhya Pradesh and Kerala. *Indian J Med Res* **105**, 111–116.

18 Serjeant GR and Sergeant BE. *Sickle Cell Disease*, 3rd edn. Oxford University Press, Oxford, 2001.

19 Monplaisir N, Merault G, Poyart C, Rhoda MD, Craescu C, Vidaud M *et al.* (1986) Hb S-Antilles: a new variant with a lower solubility than Hb S and producing sickle cell disease in heterozygotes. *Proc Natl Acad Sci USA* **83**, 9363–9367.

20 Kutlar F, Lallinger RR, Wright F, Holley L, Harbin J, Elam D and Kutlar A (2002) Hb S-Wake $\beta$(6Glu→Val +$\beta$139 Asp→Ser): a new sickling variant found in a compound heterozygous state with Hb S resulting in a severe sickling disorder. *Blood* **100**, 26b.

21 Geva A, Clark JJ, Zhang Y, Popowicz A, Manning JM and Neufeld EJ (2004) Hemoglobin Jamaica Plain — a sickling hemoglobin with reduced oxygen affinity. *N Engl J Med* **351**, 1532–1538.

22 Luo HY, Adewoye AH, Eung SH, Skelton TP, Quillen K, McMahon L *et al.* (2004) A novel sickle

hemoglobin: hemoglobin S-South End. *J Pediatr Hematol Oncol* **26**, 773–776.

23 Steinberg MH and Nagel RL. New and recombinant mutant hemoglobins of biological interest. In: Steinberg MH, Forget BG, Higgs DR and Nagel RL, eds. *Disorders of Hemoglobin: Genetics, Pathophysiology, and Clinical Management*. Cambridge University Press, Cambridge, 2001, pp. 1195–1211.

24 Witkowska HE, Lubin BH, Beuzard Y, Baruchel S, Esseltine DW, Vichinsky EP *et al*. (1991) Sickle cell disease in a patient with sickle cell trait and compound heterozygosity for hemoglobin S and hemoglobin Quebec-Chori. *N Engl J Med* **325**, 1150–1154.

25 Wong YS, Tanaka KR, Greenberg LH and Okada T (1969) Hematuria associated with haemoglobin CHarlem: a sickling hemoglobin variant. *J Urol* **102**, 762–764.

26 Cohen-Solal M, Préhu C, Wajcman H, Poyart C, Bardakdjian-Michau J, Kister J *et al*. (1998) A new sickle cell disease phenotype associating Hb S trait, severe pyruvate kinase deficiency (PK Conakry), and an α2 globin gene variant (Hb Conakry). *Br J Haematol* **103**, 950–956.

27 Nagel RL, Daar S, Romero JR, Suzuka M, Gravell D, Bouhassira E *et al*. (1998) HbS-Oman heterozygote: a new dominant sickle syndrome. *Blood* **92**, 4375–4382.

28 Jones SR, Binder RA and Donowho EM (1970) Sudden death in sickle-cell trait. *N Engl J Med* **28**, 323–325.

29 Koppes GM, Daly JJ, Coltman CA and Butkus DE (1977) Exertion-induced rhabdomyolysis with acute renal failure and disseminated intravascular coagulation in sickle cell trait. *Am J Med* **63**, 313–317.

30 Drehner D (1999) Death among U.S. Air Force basic trainees, 1956–1996. *Mil Med* **164**, 841–847.

31 Gupta AK, Kirchner KA, Nicholson R, Adams JG, Schechter AN, Noguchi CT and Steinberg MH (1991) Effects of alpha-thalassemia and sickle polymerization tendency on the urine-concentrating defect of individuals with sickle cell trait. *J Clin Invest* **88**, 1963–1968.

32 Domingues MC, Domingues LAW, Ostonoff M, Matias C, Araujo AS, Florêncio R *et al*. (2003) Report of a rare case of splenic sequestration in a patient with sickle cell trait. *Blood* **102**, 31b.

33 Rimer BA (1975) Sickle-cell trait and pregnancy: a review of a community hospital experience. *Am J Obstet Gynecol* **123**, 6–9.

34 Larrabee KD and Monga M (1997) Women with sickle cell trait are at increased risk of preeclampsia. *Am J Obstet Gynecol* **177**, 425–428.

35 Adsay NV, deRoux SJ, Sakr W and Grignon D (1999) Cancer as a marker of genetic medical disease: an unusual case of medullary carcinoma of the kidney. *Am J Surg Pathol* **22**, 260–264.

36 Steinberg MH and Embury SH (1986) β-Thalassaemia in blacks: genetic and clinical aspects and interactions with sickle hemoglobin gene. *Blood* **69**, 985–990.

37 Felice AE, Altay CA, Milner PF and Huisman THJ (1981) The occurrence and identification of α-thalassemia-2 among hemoglobin S heterozygotes. *Am J Clin Pathol* **76**, 70–73.

38 Higgs DR, Aldridge BE, Lamb J, Clegg JB, Weatherall DJ, Hayes RJ *et al*. (1982) The interaction of alpha-thalassaemia and homozygous sickle-cell disease. *N Engl J Med* **306**, 1441–1446.

39 Head CE, Conroy M, Jarvis M, Phelan L and Bain BJ (2004) Some observations on the measurement of haemoglobin $A_2$ and S percentages by high performance liquid chromatography in the presence and absence of thalassaemia. *J Clin Pathol* **57**, 276–280.

40 Steinberg MH (1991) The interactions of β-thalassaemia with hemoglobinopathies. *Hematol Oncol Clin North Am* **5**, 453–473.

41 Mears JG, Lachman HM, Labie D and Nagel RL (1983) Alpha-thalassemia is related to prolonged survival in sickle cell anemia. *Blood* **62**, 286–290.

42 Wilson CI, Hopkins PL, Cabello-Inchausti B, Melnick SJ and Robinson MJ (2000) The peripheral blood smear in patients with sickle cell trait: a morphologic observation. *Lab Med* **31**, 445–447.

43 Thompson GR (1963) Malaria and stress in relation to haemoglobins S and C. *Br Med J* **ii**, 976–978.

44 Bain BJ and Phelan L (1996) An evaluation of the HemoCard Hemoglobin S test and four sickle cell solubility kits (Ortho Sickledex, Dade Sickle-Sol, Microgen Bioproducts S-Test and Lorne Sickle-Check) for the detection of haemoglobin S and the HemoCard Hemoglobin A plus S test for the detection of haemoglobins A and S. *MDA Evaluation Report MDA/96/56*, Medical Devices Agency, London.

45 Higgs DR, Clegg JB, Weatherall DJ, Serjeant BE and Serjeant GR (1984) The interaction of the αααα glo-

bin gene haplotype and sickle haemoglobin. *Br J Haematol* **58**, 671–678.

46 Baklouti F, Ouazana R, Gonnet C, Lapillonne A, Delaunay J and Godet J (1989) β⁺-Thalassemia in *cis* of a sickle cell gene — occurrence of a promoter mutation on a β$^S$ chromosome. *Blood* **74**, 1817–1822.

47 Levere RD, Lichtman HC and Levine J (1964) Effect of iron deficiency anaemia on the metabolism of the heterogenic haemoglobins in sickle cell trait. *Nature* **202**, 499–501.

48 Heller P, Yakulis VJ, Epstein RB and Friedland S (1963) Variation in the amount of hemoglobin S in a patient with sickle cell trait and megaloblastic anemia. *Blood* **21**, 479–483.

49 Steinberg MH. Sickle cell trait. In: Steinberg MH, Forget BG, Higgs DR and Nagel RL, eds. *Disorders of Hemoglobin: Genetics, Pathophysiology, and Clinical Management*. Cambridge University Press, Cambridge, 2001, pp. 811–830.

50 Almeida AM, Henthorn JS and Davies SC (2001) Haemoglobin F levels in patients with sickle cell diseases. *Blood* **98**, 13b.

51 Matthay KK, Mentzer WC, Dozy AM, Kan YW and Bainton DF (1979) Modification of hemoglobin H disease by sickle trait. *J Clin Invest* **64**, 1024–1032.

52 Steinberg MH. Compound heterozygous and other sickle haemoglobinopathies. In: Steinberg MH, Forget BG, Higgs DR and Nagel RL, eds. *Disorders of Hemoglobin: Genetics, Pathophysiology, and Clinical Management*. Cambridge University Press, Cambridge, 2001, pp. 786–810.

53 Ustun C, Kutlat F, Holley L, Seigler N, Burgess R and Kutlar A (2003) Interaction of sickle cell trait with hereditary spherocytosis: splenic infarcts and sequestration. *Acta Haematol* **109**, 46–49.

54 Farber HW and Loscalzo J (2004) Pulmonary arterial hypertension. *N Engl J Med* **351**, 1655–1665.

55 Adekile AD, Owunwanne A, Al-Za'abi K, Haider MZ, Tuli M and Al-Mohannadi S (2002) Temporal sequence of splenic dysfunction in sickle cell disease. *Am J Hematol* **69**, 23–27.

56 King KE, Shirey RS, Lankiewicz MW, Young-Ramsaran J and Ness PM (1997) Delayed hemolytic transfusion reactions in sickle cell disease: simultaneous destruction of patients' red cells. *Transfusion* **37**, 376–381.

57 Shafeek S, Jabbar M, Strevens MJ, Oakley S, Bareford D and Smith N (2000) Two cases of post transfusion hyperhaemolysis in sickle cell disease. *Br J Haematol* **108**, Suppl. 1, 38.

58 Platt OS, Brambilla DJ, Rosse WF, Milner PF, Castro O, Steinberg MH and Klug PP (1994) Mortality in sickle cell disease: life expectancy and risk factors for early death. *N Engl J Med* **330**, 1639–1644.

59 Ohene-Frempong K and Steinberg MH. Clinical aspects of sickle cell anemia in adults and children. In: Steinberg MH, Forget BG, Higgs DR and Nagel RL, eds. *Disorders of Hemoglobin: Genetics, Pathophysiology, and Clinical Management*. Cambridge University Press, Cambridge, 2001, pp. 611–670.

60 Neonato MG, Guilloud-Bataille M, Beauvais P, Bégue P, Belloy M, Benkerrou M *et al.* (2000) Acute clinical events in 299 homozygous sickle cell patients living in France. *Eur J Haematol* **65**, 155–164.

61 Bailey S, Higgs DR, Morris J and Serjeant GR (1991) Is the painful crisis of sickle-cell disease due to sickling? *Lancet* **337**, 735.

62 Castro O and Haddy TB (1983) Improved survival of iron-deficient sickle erythrocytes. *N Engl J Med* **308**, 527.

63 Ballas SK (1998) Sickle cell disease: clinical management. *Bailliere's Clin Haematol* **11**, 185–214.

64 Ballas SK, Gay RN and Chehab FF (1997) Is Hb A$_2$ elevated in adults with sickle-α-thalassemia (β$^S$/β$^S$;–α/–α)? *Hemoglobin* **21**, 405–450.

65 Mukherjee MB, Lu CY, Ducrocq R, Gangakhedkar RR, Colah RB, Kadam MD *et al.* (1997) Effect of α-thalassaemia on sickle cell anemia linked to the Arab–Indian haplotype in India. *Am J Hematol* **55**, 104–109.

66 Davis LR (1976) Changing blood picture in sickle-cell anaemia from shortly after birth to adolescence. *J Clin Pathol* **29**, 898–901.

67 Serjeant GR, Grandison Y, Lowrie Y, Mason K, Phillips J, Serjeant BE and Vaidya S (1981) The development of haematological changes in homozygous sickle cell disease: a cohort study from birth to 6 years. *Br J Haematol* **48**, 533–543.

68 Sherwood JB, Goldwasser E, Chilcote R, Carmichael LD and Nagel RL (1986) Sickle cell anemia patients have low erythropoietin levels for their degree of anemia. *Blood* **67**, 46–49.

69 Dover GJ, Chang VT, Boyer SH, Sergeant GR, Antonarakis S and Higgs DR (1987) The cellular basis for different fetal hemoglobin levels among sickle cell individuals with two, three and four alpha-globin genes. *Blood* **69**, 341–344.

70 Thame M, Grandison Y, Mason K, Thompson M, Higgs D, Morris J et al. (1991) The red cell distribution width in sickle cell disease — is it of clinical value? *Clin Lab Haematol* **13**, 229–237.

71 Castro O, Brambilla DJ, Thorington B, Reindorf CA, Scott RB, Gillette P et al. and the Cooperative Study of Sickle Cell Disease (1994) The acute chest syndrome in sickle cell disease: incidence and risk factors. *Blood* **84**, 643–649.

72 Wong W-Y, Zhou Y, Operskalski EA, Hassett J, Powars DR, Mosley JW and the Transfusion Safety Study Group (1996) Hematologic profile and lymphocyte subpopulations in hemoglobin SC disease: comparison with SS and black controls. *Am J Hematol* **52**, 150–154.

73 Embury SH, Dozy AM, Miller J, Davis JR, Kleman KM, Preisler H et al. (1982) Concurrent sickle-cell anemia and α-thalassemia: effect on severity of anemia. *N Engl J Med* **306**, 270–274.

74 Rabb LM, Grandison Y, Mason K, Hayes RJ, Serjeant B and Serjeant GR (1983) A trial of folate supplementation in children with homozygous sickle cell disease. *Br J Haematol* **54**, 589–594.

75 Ballas SK and Smith ED (1992) Red blood cell changes during the evolution of the sickle cell painful crisis. *Blood* **29**, 2154–2163.

76 Vichinsky E and Styles E (1996) Pulmonary complications. *Hematol Oncol Clin North Am* **10**, 1275–1287.

77 Bain BJ (1993) Blood film features of sickle cell–haemoglobin C disease. *Br J Haematol* **83**, 516–518.

78 Weinstein RS, Warth JA, Near K and Marikovsky Y (1989) Sequestrocytes: a manifestation of transcellular cross-bonding of the red cell membrane in sickle cell anemia. *J Cell Sci* **94**, 593–600.

79 Ward PC, Smith CM and White JG (1979) Erythrocytic ecdysis. An unusual morphologic finding in a case of sickle cell anemia with intercurrent cold-agglutinin syndrome. *Am J Clin Pathol* **72**, 479–485.

80 Adekile AD, Al-Zaabi K, Haider MZ and Tuli M (1997) Molecular and hematological correlates of splenic function among Arab SS patients. *Blood* **90**, Suppl. 1, 216.

81 Bunn HF. Sickle hemoglobin and other hemoglobin mutants. In: Stamatoyannopoulos G, Nienhuis AW, Majerus PW and Varmus H, eds. *The Molecular Basis of Blood Diseases*, 2nd edn. W. B. Saunders, Philadelphia, PA, 1994, pp. 207–256.

82 Warth JA and Rucknagel DL (1984) Density ultracentrifugation during and after pain crisis; increased dense echinocytes in crisis. *Blood* **64**, 507–515.

83 Steinberg MH (1998) Pathophysiology of sickle cell disease. *Bailliere's Clin Haematol* **11**, 163–184.

84 Smetanina NS, Gu L-H and Huisman THJ (1998) Comparison of the relative quantities of γ-messenger RNA and fetal hemoglobin in SS patients with different haplotypes. *Acta Haematol* **100**, 4–8.

85 US Department of Health and Human Services (1993) Guideline: laboratory screening for sickle cell disease. *Lab Med* **24**, 515–522.

86 Bain BJ and Phelan L (1996) An assessment of HemoCard Hemoglobin C and HemoCard Hemoglobin E kits for the detection of haemoglobins C and E. *MDA Evaluation Report MDA/96/57*, Medical Devices Agency, London.

87 Smith SGW, Glass UH, Acharya J and Pearson TC (1989) Pulse oximetry in sickle cell disease. *Clin Lab Haematol* **11**, 185–188.

88 Goldberg MA, Brugnara C, Dover GJ, Schapira L, Charache S and Bunn HF (1990) Treatment of sickle cell anemia with hydroxyurea and erythropoietin. *N Engl J Med* **323**, 366–372.

89 Merghoub T, Perichon B, Maier-Redelsperger M, Dibenedetto SP, Samperi P, Ducrocq R et al. (1997) Dissection of the association status of two polymorphisms in the β-globin gene cluster with variations in F-cell number in non-anemic individuals. *Am J Hematol* **56**, 239–243.

90 Gonçalves I, Ducrocq R, Lavinha J, Nogueira PJ, Peres MJ, Picanco I et al. (1998) Combined effect of two different polymorphic sequences within the β globin gene cluster on the level of Hb F. *Am J Hematol* **57**, 269–276.

91 Thomas JJ, Kutlar A, Scott DF and Lanclos KD (1998) Inhibition of gene expression by the $^Gγ$ 5′ flanking region of the Bantu $β^S$ chromosome. *Am J Hematol* **59**, 51–56.

92 Marcus SJ, Kinney TR, Schultz WH, O'Branski EE and Ware RE (1997) Quantitative analysis of erythrocytes containing fetal hemoglobin F (F cells) in children with sickle cell disease. *Am J Hematol* **54**, 40–46.

93 Chang YP, Maier-Redelsperger M, Smith KD, Contu L, Ducrocq R, de Montalembert M et al. (1997) The relative importance of the X-linked FCP locus and β-globin haplotypes in determining haemoglobin F levels: a study of SS patients

homozygous for $\beta^S$ haplotype. *Br J Haematol* **96**, 806–814.

94 Milner PF, Garbutt GJ, Nolan-Davis LB and Wilson JT (1986) The effect of hemoglobin F and α thalassaemia on the red cell indices in sickle cell anemia. *Am J Hematol* **21**, 383–395.

95 Rising JA, Sautter RL and Spicer SJ (1974) Hemoglobin G-Philadelphia/S. *Am J Clin Pathol* **61**, 92–102.

96 Dacie J. *The Haemolytic Anaemias*, Volume 2, *The Hereditary Haemolytic Anaemias*, Part 2, 3rd edn. Churchill Livingstone, Edinburgh, 1988.

97 Krauss JS, Bures K and Kenimer E (1999) The elution of αMontgomery$_2\beta$S$_2$ hybrid tetramers by the Variant™ apparatus. *Blood* **94**, Suppl. 1, 25b.

98 Nagel RL, Fabry ME and Steinberg MH (2003) The paradox of hemoglobin SC disease. *Blood Rev* **17**, 167–178.

99 Adams JG and Heller P (1977) Hemoglobin Arlington Park. A new hemoglobin variant with two amino acid substitutions in the beta chain. *Hemoglobin* **1**, 419–426.

100 Nisbet-Brown E, Stehmaier K, Walker L, Waye JS and Chui DHK (2000) Sickle cell disease in a four year old child with apparent HbS trait. *Blood* **96**, 20b.

101 Powars DR, Hiti A, Ramicone E, Johnson C and Chan L (2002) Outcome in hemoglobin SC disease: a four-decade observational study of clinical, hematologic, and genetic factors. *Am J Hematol* **70**, 206–215.

102 Ware M, Tyghter D, Staniforth S and Serjeant G (1998) Airline travel in sickle cell disease. *Lancet* **352**, 652.

103 Zimmerman SA and Ware RE (2000) Palpable splenomegaly in children with haemoglobin SC disease: haematological and clinical manifestations. *Clin Lab Haematol* **22**, 145–150.

104 Serjeant GR and Serjeant BE (1972) A comparison of erythrocytic characteristics in sickle cell syndromes in Jamaica. *Br J Haematol* **23**, 205–213.

105 Lee K, Préhu C, Mérault G, Kéclard L, Roudot-Thoroval F, Bachir D *et al.* (1998) Genetic and hematological studies in a group of 114 adult patients with SC sickle cell disease. *Am J Hematol* **59**, 15–21.

106 Ballas SK, Larner J, Smith ED, Surrey S, Schwartz E and Rappaport EF (1987) The xerocytosis of SC disease. *Blood* **69**, 124–128.

107 Ballas SK and Kosher W (1988) Erythrocytes in Hb SC disease are microcytic and hyperchromic. *Am J Hematol* **28**, 37–39.

108 Steinberg MH and Hebbel RP (1983) Clinical diversity of sickle cell anemia: genetic and cellular modulation of disease severity. *Am J Hematol* **14**, 405–416.

109 Diggs LW and Bell A (1965) Intraerythrocytic hemoglobin C crystals in sickle cell–hemoglobin C disease. *Blood* **25**, 218–223.

110 Bertles JF, Rabinowitz R and Dobler J (1970) Hemoglobin interaction: modification of solid phase composition in the sickling phenomenon. *Science* **169**, 375–377.

111 Lin MJ, Nagel RL and Hirsch RE (1989) Acceleration of hemoglobin C crystallization by hemoglobin S. *Blood* **74**, 1823–1825.

112 Lawrence C, Fabry ME and Nagel RL (1991) The unique red cell heterogeneity of SC disease. *Blood* **78**, 2104–2112.

113 Rucknagel DL and Rising JA (1975) A heterozygote for Hb$^S_\beta$, Hb$^C_\beta$ and Hb$^{G\ Philadelphia}_\alpha$ in a family presenting with evidence of heterogeneity of hemoglobin alpha chain loci. *Am J Med* **59**, 53–60.

114 Lawrence C, Hirsch RE, Fatalieo NA, Patel S, Fabry ME and Nagel RL (1997) Molecular interactions between α-G Philadelphia, Hb C, and Hb S: phenotypic implications for SC α-G Philadelphia disease. *Blood* **90**, 2819–2825.

115 Serjeant GR, Ashcroft MT, Serjeant BE and Milner PF (1973) The clinical features of sickle cell/β thalassaemia in Jamaica. *Br J Haematol* **24**, 19–30.

116 Serjeant GR, Sommereaux A-M, Stevenson M, Mason K and Serjeant B (1979) Comparison of sickle cell–β$^0$ thalassaemia with homozygous sickle cell disease. *Br J Haematol* **41**, 83–93.

117 Gonzales-Redondo JM, Kutlar F, Kutlar A, Stoming TA, de Pablos JM, Kilione Y and Huisman THJ (1988) Hb S(C)–β$^+$-thalassaemia: different mutations are associated with different levels of normal HbA$_2$. *Br J Haematol* **70**, 85–89.

118 Yang Y-M, Donnell CA, Farrer JH and Mankad VN (1990) Molecular characterization of β-globin gene mutations in Malay patients with Hb E–β-thalassaemia and thalassaemia major. *Br J Haematol* **72**, 73–80.

119 Christakis J, Vavatsi N, Hassapopoulou H, Angeloudi M, Papadopoulou M, Loukopoulos D *et al.* (1991) A comparison of sickle cell syn-

dromes in northern Greece. *Br J Haematol* **77**, 386–391.

120  Kuloziz AE, Bail S, Kar BC, Serjeant BE and Serjeant GR (1991) Sickle cell–$\beta^+$ thalassaemia in Orissa state, India. Its interactions with the sickle cell gene. *Br J Haematol* **77**, 215–220.

121  Serjeant BE, Mason KP and Serjeant GR (1978) The development of haemoglobin A$_2$ in normal Negro infants and in sickle cell disease. *Br J Haematol* **39**, 259–263.

122  Tadmouri GO, Yüksel L and Basak AN (1998) HbS/$\beta^{del}$-thalassaemia associated with high levels of hemoglobins A$_2$ and F in a Turkish family. *Am J Hematol* **59**, 83–86.

123  McCurdy PR and Gieschen MM (1960) Clinical and physiologic studies in a Negro with sickle-cell hemoglobin D disease. *N Engl J Med* **262**, 961–964.

124  Charache S and Conley CL (1964) Rate of sickling of red cells during deoxygenation of blood from persons with various sickling disorders. *Blood* **24**, 25–48.

125  Schneider RD, Ueda S, Alperin JB, Levin WC, Jones RT and Brimhall B (1968) Hemoglobin D Los Angeles in two Caucasian families: hemoglobin SD disease and hemoglobin D thalassemia. *Blood* **32**, 250–259.

126  Özsoylu S (1969) Haemoglobin S-D disease in a Turkish family. *Scand J Haematol* **6**, 10–14.

127  Huisman THJ (1997) Combinations of β chain abnormal hemoglobins with each other and with β-thalassemia determinants with known mutations: influence on phenotype. *Clin Chem* **43**, 1850–1856.

128  Milner PF, Miller C, Grey R, Seakins M, Dejong WW and Went LM (1970) Hemoglobin O Arab in four negro families and its interaction with hemoglobin S and hemoglobin C. *N Engl J Med* **283**, 1417–1425.

129  Charache S, Zinkham WH, Dickerman JD, Birmhall B and Dover GJ (1977) Hemoglobin SC, SS/G Philadelphia and SO Arab diseases. Diagnostic importance of an integrative analysis of clinical, hematologic and electrophoretic findings. *Am J Med* **62**, 439–446.

130  Zimmerman SA, O'Branski EE, Rosse WF and Ware RE (1999) Hemoglobin S/O(Arab): thirteen new cases and review of the literature. *Am J Hematol* **60**, 279–284.

131  Silvestroni E, Bianco I and Baglioni C (1965) Interaction of hemoglobin Lepore with sickle cell trait and microcythemia (thalassemia) in a southern Italian family. *Blood* **25**, 457–469.

132  Fairbanks VF, McCormick DJ, Kubik KS, Rezuke WN, Black D, Ochaney MS and Schwartz D (1997) Hb S/Hb Lepore with mild sickling symptoms: a hemoglobin variant with mostly δ-chain sequences ameliorates sickle-cell disease. *Am J Hematol* **54**, 164–165.

133  Aksoy M (1960) The hemoglobin E syndromes. II. Sickle-cell–hemoglobin E disease. *Blood* **15**, 610–613.

134  Schroeder WA, Powars D, Reynolds RD and Fisher JI (1976) Hb-E in combination with Hb-S and Hb-C in a black family. *Hemoglobin* **1**, 287–289.

135  Bird AR, Wood K, Leisegang F, Mathew CG, Ellis P, Hartley PS and Karabus CD (1984) Haemoglobin E variants: a clinical, haematological and biosynthetic study of 4 South African families. *Acta Haematol* **72**, 135–137.

136  Gupta R, Jarvis M and Yardumian A (2000) Compound heterozygosity for haemoglobin S and haemoglobin E. *Br J Haematol* **108**, 463.

137  Zertal-Zidani S, Ducrocq R, Weil-Oliver C, Elion J and Krishnamoorthy R (2001) A novel δβ fusion gene expresses hemoglobin A (HbA) not Hb Lepore: Senegalese $\delta^0\beta^+$ thalassaemia. *Blood* **98**, 1261–1263.

138  Al Jahdhamy R, Makki H, Farrell G and Al Azzawi AS (2002) A case of compound heterozygosity for Hb S and Hb S Oman. *Br J Haematol* **116**, 504.

139  Kendall AG, Ojwang PJ, Schroeder WA and Huisman TH (1973) Hemoglobin Kenya, the product of a gamma–beta fusion gene: studies of the family. *Am J Hum Genet* **25**, 548–563.

140  Sweeting I, Serjeant BE, Serjeant GR, Kulozik AE and Vetter B (1998) Hb S–Hb Monroe; a sickle cell–beta-thalassemia syndrome. *Hemoglobin* **22**, 153–156.

## Answers to questions

| 4.1 | | | 4.3 | | | 4.5 | | | 4.7 | | | 4.9 | | | 4.11 | | |
|-----|---|---|-----|---|---|-----|---|---|-----|---|---|-----|---|---|------|---|---|
| | (a) | T | | (a) | T | | (a) | T | | (a) | F | | (a) | F | | (a) | T |
| | (b) | F | | (b) | F | | (b) | T | | (b) | T | | (b) | T | | (b) | T |
| | (c) | T | | (c) | F | | (c) | F | | (c) | F | | (c) | T | | (c) | F |
| | (d) | T | | (d) | F | | (d) | T | | (d) | T | | (d) | T | | (d) | T |
| | (e) | F | | (e) | T | | (e) | F | | (e) | F | | (e) | F | | (e) | T |

| 4.2 | | | 4.4 | | | 4.6 | | | 4.8 | | | 4.10 | | | 4.12 | | |
|-----|---|---|-----|---|---|-----|---|---|-----|---|---|------|---|---|------|---|---|
| | (a) | F | | (a) | F | | (a) | F | | (a) | T | | (a) | T | | (a) | T |
| | (b) | T | | (b) | T | | (b) | F | | (b) | T | | (b) | F | | (b) | T |
| | (c) | T | | (c) | F | | (c) | T | | (c) | T | | (c) | T | | (c) | T |
| | (d) | T | | (d) | F | | (d) | T | | (d) | T | | (d) | T | | (d) | T |
| | (e) | T | | (e) | T | | (e) | F | | (e) | T | | (e) | T | | (e) | T |

# 5 Other significant haemoglobinopathies

Variant haemoglobins may be clinically significant, but many are clinically silent. The recognition of those that are clinically silent may, nevertheless, be important in the diagnostic laboratory as their presence can lead to diagnostic confusion. Problems of two types can arise. Clinically irrelevant variant haemoglobins can be confused with clinically significant variants because of similar electrophoretic mobility or high performance liquid chromatography (HPLC) retention time. In addition, there may be coinheritance of two variants, leading to the presence of multiple bands on electrophoresis that can be difficult to interpret. This chapter therefore deals with both clinically relevant haemoglobinopathies and other variant haemoglobins that can cause diagnostic confusion.

The majority of recognized variant haemoglobins are $\alpha$ or $\beta$ chain variants. A variant $\alpha$ chain leads to variant forms of haemoglobins A, $A_2$ and F. A variant $\beta$ chain leads to a variant of haemoglobin A. $\delta$ and $\gamma$ chain variants also occur. Functional abnormalities of haemoglobin that can result from mutations in globin genes are shown in Table 5.1.

It should be noted that, although low-oxygen-affinity haemoglobins lead to anaemia and sometimes cyanosis, there is no clinically significant abnormality as there is normal oxygen delivery to tissues. The anaemia is consequent on a reduced erythropoietic drive.

The variant haemoglobins that are of diagnostic but not clinical significance are mainly haemoglobins with the mobility of either S or C/E on cellulose acetate electrophoresis at alkaline pH. There are also other, less common, variant haemoglobins that are diagnostically important because they have similar retention times to S, C, E, D-Punjab or glycosylated haemoglobin A on HPLC. If cellulose acetate electrophoresis is the primary method, it is important to distinguish haemoglobins such as haemoglobin G-Philadelphia or haemoglobin D-Iran, which are not clinically important, from haemoglobin D-Punjab/Los Angeles, which is of importance because of its interaction with haemoglobin S. If HPLC is the primary method, the uncommon variant haemoglobins that have a similar retention time to clinically important variants must similarly be distinguished from each other, e.g. haemoglobin E from haemoglobin Lepore and haemoglobin D-Punjab from haemoglobin G-Philadelphia (see Table 2.3).

A $\beta$ chain variant would be expected to comprise about 50% of total haemoglobin. However, if the abnormal $\beta$ chain is synthesized at a reduced rate or if there is preferential combination of $\alpha$ chains with the normal rather than the variant $\beta$ chain, the proportion will be less. Amongst the variant $\beta$ chains synthesized at a considerably reduced rate is $\beta^E$, with the result that the proportion of haemoglobin E in heterozygotes does not usually exceed 30%. Variant chains with a reduced affinity for the $\alpha$ chain, in comparison with $\beta^A$, include $\beta^S$ and $\beta^C$, probably because they are more electropositive than the normal $\beta$ chain [1,2]; as a result of the reduced affinity, the percentage of the variant is somewhat less than 50%. The converse is seen with variant $\beta$ chains, including $\beta^{J\text{-Baltimore}}$ and $\beta^{J\text{-Iran}}$, which are more electronegative [1,2] and have a greater affinity than the normal $\beta$ chain for $\alpha$ chains; the percentage of the variant is therefore greater than 50%. When there is coexisting $\alpha$ thalassaemia, a positively charged variant chain, such as $\beta^S$ or $\beta^C$, competes less well than $\beta$ for the reduced number of $\alpha$ chains, so that the percentage of the variant is lower than in individuals with a full complement of $\alpha$ genes. The converse is seen with variants such as J-Baltimore, when the negatively charged variant chain is more able to compete for the reduced pool of $\alpha$ chains and the variant is present in an even higher percentage [1].

**Table 5.1** Types of functional abnormality that can occur as a result of mutations in globin genes.

| Functional abnormality | Example |
| --- | --- |
| Polymerization leading to sickle cell formation | Haemoglobin S, haemoglobin C-Harlem |
| Interaction with haemoglobin S, permitting sickling in compound heterozygotes | Haemoglobin D-Punjab/D-Los Angeles, haemoglobin C, haemoglobin O-Arab |
| Reduced solubility leading to crystal formation and haemolytic anaemia | Haemoglobin C |
| Increased oxygen affinity leading to polycythaemia | Haemoglobin Chesapeake, haemoglobin Kempsey |
| Reduced oxygen affinity leading to anaemia | Haemoglobin S, haemoglobin Kansas |
| Haemoglobin instability leading to a Heinz body haemolytic anaemia | Haemoglobin Köln |
| Extreme instability leading to a thalassaemic phenotype | Haemoglobin Terre Haute |
| Reduced rate of synthesis leading to a thalassaemic phenotype | Haemoglobin Lepore, haemoglobin E |
| Increased tendency to oxidation leading to methaemoglobin formation and cyanosis | Haemoglobin M-Saskatoon, haemoglobin M-Hyde Park |

Predicting the percentage of an $\alpha$ chain variant is more complex as not only are there four $\alpha$ genes, but the $\alpha 2$ globin gene is transcribed at a higher rate than the $\alpha 1$ globin gene. The two allelic $\alpha 2$ genes normally contribute between them about 75% of $\alpha$ chains. An $\alpha$ chain variant would therefore be expected to comprise either about 37.5% or about 12.5% of total haemoglobin. Proportions may differ if: (i) the variant $\alpha$ chain is synthesized at a reduced rate; (ii) the variant $\alpha$ chain shows a greater or lesser affinity for the $\beta$ chain than does the normal $\alpha$ chain; (iii) the variant haemoglobin is also unstable; or (iv) there is coexisting $\alpha$ thalassaemia. As for $\beta$ globin variants, charge may influence the affinity of the variant $\alpha$ chain for the normal $\beta$ chain. For example, $\alpha^{M\text{-Iwate}}$, which is more electropositive than the normal $\alpha$ chain, combines preferentially with electronegative $\beta$ chains so that haemoglobin M-Iwate comprises 22–27% of total haemoglobin, even though it is an $\alpha 1$ variant [2]. Haemoglobin G-Philadelphia (see p. 211) illustrates the complexity of the interaction between an $\alpha$ chain variant and $\alpha$ thalassaemia. The $\alpha^{G\text{-Philadelphia}}$ gene can occur either as one of two $\alpha$ genes on a chromosome ($\alpha^G\alpha$) or as the only $\alpha$ gene on a chromosome ($-\alpha^G$) as a result of the mutation having occurred in an $\alpha 2\alpha 1$ fusion gene on a chromosome with a 3.7-kilobase (kb) deletion. The former mutation would be expected to lead to the variant being about 12.5% of total haemoglobin and the latter to the variant being somewhat more than one-third of total haemoglobin. A further complicating factor is that the same ethnic group may have both haemoglobin G-Philadelphia and a high prevalence of unlinked $\alpha$ thalassaemia. There may then be $\alpha$ thalassaemia in *trans* to the variant $\alpha$ gene, giving the genotype $-\alpha^G/-\alpha$, with haemoglobin G-Philadelphia being about 45% of total haemoglobin.

## Haemoglobin C

Haemoglobin C is a variant haemoglobin with a mutation in the $\beta$ globin gene at the same site as the mutation in the sickle cell haemoglobin. It was first recognized by Itano and Neel in 1950 [3]. Its structure is $\alpha_2\beta_2^{6\text{Glu}\to\text{Lys}}$. It may be present in the heterozygous state (haemoglobin C trait), in the homozygous state (haemoglobin C disease) and in a variety of compound heterozygous states, such as sickle cell/haemoglobin C disease and haemoglobin C/$\beta$ thalassaemia. Sickle cell/haemoglobin C disease has been discussed in Chapter 4 (see p. 164). Other haemoglobinopathies with haemoglobin C are discussed in this chapter.

Haemoglobin C is thought to have originated in West Africa, west of the Niger River (Fig. 5.1) (see Table 4.1). In northern Ghana, the proportion of indi-

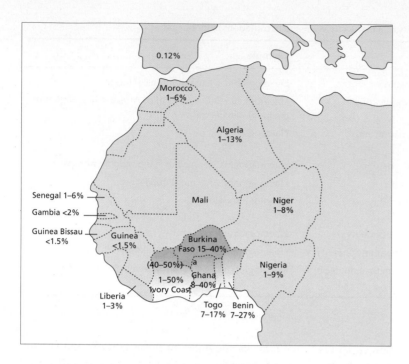

**Fig. 5.1** Distribution of haemoglobin C in north-west Africa.

viduals with haemoglobin C is as high as 40% and, in northern Côte d'Ivoire (Ivory Coast), up to 50%. In Burkina Faso (previously Upper Volta), it is 15–40%. It would appear that haemoglobin C arose in the region spanning Burkina Faso and the north of Côte d'Ivoire and Ghana. It is found in individuals of African descent in the Caribbean (3.5% prevalence), USA (2% prevalence amongst US blacks), Canada and the UK. A high incidence has been noted in a Bedouin tribe in northern Israel. There is also a significant incidence of haemoglobin C in North Africa and southern Europe. However, it should be noted that some early reports of the presence of haemoglobin C based only on electrophoresis at alkaline pH may have been a misidentification of haemoglobin O-Arab as haemoglobin C. Haemoglobin C appears to have had an independent origin in Oman and Thailand [4,5].

Haemoglobin C appears to protect against severe falciparum malaria [6], with homozygosity giving very high protection and heterozygosity giving moderate protection [7].

Oxyhaemoglobin C is prone to crystallization, but crystals dissolve on deoxygenation, so that obstruction of capillaries by cells containing crystals is not likely. In comparison with haemoglobin A, crystallization is inhibited by haemoglobins F and $A_2$ [4].

## Haemoglobin C trait

Haemoglobin C trait describes the heterozygous condition in which there is one normal β gene and one $β^C$ gene. It is of no clinical significance, but is of importance in counselling prospective parents. This is largely because of the possibility of sickle cell/haemoglobin C disease if one parent has haemoglobin C trait and the other has sickle cell trait.

*Clinical features*

There are no clinical features.

*Laboratory features*

*Blood count.* The haemoglobin is usually normal, but microcytosis is common. There is conflicting data as to whether this results from coexisting α thalassaemia trait. In one study, individuals with haemoglobin C trait and with the normal complement of four α globin genes had a mean cell volume (MCV), on average, around the bottom of the normal range [8], whereas, in another study, there was no difference between haemoglobin C trait and normal [9]. The mean cell haemoglobin concentration (MCHC) is, on average, higher than normal, usually around the top of the normal range. The red cell distribution width (RDW) is increased.

*Blood film.* The blood film (Fig. 5.2) may be completely normal or may show microcytosis, target cells, irregularly contracted cells or any combination of these features.

*Other investigations.* Haemoglobin electrophoresis (Fig. 5.3) or HPLC shows haemoglobin A to constitute slightly more than 50% of haemoglobin and haemoglobin C slightly less. The proportion of haemoglobin C is lower in those with coexisting $\alpha$ thalassaemia trait. In one study, the mean percentage of haemoglobin C (plus $A_2$) was around 44% in those thought likely to have four $\alpha$ genes, around 37.5% in those thought likely to have three $\alpha$ genes and around 32% in those thought likely to have two $\alpha$ genes [10]. In another study, the mean levels were 37% and 32% in those with four and three $\alpha$ genes,

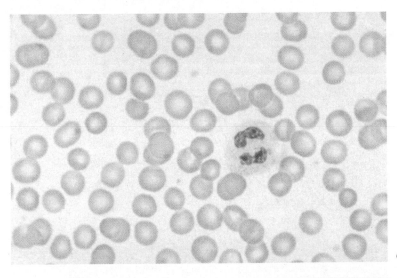

(a)

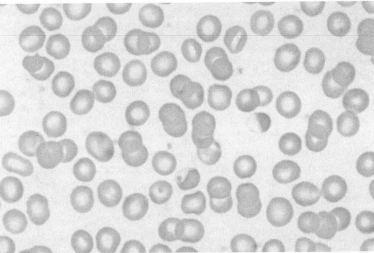

(b)

**Fig. 5.2** Blood films from four patients with haemoglobin C trait showing the range of features that may be observed: (a) normal film; (b) one irregularly contracted cell and one 'hemi-ghost'. (*Continued on p. 194.*)

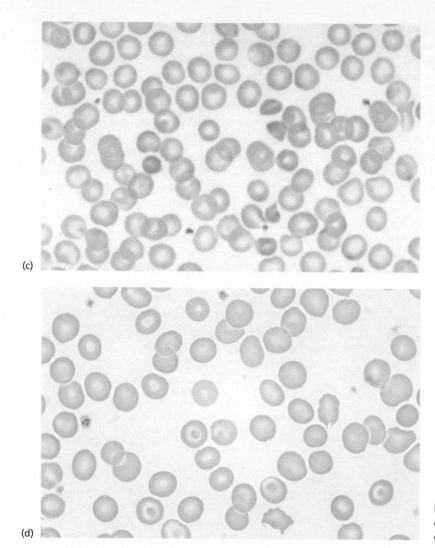

(c)

(d)

**Fig. 5.2** *Continued.* (c) irregularly contracted cells; (d) target cells and other poikilocytes.

respectively [9]. In a single patient with haemoglobin C trait and haemoglobin H disease, the haemoglobin C was 24% [4]. In subjects with five α genes, the haemoglobin C percentage tends to be higher than in those with four α genes [11]. On cellulose acetate at alkaline pH, haemoglobin C has the same mobility as haemoglobins E, A$_2$ and O-Arab. On citrate agar or agarose gel, it can be separated from haemoglobins E and A$_2$ (same mobility as haemoglobin A) and from haemoglobin O-Arab (similar mobility as haemoglobin S). On HPLC, haemoglobin C can be separated from haemoglobin E and haemoglobin O-Arab but, depending on the specific instrument/reagent system, there may be overlap with haemoglobin A$_2$ and haemoglobin Lepore. Haemoglobin C can be detected immunologically [12].

The red cell density is increased as a result of increased potassium/chloride (K$^+$/Cl$^-$) cotransport, the loss of intracellular potassium and resultant cellular dehydration [7]. The osmotic fragility is decreased. Red cell survival is normal or slightly reduced.

## Diagnosis

The diagnosis is dependent on the identification of haemoglobin A and haemoglobin C by at least two independent techniques, with haemoglobin C being present in a lower amount than haemoglobin A.

## Haemoglobin C disease

Haemoglobin C disease describes the homozygous state in which there are two $\beta^C$ genes and no normal $\beta$ gene. As a consequence, about 95% of total haemoglobin is haemoglobin C, with the remainder being haemoglobins $A_2$ and F. Homozygosity for haemoglobin C leads to a clinically mild, chronic, haemolytic anaemia.

## Clinical features

Individuals with haemoglobin C disease either have a normal haemoglobin concentration or are mildly or moderately anaemic. Because of the chronic haemolysis, there is an increased incidence of gallstones. The spleen may be enlarged.

## Laboratory features

*Blood count.* The haemoglobin ranges from about 8 g/dl up to a normal concentration. There is often marked microcytosis. In one study, patients with a normal complement of four α genes had an average MCV of 55 fl [8]. The MCHC is, on average, around the top of the normal range and the proportion of hyperdense cells is increased. The cause of the microcytosis and increased MCHC is activation of the $K^+/Cl^-$ cotransporter, which leads to the loss of water from the cell; cells are therefore smaller, denser and less deformable than normal [4]. The reticulocyte count is mildly elevated, usually 2–4%.

*Blood film.* The blood film (Fig. 5.4) characteristically shows numerous target cells and numerous irregularly contracted cells [13]. There is also microcytosis. There may be occasional nucleated red blood cells (NRBCs). Occasional cells may contain haemoglobin

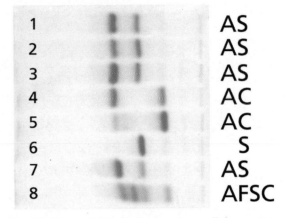

**Fig. 5.3** Haemoglobin electrophoresis on cellulose acetate at alkaline pH showing haemoglobin C trait (lane 4) and haemoglobin C/$\beta^+$ thalassaemia compound heterozygosity (lane 5); AFSC, control sample containing haemoglobins A, F, S and C.

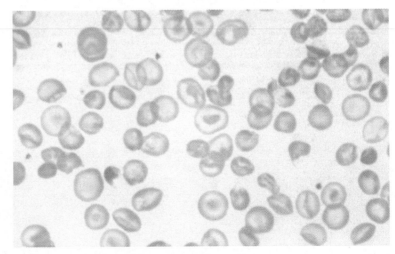

**Fig. 5.4** Blood films from four patients with haemoglobin C disease showing the range of features that may be observed: (a) target cells and irregularly contracted red cells. (*Continued on p. 196.*)

(a)

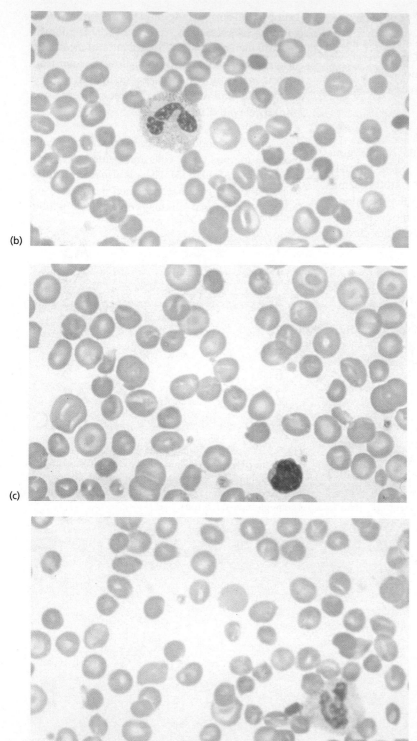

(b)

(c)

(d)

**Fig. 5.4** *Continued.* (b) irregularly contracted cells and only an occasional target cell; (c) target cells and irregularly contracted cells; (d) irregularly contracted cells and one haemoglobin C crystal (adjacent to the neutrophil).

C crystals. Crystals may be tetragonal or hexagonal. Usually all the haemoglobin in a cell has been incorporated into the crystal, so that the crystal is in a cell which otherwise appears to be empty of haemoglobin. The majority of crystals are 6–10 μm in length and 2–3 μm in diameter with pointed ends. Crystals may be present *in vivo*, but can also form *in vitro*, particularly if the film dries slowly [14].

Both crystals and NRBCs are more often seen in patients who have been splenectomized.

*Other investigations.* Haemoglobin electrophoresis (Fig. 5.5) and HPLC (Fig. 5.6) show that haemoglobin C comprises almost all the haemoglobin. Haemoglo-

bin F may be slightly elevated, but does not usually exceed 3%.

The percentage of dense cells is markedly increased. The osmotic fragility is markedly reduced. The bilirubin concentration is normal or increased. Oxygen affinity is reduced as a result of a reduction in intracellular pH, rather than any alteration of the oxygen affinity of haemoglobin C [4]. Red cell survival is reduced to about one-third of normal [4].

The bone marrow shows erythroid hyperplasia and characteristic dyserythropoietic features with an irregular nuclear membrane (Fig. 5.7). On ultrastructural examination, there may also be duplication of the nuclear membrane (Fig. 5.8).

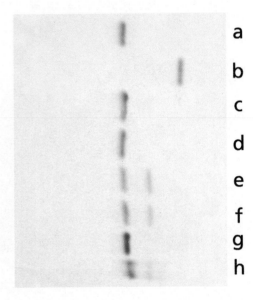

**Fig. 5.5** Haemoglobin electrophoresis on cellulose acetate at alkaline pH in haemoglobin C disease (lane b); other lanes show either haemoglobin A alone or haemoglobin A plus haemoglobin S.

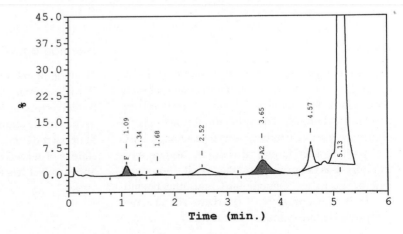

**Fig. 5.6** High performance liquid chromatography (HPLC) chromatogram in haemoglobin C homozygosity; from left to right, the peaks are haemoglobin F, unidentified, haemoglobin A2, glycosylated haemoglobin C and haemoglobin C.

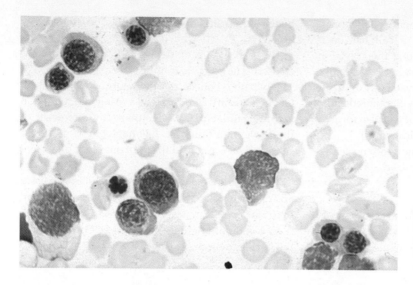

**Fig. 5.7** Bone marrow aspirate from a patient with haemoglobin C disease showing erythroid hyperplasia and an irregular nuclear margin (stained with May–Grünwald–Giemsa stain).

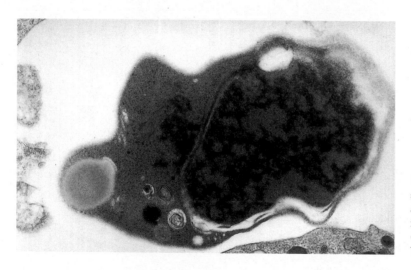

**Fig. 5.8** Ultrastructural examination showing the characteristic abnormality of the nuclear membrane in homozygosity for haemoglobin C. (By courtesy of Professor S. N. Wickramasinghe.)

*Diagnosis*

The diagnosis is dependent on the identification of haemoglobin C as the sole variant haemoglobin, in the absence of haemoglobin A, by at least two independent techniques. The differential diagnosis includes compound heterozygosity for haemoglobin C and $\beta^0$ thalassaemia and, if cellulose acetate electrophoresis is the primary method used, compound heterozygosity for haemoglobin C and either haemoglobin E or haemoglobin C-Harlem. The last two compound heterozygous states are rare.

## Haemoglobin C/β thalassaemia

Haemoglobin C may be coinherited with either $\beta^0$ or $\beta^+$ thalassaemia. The latter is more common because $\beta^+$ thalassaemia is more common than $\beta^0$ thalassaemia in the ethnic groups that are most likely to inherit haemoglobin C. This compound heterozygous state is observed particularly in those with African ancestry, but has also been reported in Italians and Turks.

## Clinical features

Compound heterozygosity for haemoglobin C and β thalassaemia leads to a moderately severe anaemia with splenomegaly. The clinical picture if haemoglobin C is coinherited with $β^0$ thalassaemia or severe $β^+$ thalassaemia resembles thalassaemia intermedia, with moderately severe anaemia, splenomegaly and sometimes hypersplenism. Worsening anaemia consequent on aplastic crises has been observed. If haemoglobin C is coinherited with mild $β^+$ thalassaemia, the features are similar to those of homozygosity for haemoglobin C. There is a mild to moderate haemolytic anaemia and some splenomegaly.

## Laboratory features

*Blood count.* The haemoglobin concentration varies from 7 to 10 g/dl in haemoglobin C/$β^0$ thalassaemia. In haemoglobin C/$β^+$ thalassaemia, the haemoglobin may be reduced or, occasionally, normal. The MCV is markedly reduced. The reticulocyte count is moderately elevated.

*Blood film.* The blood film (Fig. 5.9) shows hypochromia, microcytosis, target cells and irregularly contracted cells. There is more anisocytosis and poikilocytosis than in haemoglobin C disease, particularly in cases of haemoglobin C/$β^0$ thalassaemia. Haemoglobin C crystals are sometimes present.

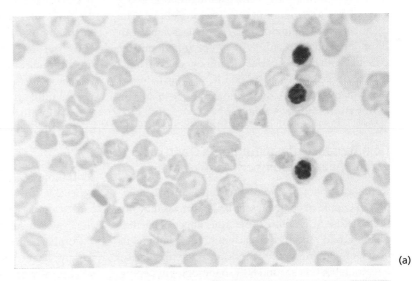

(a)

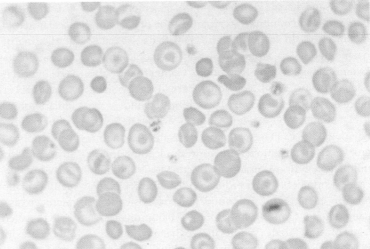

(b)

**Fig. 5.9** Blood films from two patients with haemoglobin C/β thalassaemia compound heterozygosity: (a) haemoglobin C/$β^0$ thalassaemia compound heterozygosity showing hypochromia, irregularly contracted cells, three nucleated red blood cells and a cell containing a haemoglobin C crystal; (b) haemoglobin C/$β^+$ thalassaemia compound heterozygosity showing irregularly contracted cells and target cells; the electrophoretic pattern of this patient is shown in Fig. 5.3 (lane 5).

*Other investigations.* The major haemoglobin is haemoglobin C, with haemoglobin F usually comprising 2–10% (most often greater than 5%). Haemoglobin A may be totally absent (haemoglobin C/$\beta^0$ thalassaemia) or, when haemoglobin C is coinherited with a mild $\beta^+$ thalassaemia, usually 20–30% of total haemoglobin. The osmotic fragility is markedly reduced.

*Diagnosis*

The diagnosis of haemoglobin C/$\beta^+$ thalassaemia is straightforward, being dependent on the identification of haemoglobin A and haemoglobin C by two independent techniques, with haemoglobin C being present in a larger amount than haemoglobin A. The diagnosis of haemoglobin C/$\beta^0$ thalassaemia can be more problematical, as it is not infrequent for patients with haemoglobin C homozygosity to have microcytosis, often as a result of coexisting $\alpha$ thalassaemia trait. A distinction may be made by family studies or DNA analysis.

## Coinheritance of haemoglobin C and other variant haemoglobins or thalassaemias

Coinheritance of haemoglobin C and either haemoglobin Lepore or $\delta\beta$ thalassaemia leads to a clinically mild disease resembling the coinheritance of haemoglobin C and mild $\beta^+$ thalassaemia. In haemoglobin C/haemoglobin Lepore compound heterozygosity, haemoglobin C is around 80%, haemoglobin Lepore 10–15% and haemoglobin F 6–12%. Haemoglobin Lepore-Boston inhibits the crystallization of haemoglobin C [4]. In haemoglobin C/$\delta\beta$ thalassaemia, haemoglobin C is around 75% and haemoglobin F around 25% of total haemoglobin. Coinheritance of haemoglobin C and deletional hereditary persistence of fetal haemoglobin is also clinically mild.

Haemoglobin C crystallization is accelerated in haemoglobin C heterozygotes who are also heterozygous for haemoglobin Korle Bu, leading to a mild haemolytic anaemia with microcytosis and increased numbers of hyperdense cells [15,16]. Crystals are cubic [15]. Compound heterozygosity for haemoglobin C and haemoglobin N-Baltimore also leads to accelerated crystallization of haemoglobin C in comparison with that in haemoglobin C trait [16].

The phenotype may be intermediate in severity between heterozygosity and homozygosity for haemoglobin C. If haemoglobin Riyadh is coinherited with haemoglobin C, crystallization is retarded and microcytosis is usually the only feature [16,17]. Haemoglobin C coinherited with haemoglobin K-Woolwich or haemoglobin P-Galveston does not differ in severity from haemoglobin C trait [18].

The coinheritance of haemoglobins C and E has been described [5,19,20]. It has been noted that the haemoglobin E percentage tends to be higher than in haemoglobin E trait [5,20]. For example, three children had haemoglobin E plus $A_2$ of 33–37% (cf. 25–30% in haemoglobin E simple heterozygotes), haemoglobin C of 54–56% and haemoglobin F of 2.1–5.8% [5]. In one patient, who was clinically well, the haematocrit and reticulocyte count were normal [19]; the red cells were normocytic and normochromic, but showed cytoplasmic folding and stomatocyte formation. In a second patient, there was a mild anaemia (haemoglobin concentration 9.9 g/dl) with red cell indices suggestive of thalassaemia trait. Haemoglobin C was 60% and haemoglobin E 39% [20]. Two of the three children mentioned above were anaemic (haemoglobin concentrations of 7.5 and 9.5 g/dl) and markedly microcytic (MCVs of 52 and 61 fl) in the absence of coexisting $\alpha$ thalassaemia trait (although iron deficiency was not excluded) [5].

Coinheritance of haemoglobin C and the $\alpha$ chain variant, haemoglobin G-Philadelphia, does not differ clinically or haematologically from haemoglobin C trait, although haemoglobin C crystallization is accelerated [4]. Electrophoresis on cellulose acetate at alkaline pH shows four bands: haemoglobin A, haemoglobin G, haemoglobin C and a slow-moving G–C hybrid haemoglobin (Fig. 5.10). On agarose gel at acid pH, there are only two bands: A plus G-Philadelphia and C plus C–G hybrid (Fig. 5.11).

Coexistence of haemoglobin C heterozygosity and the genotype of haemoglobin H disease leads to an atypical form of haemoglobin H disease. One reported case had a chronic haemolytic anaemia and significant splenomegaly [21]. There was marked microcytosis. Only haemoglobins A and C (20%) were detected on haemoglobin electrophoresis and only occasional inclusion-containing cells were found on a haemoglobin H preparation.

As is the case with the sickle cell mutation, the haemoglobin C mutation can occur as one of two mutations on a chromosome. Haemoglobin Arlington Park is $\alpha_2\beta_2{}^{6Glu\rightarrow Lys,95Lys\rightarrow Glu}$. There is no net change in charge relative to haemoglobin A, so that this variant haemoglobin is electrophoretically silent. Nevertheless, it interacts in the same manner as haemoglobin C with haemoglobin S to give a clinically significant sickling disorder.

## Haemoglobin E

Haemoglobin E is a $\beta$ chain variant, $\alpha_2\beta^{26Glu\rightarrow Lys}$, which is common in South-East Asia (Table 5.2) [22–28]. It was first described by Chernoff and colleagues in 1954 [29] and independently in the same year by Itano and colleagues [30]. The highest prevalence occurs in some parts of Thailand, Kampuchea (previously Cambodia) and Laos. Thailand and Myanmar (previously Burma) have an overall preva-

**Table 5.2** Prevalence of haemoglobin E carriers in various countries. (From references [22–28] and other sources.)

| Country | Percentage |
|---|---|
| India | 0–3.5* |
| Pakistan | 0.5–1 |
| Bangladesh | 4 |
| Bhutan | 1.5–6.5 |
| Nepal | <1 |
| Sri Lanka | 0–13† (overall 0.5) |
| Myanmar (previously Burma) | 1–33 |
| Thailand | 8–40‡ |
| Laos | 20–40‡ |
| Cambodia | 15–30‡ |
| Malaysia | 7–23 |
| Vietnam | 2–4§ |
| Southern China | 1–2.5 |
| Malaysia | 1–40¶ |
| Indonesia | 1–13 |
| Philippines | ≈1 |
| Turkey | 0.5–1 |
| Jamaica | 0.007 |

*But 22% in Calcutta and 50–80% in Assam.
†Common in the Veddah.
‡Haemoglobin E occurs in 70% of the So people of north-east Thailand, in 50% of the Khymer people on the borders of Laos, Thailand and Cambodia, and in 50% of the Kachari people in Assam [27].
§Much higher incidence amongst the Khymer population in Vietnam (20–30%) and in certain other ethnic groups including the Ede and the Vân Kiêv (5–50%).
¶More frequent in the aboriginal population than in the Malays [24].

## Hb electrophoresis
### double heterozygote G<sup>Ph</sup>/C

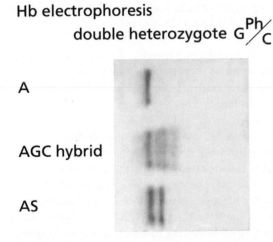

**Fig. 5.10** Haemoglobin electrophoresis on cellulose acetate at alkaline pH in a patient with heterozygosity for both haemoglobin C and the α chain variant, haemoglobin G-Philadelphia; four bands are apparent.

**Fig. 5.11** Haemoglobin electrophoresis on agarose gel at acid pH in a patient with heterozygosity for both haemoglobin C and the α chain variant, haemoglobin G-Philadelphia; at this pH, only two bands are apparent (apart from a faint haemoglobin F band); FASC, control sample containing haemoglobins F, A, S and C.

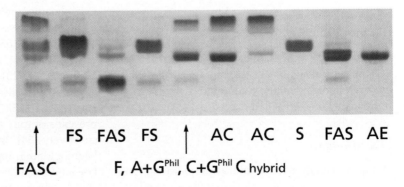

lence of around 14–15%. Gene frequency in Thailand varies from 8% to 50–70%, being highest in north-eastern Thailand. Haemoglobin E is also found in Sri Lanka, north-eastern India (Bengal and Assam), Bangladesh, Pakistan, Nepal, Vietnam, Malaysia, the Philippines, Indonesia and Turkey. Although haemoglobin E is prevalent in Sri Lanka, it is not prevalent in southern India; it is thought to have reached Sri Lanka during migration from north-eastern India during the 5th century BC. Occasional cases have been observed in individuals of apparent Northern European Caucasian descent and a single affected family has been observed in the former Czechoslovakia.

The $\beta^E$ chain is synthesized at a reduced rate in comparison with $\beta^A$. This is because the mutation creates a false splicing site towards the 3' end of exon 1 so that there is a proportion of abnormally spliced messenger RNA (mRNA). Post-transcriptional processing of the latter is abnormal. The result of the reduced rate of synthesis of the $\beta^E$ chain, and therefore of haemoglobin E, is that heterozygotes, compound heterozygotes and homozygotes show some thalassaemic features. Haemoglobin E may therefore be regarded as a thalassaemic haemoglobinopathy. The $\alpha$:non-$\alpha$ chain synthesis ratio is 1.2–2.1 in heterozygotes [31]. Haemoglobin E also has weakened $\alpha_1\beta_1$ contacts, leading to instability in conditions of increased oxidant stress. The most significant clinical consequences occur if haemoglobin E is coinherited with $\beta$ thalassaemia trait, leading to thalassaemia major or thalassaemia intermedia. Homozygosity for haemoglobin E produces a clinically mild condition and is thus of much less significance.

Haemoglobin E may protect against severe falciparum malaria [32].

## Haemoglobin E trait

Haemoglobin E trait is an asymptomatic condition with no clinical significance, except for the possibility of homozygous or compound heterozygous states in the children of heterozygotes.

### Clinical features

There are usually no clinical features, although in-creased susceptibility to oxidant-induced haemolysis has been suspected.

### Laboratory features

*Blood count.* Some patients have a normal blood count. Others have an increased red cell count (RBC) and reduced MCV and mean cell haemoglobin (MCH), with or without mild anaemia. Haemoglobin does not usually fall much below 12 g/dl. The MCHC is normal or, occasionally, increased. The red cell indices not infrequently resemble those of thalassaemia trait [33]. It is not uncommon for individuals with haemoglobin E trait to also have a deletion of one or two $\alpha$ genes. However, even those with a full complement of $\alpha$ genes may be microcytic and mildly anaemic. In a report of 34 such cases, the average haemoglobin concentration was 12.4 g/dl, the MCV 79.7 fl and the MCH 26.2 pg [34].

*Blood film.* The blood film (Fig. 5.12) may be normal or may show hypochromia, microcytosis, target cells, irregularly contracted cells, basophilic stippling or any combination of these features.

*Other investigations.* Haemoglobin electrophoresis at alkaline pH (Fig. 5.13) shows that the variant haemoglobin has the same mobility as haemoglobins C and $A_2$. On citrate agar or agarose gel at acid pH, the mobility of haemoglobin E is the same as that of haemoglobin A and $A_2$. Haemoglobin E has a characteristic mobility on isoelectric focusing, being well separated from haemoglobin A and moving close to haemoglobins C and $A_2$. On HPLC, it is easily separated from haemoglobins A and C, but co-elutes with haemoglobin $A_2$ (Fig. 5.14). Haemoglobin E can also be detected by immunoassay [12].

In haemoglobin E heterozygotes, the variant usually comprises 30% or less of total haemoglobin. More than 39% of haemoglobin E suggests the diagnosis of haemoglobin E/$\beta$ thalassaemia not haemoglobin E trait [31]. A trimodal distribution of the variant haemoglobin is found, with modal percentages of 29.1%, 27.3% and 17.4% correlating with the presence of four, three and two $\alpha$ globin genes, respectively [34]. Individuals with less than 25% of haemoglobin E almost always have coexisting $\alpha$ thalassaemia trait [34]. When an individual is heterozy-

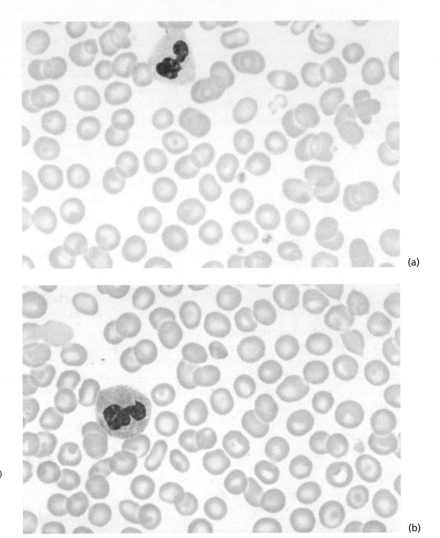

(a)

(b)

**Fig. 5.12** Blood films from two patients with haemoglobin E trait: (a) microcytosis, minimal hypochromia and one target cell; (b) microcytosis (the mean cell volume was 72 fl) and target cells.

gous for haemoglobin E and also has the genotype of haemoglobin H disease, the percentage of haemoglobin E is even lower, sometimes as low as 10%. On the basis of extensive experience in Thailand, Fucharoen [31] has further reported that heterozygotes have 25–30% of haemoglobin E when three or four α genes are present, 19–21% when two α genes are present and 13–15% when the genotype is that of haemoglobin H disease. The percentage of haemoglobin E can also be lowered by coexisting iron deficiency. It should be noted that the percentages of haemoglobin E reported in various haemoglobin E syndromes are likely to represent haemoglobin E plus haemoglobin $A_2$.

Haemoglobin E is slightly unstable on heat and isopropanol stability tests. Red cell protoporphyrin, often used as a screening test for iron deficiency, can be elevated in haemoglobin E heterozygosity [35]. The osmotic fragility of red cells is reduced. Pyrimidine 5′ nucleotidase 1 is reduced to levels comparable with those seen in heterozygotes for inherited deficiency [36].

### Diagnosis

The diagnosis is dependent on the demonstration of the presence of haemoglobin E and haemoglobin A by two independent techniques, with haemoglobin E comprising about one-third of total haemoglobin. If the primary diagnostic method is cellulose acetate electrophoresis at alkaline pH, the differential diagnosis is mainly with haemoglobin C trait. If HPLC is the primary diagnostic method, the differential diagnosis is with heterozygosity for haemoglobin Lepore or other uncommon haemoglobins, such as haemoglobin D-Iran (Fig. 5.15) and haemoglobin G-

Coushatta (Fig. 5.16). The percentage of the variant and the precise retention time are useful. Although the last two variant haemoglobins elute in the E window, the shape of the chromatogram differs from that of haemoglobin E and the percentage is much higher.

## Haemoglobin E homozygosity ('haemoglobin E disease')

Individuals with the genotype $\beta^E\beta^E$ are usually completely asymptomatic. It has therefore been suggested that the term 'haemoglobin E homozygosity' is preferable to the term 'haemoglobin E disease'.

### Clinical features

There is usually no anaemia and rarely any evidence of haemolysis [23,24,37]. The spleen is not usually enlarged.

### Laboratory features

*Blood count.* The blood count often resembles that of β thalassaemia trait, with a normal haemoglobin concentration or very mild anaemia, an increased red cell count and reduced MCV and MCH. The MCHC is usually normal. The reticulocyte count is usually normal, but may be slightly elevated.

*Blood film.* The blood film (Fig. 5.17) usually shows hypochromia and microcytosis with variable numbers of target cells and irregularly contracted cells.

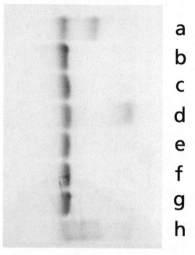

**Fig. 5.13** Haemoglobin electrophoresis on cellulose acetate at alkaline pH in a patient with haemoglobin E trait (lane d). Note that the variant haemoglobin comprises only about 30% of total haemoglobin; lanes b–g contain haemoglobin A only; faint control bands (A and S) are apparent in lane h.

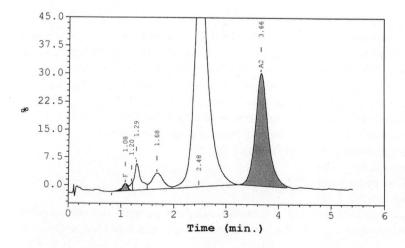

**Fig. 5.14** HPLC chromatogram from a patient with haemoglobin E heterozygosity. Haemoglobin E appears in the 'A₂ window' and was 30.2% with a retention time of 3.66 min (Bio-Rad Variant II); from left to right, the peaks are haemoglobin F, post-translationally modified haemoglobin A (two peaks), haemoglobin A and haemoglobin E plus haemoglobin A₂.

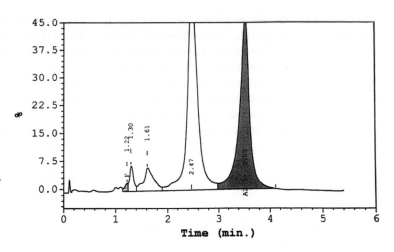

**Fig. 5.15** HPLC chromatogram from a patient with haemoglobin D-Iran heterozygosity. Haemoglobin D-Iran appears in the 'A$_2$ window' and was 46.6% with a retention time of 3.53 min (Bio-Rad Variant II); from left to right, the peaks are haemoglobin F, post-translationally modified haemoglobin A (two peaks) and haemoglobins A and D-Iran plus A$_2$.

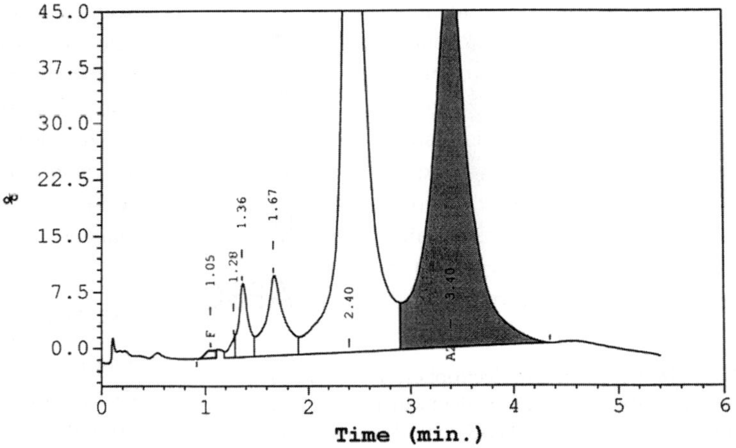

**Fig. 5.16** HPLC chromatogram from a patient with haemoglobin G-Coushatta heterozygosity. Haemoglobin G-Coushatta appears in the 'A$_2$ window' and was 51.5% with a retention time of 3.40 min (Bio-Rad Variant II); from left to right, the peaks are haemoglobin F, post-translationally modified haemoglobin A (two peaks) and haemoglobins A and G-Coushatta plus A$_2$.

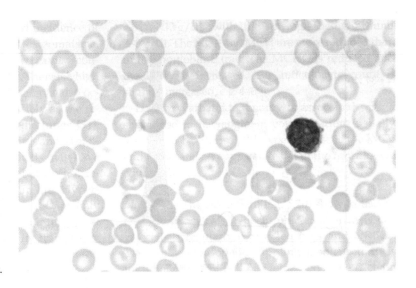

**Fig. 5.17** Blood film from a patient with haemoglobin E homozygosity showing microcytosis and target cells.

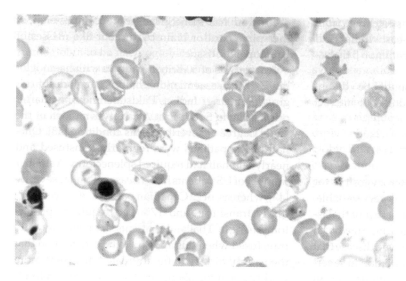

**Fig. 5.20** Blood film from a patient with haemoglobin E/β thalassaemia compound heterozygosity severe enough to have required splenectomy showing poikilocytosis, some hypochromic cells, Pappenheimer bodies, a nucleated red blood cell and erythrocytes containing precipitates that are likely to represent precipitated α chain.

inclusions [46], in addition to the usual post-splenectomy changes.

*Other investigations.* Haemoglobin electrophoresis and HPLC show haemoglobins E, $A_2$ and F in the case of haemoglobin E/$\beta^0$ thalassaemia and E, A, $A_2$ and F in the case of haemoglobin E/$\beta^+$ thalassaemia. Compound heterozygotes for E and $\beta^0$ thalassaemia have haemoglobin E representing 40–60% of total haemoglobin; there is little overlap with homozygous haemoglobin E where the percentage is usually 85–99%. Conversely, haemoglobin F is 30–60% in haemoglobin E/$\beta^0$ thalassaemia, whereas, in homozygous haemoglobin E, it is less than 15% and usually less than 5%. Overall, haemoglobin F is very variable, from 5% to 87% [40]. The increase in haemoglobin F is attributable to erythropoietin-driven bone marrow expansion and possibly increased F-cell production combined with preferential survival of F cells [47]. When haemoglobin A is present, it usually constitutes around 10% of total haemoglobin.

Hydroxycarbamide therapy is associated with a significant rise in haemoglobin F percentage and a reciprocal fall in haemoglobin E percentage [45]. Regular blood transfusion is associated with a greater decrease in haemoglobin F synthesis than haemoglobin E synthesis [47].

Tests for haemoglobin instability are weakly positive. The osmotic fragility is reduced. The red cell life span is reduced. The bone marrow shows erythroid hyperplasia, dyserythropoiesis, increased macrophage activity and increased storage iron. The serum transferrin receptor concentration is increased, reflecting the expanded erythropoiesis.

*Diagnosis*

The differential diagnosis is as for haemoglobin E homozygosity (see p. 206).

## Coinheritance of haemoglobin E and other variant haemoglobins, thalassaemias and haematological disorders

The coinheritance of haemoglobins S and E has been described on p. 178 and the interaction with β thalassaemia, α thalassaemia trait and haemoglobin C above.

Because both are relatively common in South-East Asia, haemoglobin E heterozygosity or homozygosity may coexist with the genotype of haemoglobin H disease. In one series of patients, individuals with heterozygosity for haemoglobin E and the genotype of haemoglobin H disease had a condition that was clinically similar to uncomplicated haemoglobin H disease, with the average haemoglobin concentration being around 7–8 g/dl and the MCV averaging 67 fl [48]. In another series of patients, the haemoglobin concentration was around 7–9 g/dl (similar to uncomplicated haemoglobin H disease), but the MCV was lower at 52–58 fl [49]. The haemoglobins present are A, E and Bart's, with more A than E and more E than Bart's [50]. Only a small percentage of cells (1–5%) [48], if any [49], contain haemoglobin H inclusions and haemoglobin H is usually not detected on electrophoresis [49]. Haemoglobin F is increased to 3–13%, whereas, in uncomplicated haemoglobin H disease, it averages 1–2% [49]. It appears that the reduced quantity of the α chain combines preferentially with the normal β chain rather than with $\beta^E$ [48], with the percentage of haemoglobin E plus $A_2$ being as low as 8–16% [49]. The designation AEBart's disease has been used. Coinheritance of haemoglobin E heterozygosity and $--/\alpha^{CS}\alpha$ has a more severe clinical phenotype than coinheritance of haemoglobin E heterozygosity and $--/-\alpha$ [31].

Homozygosity for haemoglobin E coinherited with the genotype of haemoglobin H disease gives a severe thalassaemia intermedia phenotype with a haemoglobin concentration similar to that in AEBart's disease, but, on average, a lower MCV (mean 61 fl). The haemoglobins present are usually E, Bart's and F, comprising c. 80%, 1–25% (average 10%) and 1–7%, respectively, of total haemoglobin [48,51]. No inclusions are detected in haemoglobin H preparations, suggesting that the $\beta^E$ chains do not form tetramers. The designation EFBart's disease has been used, but it should be noted that some patients have been described with no haemoglobin F or Bart's [51]. Closely related clinical phenotypes result from the coinheritance of either $\beta^E\beta^E$ or $\beta^E\beta^0$ and either $--/-\alpha$ or $--/\alpha^{CS}\alpha$.

The interaction of haemoglobin E and haemoglobin Lepore [20] can cause significant anaemia with the phenotype of thalassaemia intermedia.

Coinheritance of haemoglobin E and deletional hereditary persistence of fetal haemoglobin leads to red cell indices similar to those of thalassaemia trait, but no clinical abnormality [18].

Coinheritance of haemoglobin E and the elongated β chain variant, haemoglobin Tak, has been reported in one patient. A mild polycythaemia was observed [50].

A single individual has been reported in whom coinheritance of haemoglobin E disease and pyrimidine 5′ nucleotidase 1 deficiency led to a clinically severe phenotype with reticulocytosis and a haemoglobin concentration of less than 3 g/dl [43].

## Haemoglobin D-Punjab/D-Los Angeles

Haemoglobin D-Punjab is a β chain variant, $\alpha_2\beta_2^{121Glu\rightarrow Gln}$, initially described under the name of haemoglobin D-Los Angeles. The latter is the correct designation and is used in North America, whereas in the UK the designation D-Punjab tends to be employed. This variant haemoglobin has also been designated haemoglobin D-Cyprus, D-Conley, D-Chicago, D-North Carolina, D-Portugal and haemoglobin Oak Ridge [52]. Its only major importance is because of its interaction with haemoglobin S (see p. 174). Its highest incidence is amongst Sikhs in the Punjab who show a prevalence of 2–3%. Gujeratis have a prevalence of about 1% and a similar prevalence is found in British Pakistanis. There is a low but significant prevalence amongst Afro-Americans (0.4%) [53] and Afro-Caribbeans (0.01%) [26]. It has also been reported in individuals with American Indian ancestry. There is a low prevalence amongst Caucasian populations in England, France and Portugal who have had a close contact with India. In England, the highest prevalence is in Norfolk where it has been attributed to the sojourn of the IXth Foot Regiment in India. Haemoglobin D-Punjab is also found in Pakistan, Afghanistan, Iran, China, Turkey, Yugoslavia, Greece, Holland, Australia and North Africa.

It is important to distinguish haemoglobin D-Punjab from other α and β chain variants with similar electrophoretic properties, but with less or no clinical significance. Other β chain variants with similar electrophoretic mobility to haemoglobin D-Punjab on cellulose acetate at alkaline pH include haemoglobin D-Ibadan, $\alpha_2\beta_2^{87Thr\rightarrow Lys}$, haemoglobin D-Iran (Fig. 5.15), $\alpha_2\beta_2^{22Glu\rightarrow Gln}$, haemoglobin G-Coushatta (Fig. 5.16), $\alpha_2\beta_2^{22Glu\rightarrow Ala}$, and haemoglobin Korle Bu, $\alpha_2\beta_2^{73Asp\rightarrow Asn}$, none of which appear to be of clinical significance. Haemoglobin Korle Bu, initially described as haemoglobin G and then as haemoglobin G-Accra, originated in West Africa (Ghana or Ivory Coast) [54]. It moves slightly on the A side of S on electrophoresis at acid pH and has the same retention time as haemoglobin $A_2$ on HPLC. The most common α chain variant with the potential to be confused with haemoglobin D-Punjab is haemoglobin G-Philadelphia (see below).

Haemoglobin D has a normal stability and a normal or slightly increased oxygen affinity.

## Haemoglobin D-Punjab trait

Heterozygosity for haemoglobin D is of genetic but no other clinical significance.

### Clinical features

Haemoglobin D heterozygotes are clinically normal.

### Laboratory features

*Blood count.* The blood count is normal [55], unless there is coexisting α thalassaemia trait. The reticulocyte count is normal.

*Blood film.* The blood film may be normal or show some target cells.

*Other investigations.* On cellulose acetate at alkaline pH, haemoglobin D-Punjab has the same electrophoretic mobility as haemoglobin S and a variety of other α and β chain variants randomly designated haemoglobin D or G. On citrate agar or agarose gel at acid pH, haemoglobin variants designated D or G separate from S and move with or near to haemoglobin A; D/G variants cannot be separated from each other by either of these electrophoretic techniques. On isoelectric focusing, D-Punjab is easily separated from haemoglobins A and S and from the other relatively common D/G variants, including G-Philadelphia. It can be separated from haemoglobins S, A, G-Ibadan, G-Coushatta, D-Iran and Korle Bu by HPLC. Although G-Philadelphia elutes in the D-Punjab window, the two can be distinguished on HPLC by the presence of the minor $G_2$ fraction in association with haemoglobin G-Philadelphia.

In heterozygotes, haemoglobin D is somewhat less than 50% of total haemoglobin. Coexisting α thalassaemia reduces the percentage of the variant [56]. The osmotic fragility and red cell survival are normal.

### Diagnosis

The diagnosis requires the identification of haemoglobins A and D-Punjab by two independent techniques. It should be noted that a reliable identification of haemoglobin D-Punjab by a combination of cellulose acetate electrophoresis at alkaline pH and acid agarose electrophoresis is not possible. Isoelectric focusing and HPLC are more useful. Confirmation by DNA analysis is possible.

## Haemoglobin D-Punjab disease

Haemoglobin D-Punjab homozygosity (haemoglobin D disease) is associated with a clinically mild phenotype.

### Clinical features

There may be mild haemolysis and sometimes a mild haemolytic anaemia [55,57,58]. Some homozygotes have splenomegaly.

### Laboratory features

*Blood count.* The reported haemoglobin concentration has ranged from 9–10 g/dl up to normal levels. The red cell indices may be suggestive of thalassaemia with an elevated red cell count and reduced MCV and MCH. The reticulocyte count may be normal or elevated to 2–4%.

*Blood film.* The blood film shows infrequent or numerous target cells and may show irregularly contracted cells.

*Other investigations.* The osmotic fragility is reduced. The red cell survival is slightly reduced. Haemoglobin electrophoresis and HPLC show normal amounts of haemoglobin $A_2$ and F with the rest of the haemoglobin being haemoglobin D.

### Diagnosis

The diagnosis is dependent on the identification of haemoglobin D-Punjab as the sole variant haemoglobin, in the absence of haemoglobin A, by two reliable independent techniques. If there is microcytosis, the

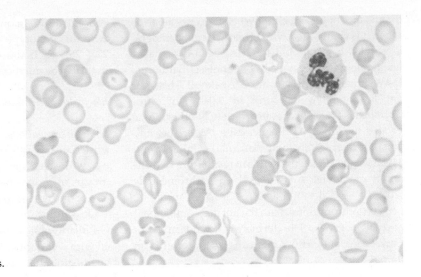

**Fig. 5.21** Blood film from a patient with haemoglobin D-Punjab/$\beta^0$ thalassaemia compound heterozygosity showing hypochromia, microcytosis and poikilocytosis, including target cells.

differential diagnosis is with compound heterozygosity for haemoglobin D-Punjab and $\beta^0$ thalassaemia.

## Haemoglobin D-Punjab/$\beta$ thalassaemia

Compound heterozygosity for haemoglobin D-Punjab and $\beta^0$ thalassaemia produces a mild thalassaemic condition [18,59]. Haemoglobin D-Punjab/$\beta^+$ thalassaemia [52,60] is less common than haemoglobin D-Punjab/$\beta^0$ thalassaemia. Curiously, one reported case had a more severe thalassaemic phenotype than some cases of haemoglobin D-Punjab/$\beta^0$ thalassaemia [60].

### Clinical features

Compound heterozygotes more often resemble $\beta$ thalassaemia trait than $\beta$ thalassaemia intermedia. There is mild anaemia and sometimes splenomegaly.

### Laboratory features

*Blood count.* The reported haemoglobin concentrations have usually ranged from 10.5 g/dl up to normal levels, but occasional patients have been more severely anaemic. The red cell count may be elevated and there is marked reduction of the MCV and MCH. The reticulocyte count is slightly elevated.

*Blood film.* The blood film (Fig. 5.21) shows anisocytosis, poikilocytosis, hypochromia, numerous target cells and some irregularly contracted cells.

*Other investigations.* Haemoglobin electrophoresis and HPLC show almost all the haemoglobin to be haemoglobin D. Haemoglobin F is elevated in some patients. The haemoglobin $A_2$ percentage has been reported to range from high-normal levels (3%) to levels similar to those seen in $\beta$ thalassaemia trait (4.6–8%) [18,20].

## Coinheritance of haemoglobin D-Punjab and other variant haemoglobins and thalassaemias

Coinheritance of haemoglobin D-Punjab and haemoglobin S has been described on p. 174. Coinheritance with haemoglobin G-Philadelphia is discussed below.

### Diagnosis

The diagnosis and differential diagnosis are as for haemoglobin D-Punjab homozygosity.

## Haemoglobin G-Philadelphia

Haemoglobin G-Philadelphia, $\alpha_2^{68Asp \to Lys}\beta_2$, is of no clinical significance, but has the potential to cause diagnostic confusion, either when it occurs alone or when it is coinherited with other variant haemoglobins. This haemoglobin has also been designated haemoglobin Stanleyville I, D-St Louis, D-Baltimore, D-Washington, G-Bristol and G-Azakouli. This variant haemoglobin is found in 0.044% of Afro-Caribbeans [26]. It occurs in a variety of other ethnic groups including Afro-Americans, Algerians, Italians (northern Italy and Sardinia), Chinese and Melanesians. Interestingly, it can result from two different mutations: AAC→AAG on a chromosome with the $-\alpha^{3.7}$ deletion and AAC→AAA in the $\alpha 2$ gene on a chromosome with the normal complement of two $\alpha$ genes. The former is found in Afro-Caribbeans and Afro-Americans and the latter in Italians.

## Haemoglobin G-Philadelphia trait

Haemoglobin G-Philadelphia trait is of no clinical significance. In about 80% of cases, this mutated gene occurs on a $-\alpha^{3.7}$ chromosome, whereas the other 20% of cases have $\alpha^G \alpha$.

### Clinical features

There are no clinical features.

### Laboratory features

*Blood count.* In those with the genotype $-\alpha^G/\alpha\alpha$, there may be mild anaemia or a normal haemoglobin concentration. In one study [61], the MCV in adults with this genotype was 71–80 fl and the MCH was 22.7–26.8 pg. In those who also have $\alpha^+$ thalassaemia in *trans*, the microcytosis is more marked.

*Blood film.* The blood film is normal.

*Other investigations.* The variant haemoglobin comprises 20–25%, 30–35% or 45–48% of total haemoglobin, with the trimodal distribution likely to indicate groups of individuals with one $\alpha^G$ gene and three, two or one normal $\alpha$ genes, respectively.

On cellulose acetate electrophoresis, haemoglobin G-Philadelphia, being an $\alpha$ chain variant, is associated with a variant haemoglobin $A_2$, producing a split haemoglobin $A_2$ band. Similarly, at birth, there is a variant haemoglobin F. The $A_2$ variant, haemoglobin $G_2$, has been reported to be present in a smaller amount than haemoglobin $A_2$, with the total $A_2$ plus $G_2$ percentage being normal or slightly elevated [61].

Haemoglobin G-Philadelphia can be distinguished from haemoglobin D-Punjab by isoelectric focusing and HPLC (Fig. 5.22).

### Diagnosis

The diagnosis requires the identification of haemoglobin G-Philadelphia and haemoglobin A by two reliable independent techniques. It can be difficult to detect the split $A_2/G_2$ band on electrophoresis, so that diagnosis by a combination of cellulose acetate alkaline electrophoresis and agarose gel acid elec-

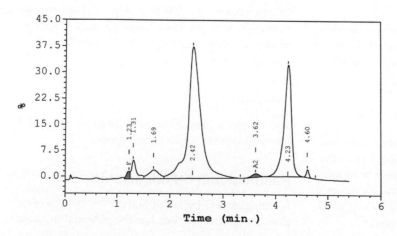

**Fig. 5.22** HPLC chromatogram from a patient with haemoglobin G-Philadelphia heterozygosity. Haemoglobin G-Philadelphia appears in the 'D window' and was 30% with a retention time of 4.23 min. Note that the $G_2$ fraction, which helps to identify this as an $\alpha$ chain variant, appears in the 'S window' (Bio-Rad Variant II); from left to right, the peaks are haemoglobin F, post-translationally modified haemoglobin A (two peaks) and haemoglobins A, $A_2$, G and $G_2$.

trophoresis is not very reliable. Isoelectric focusing and HPLC give more dependable information.

## Haemoglobin G-Philadelphia homozygosity and coinheritance of haemoglobin G-Philadelphia and other variant haemoglobins or thalassaemias

Homozygosity for $-\alpha^G$ has been reported. There is marked hypochromia and microcytosis.

Compound heterozygosity for $-\alpha^G$ and $\alpha^0$ thalassaemia leads to haemoglobin H disease with haemoglobin G-Philadelphia but no haemoglobin A.

Individuals who are heterozygous for both haemoglobin G-Philadelphia and haemoglobin D-Punjab may have a normal haemoglobin concentration or mild anaemia [62]. The blood film and reticulocyte count are normal. Haemoglobin electrophoresis at alkaline pH shows 30–40% haemoglobin A, approximately 45% haemoglobin with the mobility of S (representing haemoglobin D-Punjab and haemoglobin G-Philadelphia), approximately 15% haemoglobin with the mobility of C/E/A$_2$ (representing haemoglobin A$_2$ and the hybrid G-Philadelphia–D-Punjab haemoglobin) and about 2% of haemoglobin G$_2$. Haemoglobin electrophoresis at acid pH is normal.

Coinheritance of haemoglobin G-Philadelphia with haemoglobin S heterozygosity and homozygosity has been discussed on pp. 148 and 164, and with haemoglobin C and haemoglobin S plus C on pp. 200 and 169.

## Haemoglobin O-Arab

Haemoglobin O-Arab (also reported as haemoglobin Egypt) is a β chain variant, $\alpha_2\beta_2^{121Glu\rightarrow Lys}$. It has been found in a great variety of ethnic groups, but is not common in any of them. Despite its name, it is actually quite uncommon amongst Arabs. It appears to be of African rather than Arab origin, with a distribution similar to that of the Ottoman Empire [63]. It has been suggested that it entered the Turkish domain with Sudanese contingents of the Turkish army. In addition to its occurrence amongst Arabs (in Israel, Yemen, Egypt, Saudi Arabia, Aden), it has been reported in Greeks, Italians, in eastern Europe (Bulgaria, the former Yugoslavia, Hungary), in gypsies and amongst Africans (Kenyans, Sudanese, Moroccans, Tunisians) and those of African descent. In a survey in Jamaica, the prevalence was 0.016% [26]. Its main importance is because of possible interaction with haemoglobin S (see p. 175) and β thalassaemia.

### Haemoglobin O-Arab trait

Haemoglobin O-Arab trait is of genetic but no other clinical significance.

*Clinical features*

Haemoglobin O-Arab trait causes no clinical abnormality.

*Laboratory features*

*Blood count.* The haemoglobin concentration is normal. The MCV may be normal or borderline low.

*Blood film.* The blood film may show slight anisocytosis, poikilocytosis, hypochromia and a few target cells [18].

*Other investigations.* The percentage of dense red cells is increased [7]. Haemoglobin O-Arab comprises 38–43% of total haemoglobin. It has a mobility similar to haemoglobin C at alkaline pH (Fig. 5.23). On citrate agar at acid pH, it moves close to but slightly ahead of haemoglobin S, whereas, on agarose gel at acid pH, it moves close to but slightly behind haemoglobin S (Fig. 5.24). On HPLC, haemoglobin O-Arab has a retention time between those of haemoglobins S and C (Fig. 5.25). The relatively low percentage may result, as with haemoglobins S and C, from the positive charge of the $\beta^{O-Arab}$ chain. Individuals with coexisting α thalassaemia trait have a somewhat lower percentage of the variant haemoglobin.

*Diagnosis*

If the primary diagnostic method is cellulose acetate electrophoresis at alkaline pH, the differential diagnosis is with haemoglobins C, E and C-Harlem. The physicochemical characteristics are very similar to those of haemoglobin C-Harlem but, in simple

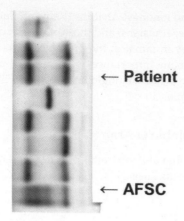

**Fig. 5.23** Cellulose acetate electrophoresis at alkaline pH in a patient with haemoglobin O-Arab heterozygosity. O-Arab has the same mobility as haemoglobins C and E, but is present at a higher percentage than haemoglobin E; AFSC, control sample containing haemoglobins A, F, S and C.

heterozygotes, the distinction can be made easily because C-Harlem has a positive sickle solubility test. If the primary diagnostic method is HPLC, haemoglobin C-Harlem must again be considered.

## Haemoglobin O-Arab disease

Homozygosity for haemoglobin O-Arab has been reported in Bulgaria, the former Yugoslavia (a gypsy family), Morocco, Tunisia, Sudan and Kenya [18,63–66].

### Clinical features

Homozygotes may be asymptomatic with compensated haemolysis or there may be recurrent jaundice and anaemia. The spleen may be enlarged.

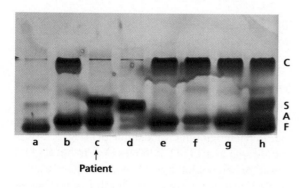

**Fig. 5.24** Agarose gel electrophoresis at acid pH in a patient with haemoglobin O-Arab heterozygosity. From left to right: (a) F plus faint S; (b) A plus C; (c) A plus O-Arab; (d) faint F and A plus S; (e, f, g) A plus C; (h) F, A, S and C (control sample). Note that haemoglobin O-Arab is slightly slower than haemoglobin S, i.e. slightly closer to C.

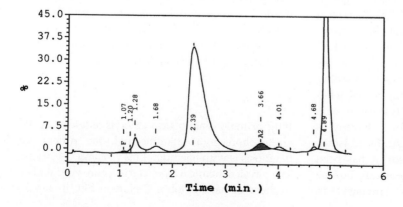

**Fig. 5.25** HPLC chromatogram from a patient with haemoglobin O-Arab heterozygosity. Haemoglobin O-Arab has a longer retention time than haemoglobin S, 4.9 min on this sample (Bio-Rad Variant II); from left to right, the major peaks are post-translationally modified haemoglobin A (two peaks) and haemoglobins A, $A_2$, and O-Arab.

*Laboratory features*

*Blood count.* The haemoglobin concentration may be normal or reduced and the MCV is reduced. The reticulocyte count is mildly increased.

*Blood film.* The blood film shows numerous target cells.

*Other investigations.* Haemoglobin O-Arab comprises almost all of the haemoglobin with a small amount of haemoglobin $A_2$. The percentage of dense cells is increased, the abnormality being comparable to that seen in homozygosity for haemoglobin C [7].

## Haemoglobin O-Arab/β thalassaemia

Haemoglobin O-Arab/$β^0$ thalassaemia has been described in Bulgaria, Hungary and Italy and haemoglobin O-Arab/$β^+$ thalassaemia in Saudi Arabia, Turkey and in an Afro-Caribbean [18,20].

*Clinical features*

This compound heterozygous state causes slight to moderate anaemia with jaundice and splenomegaly. The haemolytic anaemia may be episodic, being precipitated by intercurrent infection.

*Laboratory features*

*Blood count.* The reported haemoglobin concentration has ranged from 6 g/dl to normal levels. The MCV is reduced and the reticulocyte count is mildly increased.

*Blood film.* The blood film shows anisocytosis, poikilocytosis, hypochromia, microcytosis and target cells, which may be infrequent or numerous.

*Other investigations.* The haemoglobins present are haemoglobins O and $A_2$ with or without haemoglobin A. Haemoglobin F may be mildly increased.

## Coinheritance of haemoglobin O-Arab and other variant haemoglobins or thalassaemias

Coinheritance of haemoglobin S and haemoglobin O-Arab causes significant disease. This condition has been described on p. 175.

# Unstable haemoglobins

The term 'unstable haemoglobin' is best restricted to those variant haemoglobins that cause clinically recognizable haemolysis. Other haemoglobins, for example haemoglobin E, are unstable *in vitro*, but this probably does not contribute significantly to the associated clinical features. Both α and β chain variant haemoglobins may be unstable. Two γ chain variants have been described which led to haemoglobin instability in a neonate [67,68], and two γ chain variants that were methaemoglobins were also unstable [69]. δ chain variants can also be unstable but, because of their low concentration, this is of no clinical significance. Several patients have been described with two unstable haemoglobins, together with haemoglobin A or a $β^0$ thalassaemia determinant. This results not from three β genes in the genome, but from post-translational modification of an unstable haemoglobin. Both haemoglobin Sydney and haemoglobin Atlanta can be modified in this manner, producing haemoglobin Sydney-Coventry and haemoglobin Atlanta-Coventry, respectively. Haemoglobin instability can result from an unstable globin chain or an unstable haemoglobin molecule. The causative primary abnormality can affect the secondary structure (α helix and intervening turns), the tertiary three-dimensional structure of the monomer or the quaternary structure (relationship between monomers).

Haemoglobin instability may be consequent on:
• an abnormality of the haem pocket, so that haem is not firmly bound and water can enter the normally hydrophobic haem pocket; haem-depleted dimers and tetramers are present;
• interference with the α helical structure, often because an amino acid is replaced by the imino acid proline, or interference with the interhelical bends (abnormality of the secondary structure);
• replacement of an internal non-polar amino acid with a polar amino acid, which must be oriented

outwards and thus disrupts the molecule (interference with the tertiary structure);
• interference of the binding of α and β subunits to each other, specifically impairment of the $\alpha_1\beta_1$ dimeric bonds (interference with the quaternary structure); this can result in dissociation into monomers, favouring methaemoglobin formation;
• elongation of the β chain.

The first unstable haemoglobins identified were two β chain variants, haemoglobin Zurich and haemoglobin Köln, both reported in the early 1960s. Subsequently, a case of 'congenital non-spherocytic haemolytic anaemia', reported in the 1950s, was found to be attributable to haemoglobin Bristol. Since these early reports, more than 100 unstable haemoglobins have been described of which haemoglobin Köln appears to be the most common. Many more unstable β variants have been reported than unstable α variants, perhaps because α variants, being a lower proportion of total haemoglobin, are more likely to go unrecognized.

Unstable haemoglobins may result from:
• point mutations leading to replacement of one amino acid by another or replacement of an amino acid by the imino acid proline [18];
• point mutation followed by post-translational modification of the haemoglobin encoded; leucine in an abnormal haem pocket is modified to hydroxyleucine [70,71];
• deletions of one to eight codons leading to the deletion of a small number of amino acids, e.g. haemoglobin Gun Hill has a β chain which lacks five amino acids including the haem-binding site [72], and haemoglobin J-Biakra (unstable only *in vitro*) has an α chain which lacks eight amino acids [73];
• tandem duplication of codons leading to duplication of a small number of amino acids, e.g. haemoglobin Fairfax has five extra amino acids [74], the same amino acids that are deleted in haemoglobin Gun Hill;
• frame shift or stop codon mutations leading to the synthesis of an elongated β chain.

Of these various mechanisms, by far the most common is a single amino acid substitution.

Unstable haemoglobins show a greater or lesser tendency to Heinz body formation. Heinz bodies are composed of hemichromes, which are derivatives of ferric haemoglobin (methaemoglobin) in which the haem has been lost from the haem pocket and has bound elsewhere to denatured globin [68]. Heinz bodies bind to the inner surface of the red cell membrane, probably by hydrophobic interactions rather than covalent bonds [68]. The membrane can also be damaged by free haem and free iron. The cell becomes less deformable.

Most unstable haemoglobins cause haematological abnormalities in heterozygotes, but homozygosity has not been described. An exception to this generalization is haemoglobin Bushwick, which is only slightly unstable; it causes no significant abnormality in heterozygotes, but caused significant haemolytic anaemia in the one homozygote described [75]. Unstable haemoglobins have been described in a great variety of different ethnic groups, and sometimes an identical mutation has been found in a small number of individuals in very different parts of the world, suggesting that independent mutations have occurred. A significant proportion of unstable haemoglobins, probably about one-third, are new mutations, so that both parents are normal.

Unstable haemoglobins may, in addition to being unstable, show either increased or decreased oxygen affinity. Interaction with 2,3-DPG may be impaired. They may also be increasingly prone to oxidation to methaemoglobin. Haemoglobin Zurich has an unusual abnormality of the haem pocket, which is associated with an increased affinity for carbon monoxide and an increase in carboxyhaemoglobin; paradoxically, this reduces the instability, so that Heinz body haemolytic anaemia is less likely in smokers with haemoglobin Zurich than in non-smokers [1,68]. Some unstable haemoglobins, e.g. haemoglobin Köln, are synthesized at a reduced rate [76].

The proportion of abnormal haemoglobin for unstable β chain variants is very variable, ranging from 35–40% in the case of haemoglobin Hammersmith, through 10–15% in the case of haemoglobin Köln to almost undetectable in the case of very unstable haemoglobins such as haemoglobin Cagliari. The proportion of the variant haemoglobin is determined by:
• the rate of synthesis of the variant chain;
• the rate of breakdown of the $\beta^{variant}$ chain before association with the α chain can occur;

- the rate of association of $\alpha$ and $\beta^{variant}$ chains in comparison with the rate of association of $\alpha$ chains and normal $\beta^A$ chains;
- the rate of breakdown of $\alpha\beta^{variant}$ dimers before assembly of dimers to tetramers can occur;
- the rate of denaturation of unstable haemoglobin (with consequent removal as Heinz bodies).

In the case of unstable $\alpha$ chain variants, the proportion of variant haemoglobin is usually less than 15%, but may be 1–2% or even less. The explanation for the variable proportion of the variant haemoglobin is the same as for the $\beta$ chain variants.

In some instances, the proportion of an unstable haemoglobin is also affected by the fact that the mutation occurs in *cis* to an $\alpha$ thalassaemia determinant (haemoglobin Suan-Dok, haemoglobin Petah Tikva) or a $\beta$ thalassaemia determinant (haemoglobin Leiden) [68].

Depending on the degree of instability of a variant globin chain or variant haemoglobin, various degrees of abnormality are possible: (i) a very unstable $\alpha$ or $\beta$ chain is destroyed so rapidly that no variant globin chain or haemoglobin is detectable and the phenotype is that of thalassaemia; (ii) an unstable globin binds haem, but cannot bind to other globin chains, so that it precipitates as Heinz bodies in erythroid precursors; this leads to dyserythropoietic and ineffective erythropoiesis, as in dominant $\beta$ thalassaemia intermedia resulting from heterozygosity for a hyperunstable $\beta$ chain; (iii) a lesser degree of instability permits a variant haemoglobin to be synthesized, leading to a haemolytic anaemia and the clinical features recognized in association with an unstable haemoglobin. Highly unstable $\alpha$ chain variants are usually clinically silent but, if they interact with an $\alpha$ thalassaemia determinant, the phenotype may be either that of haemoglobin H disease or a haemolytic anaemia or may simulate $\beta$ thalassaemia intermedia; in the latter instance, there is no haemoglobin H detectable, there is dyserythropoiesis and globin chain synthesis studies show a paradoxically increased $\alpha : \beta$ ratio [77]. A phenotype with features of both thalassaemia and a Heinz body haemolytic anaemia can be produced either by a reduced rate of synthesis of an unstable variant or by marked instability leading to destruction of the variant globin chain or of $\alpha\beta$ dimers before assembly of haemoglobin tetramers can occur.

Patients with a very unstable haemoglobin are sometimes treated by splenectomy. Although this may lead to a reduction in haemolysis, there may also be an increase in the platelet count, leading to thrombotic complications. They are also sometimes treated with hydroxycarbamide, leading to a beneficial increase in haemoglobin F percentage and a fall in the percentage of the unstable variant.

## Clinical features

An unstable haemoglobin may cause severe, moderate or mild anaemia. Depending on the severity of the abnormality and the chain that is abnormal, presentation may be in infancy, childhood or adult life. One $\alpha$ chain variant, haemoglobin Hasharon, causes significant haemolysis in neonates but not in adult life, suggesting that $\alpha_2^{Hasharon}\gamma_2$ is more unstable than $\alpha_2^{Hasharon}\beta_2$ [1]. There may be intermittent or constant jaundice and the passage of dark brown or almost black urine, the latter attributable to the excretion of dipyrroles, which are abnormal breakdown products of haem. The incidence of gallstones is increased. The spleen may be enlarged and hypersplenism sometimes occurs. Anaemia may be intermittent or may intermittently worsen. Such deterioration is often attributable to intercurrent infection or exposure to oxidant drugs. In the case of haemoglobin Zurich, haemolysis may occur only on exposure to oxidants, and smokers, for the reason described on p. 216, exhibit less haemolysis than non-smokers. Aplastic crises and acute deterioration caused by folic acid deficiency or by parvovirus B19 infection have also been recognized. When an unstable haemoglobin is abnormally prone to oxidation to methaemoglobin, the patient may be cyanosed. Low oxygen affinity of an unstable haemoglobin may also cause cyanosis.

Some variant haemoglobins are only slightly unstable so that, although *in vitro* tests for instability are positive, there is usually no associated clinical abnormality.

## Laboratory features

*Blood count.* The haemoglobin concentration may be normal, except during episodic haemolysis, or may be mildly, moderately or severely reduced. On average, the haemoglobin concentration is higher when the unstable haemoglobin also has increased oxygen affinity. The MCV may be elevated and the MCH and MCHC may be reduced. The reduction of the MCH and MCHC may be attributable to the removal of Heinz bodies by the spleen. A low MCHC despite normocytic cells on a blood film can also be caused by the loss of haem from the haem pocket; the staining of the red cells in a blood film is attributable to the globin content, whereas the chemical measurement of haemoglobin is dependent on the haem molecule [72]. The reticulocyte count may be elevated constantly or intermittently. The degree of elevation of the reticulocyte count is not necessarily proportional to the reduction in the haemoglobin concentration because of the effect of altered oxygen affinity. If an unstable haemoglobin has a high oxygen affinity, the reticulocyte count will be higher, in relation to the haemoglobin concentration, than is the case for an unstable haemoglobin with a low oxygen affinity. There may be thrombocytopenia, which is sometimes disproportionate to the degree of splenomegaly and is not readily explicable.

Most unstable haemoglobins are synthesized at a normal rate, but some, e.g. haemoglobin Leiden (a β chain variant) and haemoglobin Petah Tikva (an α chain variant), have a reduced rate of synthesis because of a thalassaemia mutation in *cis* and have red cell indices similar to those of thalassaemia trait. Thalassaemic features can also result from a very unstable globin chain that is not incorporated into haemoglobin tetramers (see above).

Occasionally, when an unstable haemoglobin has increased oxygen affinity, there is polycythaemia rather than anaemia. Polycythaemia has also occasionally been observed to develop following splenectomy.

During haemolytic crises, there is a fall in the haemoglobin concentration and a rise in the reticulocyte count. The white cell count and the neutrophil count usually also rise.

*Blood film.* The blood film (Fig. 5.26) may show anaemia, macrocytosis, polychromatic macrocytes, mild hypochromia, basophilic stippling and the presence of irregularly contracted cells and keratocytes ('bite cells'). Although it is often considered that Heinz bodies cannot be detected on a Romanowsky-stained film, it has been pointed out that they can in fact be identified in patients who have required splenectomy because of the presence of an unstable haemoglobin (and also in other patients with severe oxidant-induced haemolytic anaemia) [18].

During haemolytic crises, there is an increase in polychromasia and in the number of irregularly contracted cells and keratocytes. Functional hyposplenism, consequent on reticuloendothelial overload, can lead to the appearance of Howell–Jolly bodies.

*Other investigations.* Haemoglobin electrophoresis may be abnormal (Fig. 5.27), but is basically normal in more than one-half of the reported unstable haemoglobins, specifically in those with no change in charge [1]. If the variant haemoglobin has a normal electrophoretic mobility, there may nevertheless be a tail behind the main haemoglobin band, representing either denatured haemoglobin or haemoglobin with a variable degree of haem depletion [78]; such bands are more likely if the specimen is not fresh. The disappearance of an abnormal band when haemin is added demonstrates that it results from haem depletion. In the case of unstable β chain variants, free α chains may form a discrete band near the origin, just behind haemoglobin $A_2$. Occasionally, two abnormal bands have been reported, for example in the case of haemoglobin Rush, apparently representing migration of asymmetric hybrids ($\alpha_2\beta\beta^{Rush}$) as well as haemoglobin A and haemoglobin Rush [1].

Some unstable haemoglobins appear as a discrete peak on HPLC; in others, there is a minor component apparent, representing degraded haemoglobin (Fig. 5.28). Sometimes standard electrophoretic and HPLC techniques all give normal results and DNA analysis or mass spectrometry is required for the demonstration of the variant haemoglobin.

When the unstable haemoglobin is a β chain variant, the concentration of haemoglobin $A_2$ may be increased, as a consequence of selective denaturation and removal of the unstable variant. The haemoglobin F concentration may be moderately increased, e.g. to 10–12%. Methaemoglobin may be present in fresh blood or, more often, appears abnormally rapidly as the specimen ages.

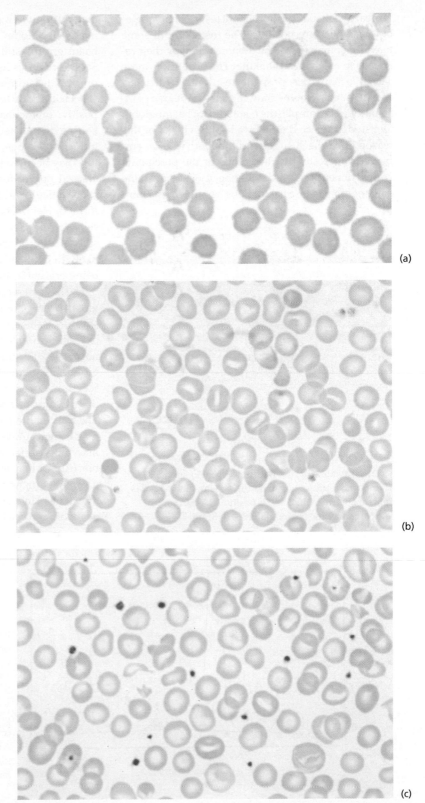

(a)

(b)

(c)

**Fig. 5.26** Blood films from three patients with unstable haemoglobins: (a) irregularly contracted cells, macrocytosis and thrombocytopenia in a patient heterozygous for haemoglobin Köln; (b) several stomatocytes and several irregularly contracted cells in a patient with haemoglobin Siriraj; (c) hypochromia and poikilocytosis in a patient with haemoglobin St Mary's.

Heat and, usually, isopropanol tests for haemoglobin instability are positive. The instability of some haemoglobins can also be demonstrated by their response to mechanical shaking. The heat test is more sensitive than the isopropanol test, and so will detect variant haemoglobins showing a lesser degree of instability. For example, the instability of haemoglobin Olmsted is detected only by a heat test [79]. For this reason, it has been suggested that both tests be employed. Interestingly, the colour of the precipitate varies, depending on the tendency of the unstable haemoglobin to lose haem. Thus haemoglobin Ham-

mersmith gives a red–brown precipitate, representing haemoglobin Hammersmith with most of its haem groups still attached, whereas haemoglobin Santa Ana loses its haem groups so readily that the precipitate is almost white [18].

A Heinz body test may be positive or may become positive on incubation of the blood at 37°C for 24 h. During acute haemolytic episodes, including those induced by drugs, a previously negative Heinz body test may become positive. This is because of an increased rate of formation of Heinz bodies and because reticuloendothelial overload means that, once formed, Heinz bodies are not being pitted from red cells by hepatic and splenic macrophages. If a splenectomy has been necessary, a Heinz body test is likely to be positive, with Heinz bodies sometimes being present in almost every red cell.

The oxygen affinity may be increased (e.g. haemoglobin Köln) or reduced (e.g. haemoglobin Hammersmith). Of the reported unstable haemoglobins, the oxygen affinity has been found to be reduced in 30%, normal in 20% and increased in 50% [1]. As these conditions are generally heterozygous, the oxygen dissociation curve is generally biphasic, representing the mixture of normal and variant haemoglobins. The red cell life span is reduced, but measurements may be inaccurate for the following reasons: (i) $^{51}$Cr may bind preferentially to the unstable haemoglobin; (ii) $^{51}$Cr may lead to denaturation of the unstable haemoglobin; and (iii) loss of $^{51}$Cr may indicate removal of a Heinz body by the spleen rather than the death of a red cell [18].

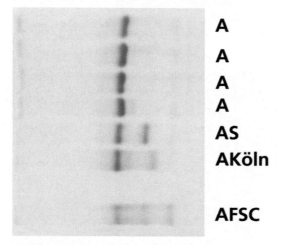

**Fig. 5.27** Haemoglobin electrophoresis on cellulose acetate at alkaline pH in a patient with haemoglobin Köln; a faint band representing denatured haemoglobin Köln is apparent between the S and C positions; AFSC, control sample containing haemoglobins A, F, S, and C.

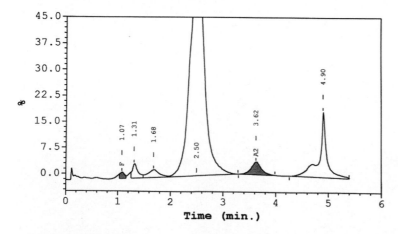

**Fig. 5.28** HPLC chromatogram from a patient with haemoglobin Köln heterozygosity showing minor components that represent denatured haemoglobin Köln (far right) (Bio-Rad Variant II); from left to right, the other peaks are haemoglobin F, post-translationally modified haemoglobin A (two peaks), haemoglobin A plus unaltered haemoglobin Köln and haemoglobin $A_2$.

Bone marrow examination (Fig. 5.29) may show erythroid hyperplasia and dyserythropoietic features, such as binuclearity/multinuclearity and nuclear irregularity or lobulation [80]; ring sideroblasts are sometimes present.

There may be an increase in bilirubin concentration (mainly unconjugated bilirubin) and lactate dehydrogenase (LDH), together with evidence of intravascular haemolysis, such as a reduced serum haptoglobin concentration, reduced serum haemopexin and the presence of serum methaemalbumin and urinary haemosiderin.

It should be noted that inaccurate (low) pulse oximeter measurements of oxygen saturation have been reported, as a result of the abnormal absorption spectrum of the variant haemoglobin, with a number of unstable haemoglobins, including haemoglobin Köln, haemoglobin Hammersmith and haemoglobin Cheverly [81,82].

### Diagnosis

Haemoglobin electrophoresis, HPLC or both should be performed. However, as other tests may all give

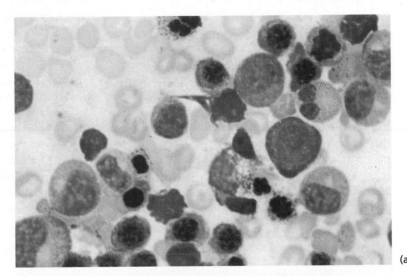

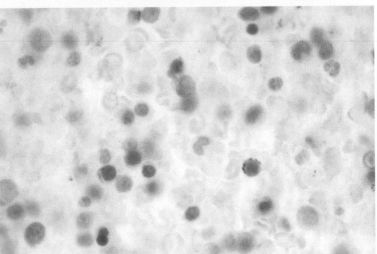

**Fig. 5.29** Bone marrow aspirate from a patient with haemoglobin St Mary's: (a) May–Grünwald–Giemsa stain showing erythroid hyperplasia and dyserythropoiesis (lobulated nuclei and basophilic stippling); (b) Perls' stain for iron showing ring sideroblasts.

(a)

(b)

normal results, diagnosis requires a specific test for an unstable haemoglobin. A blood film examination is particularly useful.

## Coinheritance of an unstable haemoglobin and other variant haemoglobins or thalassaemia

The severity of disease caused by an unstable β chain variant may be reduced by coinheritance of α thalassaemia [83]. Coinheritance of an unstable haemoglobin, e.g. haemoglobin Acharnes, haemoglobin Arta or haemoglobin Lulu Island, with β thalassaemia has been associated with the clinical picture of β thalassaemia intermedia (see Table 3.10).

## Haemoglobin M

The designation haemoglobin M is given to a variety of α, β and γ chain haemoglobin variants that show an increased tendency to oxidation to methaemoglobin, with consequent cyanosis or pseudocyanosis. The abnormal colour of the patient's skin differs from the purplish-blue of true cyanosis and has been variously described as lavender-blue, slate grey or brownish-slate. However, with haemoglobins M-Boston and M-Iwate, which have a low oxygen affinity, there is also an element of true cyanosis

[68]. In Japan, terms meaning 'black mouth', 'black blood' or 'black child' were used for carriers of haemoglobin M-Iwate. The first haemoglobin M was recognized in 1948, a year before the first description of haemoglobin S [84].

The molecular abnormality is usually the replacement of a histidine residue in the haem pocket by tyrosine, so that the iron of the haem molecule is stabilized in the ferric ($Fe^{3+}$) form. Either the proximal or the distal histidine may be involved (Fig. 5.30). The exception is haemoglobin M-Milwaukee in which the longer side-chain of glutamic acid, substituted for valine at β67, reaches the haem molecule and stabilizes an abnormal ferric state [68]. Once the variant globin chain has been oxidized, it becomes non-functional from the viewpoint of oxygen transport. In the case of the three α chain variants, M-Boston, M-Iwate and M-Milwaukee, only the β chains can bind oxygen; in the case of the two β chain variants, M-Saskatoon and M-Hyde Park, only the α chains can bind oxygen. Conversion to methaemoglobin may be accelerated by exogenous oxidants. Some M haemoglobins have a reduced oxygen affinity. Some are also unstable and instability may be aggravated by oxidant stress. Haemoglobin M-Hyde Park is an example of an unstable haemoglobin M with partial haem loss leading to haemoglobin instability and haemolysis. They all have a marked reduc-

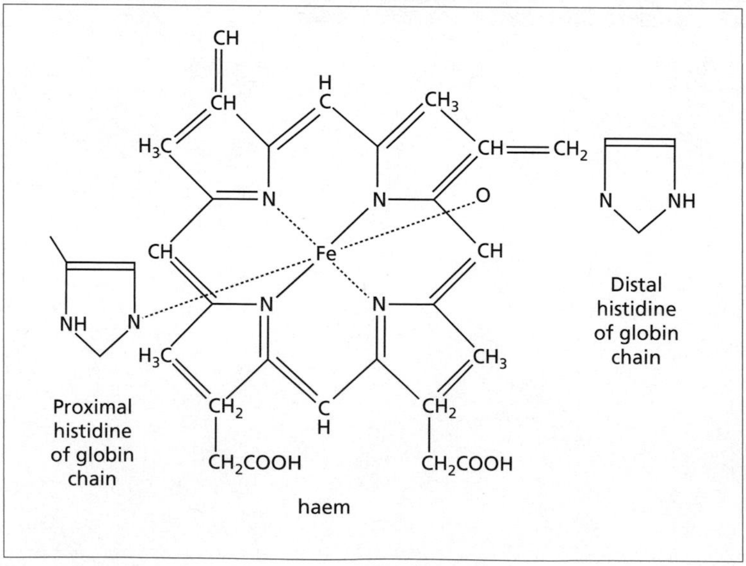

**Fig. 5.30** Diagram showing the relationship of haem to the proximal and distal histidines of the haem pocket. Mutation of either of the corresponding codons can lead to a haemoglobin M.

tion in cooperativity indicated by a low *n* number [85] (see below). These variant haemoglobins are summarized in Table 5.3.

The α chain M haemoglobins investigated to date have all been α1 variants [2]. It has been postulated that this is because, with an α2 mutation, the preferential combination of the variant α chain with normal non-α chains could lead to a haemoglobin M percentage incompatible with fetal viability.

### Clinical features

There is cyanosis from birth in the case of α chain variants and from around 3–6 months of age in the case of β chain variants. Babies with γ chain variants are mildly cyanosed at birth, but cyanosis lessens as β chain production takes over from γ [69]. When there is a significant amount of methaemoglobin present, a blood sample appears macroscopically brownish.

### Laboratory features

*Blood count.* The haemoglobin concentration may be normal or high. Occasional patients are anaemic. The reticulocyte count is sometimes elevated, particularly in the case of carriers of haemoglobin M-Hyde Park and haemoglobin M-Saskatoon, which may be associated with a compensated haemolytic state.

*Blood film.* The blood film may show poikilocytosis.

*Other investigations.* The diagnosis is usually by spectrometry as the absorbance spectrum of methaemoglobin differs from that of haemoglobin A. The absorption spectra of different haemoglobin Ms differ from each other, but not sufficiently to permit definitive diagnosis. However, if haemoglobin is first oxidized, the spectra are characteristic (Fig. 5.31). Haemoglobin electrophoresis is normal at alkaline pH, but electrophoresis at pH 7 in phosphate buffer shows abnormal mobility of haemoglobin Ms, as the mutation involves histidine which ionizes at neutral pH [86]. Other congenital and acquired causes of methaemoglobinaemia need to be excluded (see p. 244). In contrast with low-affinity haemoglobins, oxygenation of the sample *in vitro* does not restore the normal colour. Haemoglobin electrophoresis may show an abnormal band, but the normal and variant haemoglobins are more readily separated if they are both converted to methaemoglobin prior to electrophoresis. The oxygen dissociation curve may be abnormal in shape and either right or left shifted.

**Table 5.3** M haemoglobins.

| Haemoglobin | Oxygen affinity | Usual percentage of variant | *n* number* | Other features |
|---|---|---|---|---|
| *β chain variants* | | | | |
| M-Saskatoon ($\alpha_2\beta_2^{63(E7)His\rightarrow Tyr}$) | Normal | 35 | 1.2 | Mild or no haemolysis |
| M-Hyde Park ($\alpha_2\beta_2^{92(F8)His\rightarrow Tyr}$) | Normal | NA† | 1.3 | Mild haemolysis |
| M-Milwaukee ($\alpha_2\beta_2^{67(E11)Val\rightarrow Glu}$) | Reduced | 50 | 1.2 | No haemolysis |
| | | | | |
| *α chain variants* | | | | |
| M-Iwate‡ ($\alpha_2^{87(F8)His\rightarrow Tyr}\beta_2$) | Reduced | 19 | 1.1 | Not anaemic |
| M-Boston ($\alpha_2^{58(E7)His\rightarrow Tyr}\beta_2$) | Reduced | NA | 1.2 | Sometimes anaemic |
| | | | | |
| *γ chain variants* | | | | |
| F M-Osaka ($\alpha_2{}^G\gamma_2^{63(E7)His\rightarrow Tyr}$) | | | | Neonatal cyanosis |
| F M-Fort Ripley ($\alpha_2{}^G\gamma_2^{92(F8)His\rightarrow Tyr}$) | | | | Neonatal cyanosis' |

* The *n* number indicates the degree of cooperativity between haemoglobin subunits; normal haemoglobins have an *n* value of 2.7–3.0, whereas a haemoglobin with no cooperativity has an *n* value of unity [85].

† Information not available.

‡ Also known as haemoglobin Kankakee, haemoglobin M-Oldenberg and haemoglobin M-Sendai [2].

# 6 Acquired abnormalities of globin chain synthesis or haemoglobin structure

Acquired disorders of globin chain synthesis may result from: (i) mutation of a globin gene; (ii) altered methylation status of a globin gene leading to altered expression; or (iii) the influence of other genes on the expression of globin genes. Acquired somatic mutations of globin genes are very rare. Altered expression is much more common.

Post-translational modification of haemoglobin structure can also occur as a result of inherited abnormalities, other than those of globin genes, or as a result of exposure to toxic drugs or chemicals.

## Acquired thalassaemia

Alterations in the rates of globin chain synthesis, with $\alpha:\beta$ ratios similar to those observed in thalassaemia, are quite common in myeloid malignancies. This may be regarded as a mild form of acquired thalassaemia. Peters *et al.* [1] observed an increased $\alpha:\beta$ ratio in six of 11 patients with myelodysplastic syndromes ($\alpha:\beta$ chain synthesis ratio of 1.28–2.43; normal range 0.97–1.19) and in two of four patients with acute myeloid leukaemia (AML) (both cases evolved from myelodysplastic syndromes; $\alpha:\beta$ chain synthesis ratios of 1.8 and 2.1). In this study, red cell hypochromia and microcytosis were not confined to patients with abnormalities in the $\alpha:\beta$ chain synthesis ratio.

The phenotype of $\alpha$ or $\beta$ thalassaemia is much less common amongst cases of leukaemia, myelodysplastic syndrome and related disorders than is an alteration in the ratio of $\alpha$ and $\beta$ globin chain synthesis. When acquired thalassaemia occurs, the phenotype is most often that of haemoglobin H disease, although acquired $\alpha$ thalassaemia trait [2] and $\beta$ or $\delta\beta$ thalassaemia [3–6] have also been reported. It should be noted that cases described as acquired $\beta$ or $\delta\beta$ thalassaemia are not as well characterized as acquired haemoglobin H disease and it is less clear whether

this is a distinct entity. The molecular mechanism, deletion of the $\alpha$ gene cluster from one chromosome 16, was identified in a single patient with acquired $\alpha$ thalassaemia trait as a feature of a myelodysplastic syndrome [2].

More than 30 cases of acquired haemoglobin H disease have been described [7–20]. Some of the published cases are summarized in reference [18]. This syndrome has been associated with myelodysplastic syndromes, AML, idiopathic myelofibrosis, atypical chronic myeloid leukaemia and various difficult to classify atypical myeloproliferative/myelodysplastic disorders. The type of myelodysplastic syndrome most strongly associated with acquired haemoglobin H disease is refractory anaemia with ring sideroblasts (Fig. 6.1), but some cases have had refractory anaemia or refractory anaemia with excess of blasts. Cases of AML have typically been erythroleukaemia (Fig. 6.2) (French–American–British (FAB) type M6 AML), sometimes with sideroblastic erythropoiesis. Atypical myelodysplastic/myeloproliferative syndromes have included several cases of refractory anaemia, with or without ring sideroblasts, with coexisting thrombocytosis. It was demonstrated that, in acquired haemoglobin H disease, although all four $\alpha$ genes are intact and show a normal pattern of methylation, $\alpha$ chain messenger RNA (mRNA) was greatly reduced. In many patients, the defect in $\alpha$ chain synthesis was so severe that it was clear that all four $\alpha$ genes were downregulated. Interestingly, one patient with acquired haemoglobin H disease had five $\alpha$ genes, as a result of a constitutional triple $\alpha$, but, despite this, had an $\alpha:\beta$ globin chain synthesis ratio of 0.09 [18]. In this patient, all five $\alpha$ genes must have been downregulated. Clearly, a *trans*-acting factor was implicated. This was supported by the observation that the ratio of $\alpha2$ and $\alpha1$ gene transcripts was normal [19]. The hypothesis that the cause of the reduced synthesis was the downregulation of struc-

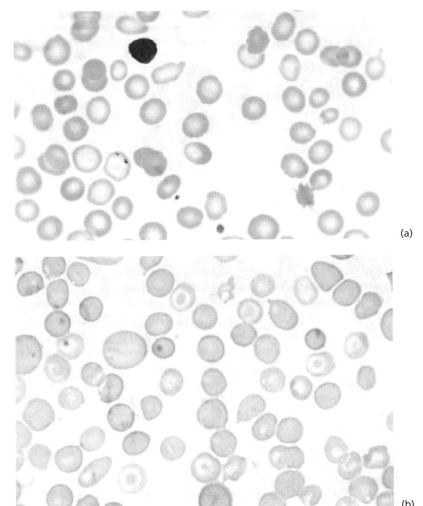

(a)

(b)

**Fig. 6.1** Blood film from a 60-year-old man with acquired haemoglobin H disease associated with refractory anaemia with ring sideroblasts. The white blood cell count (WBC) was $9.2 \times 10^9/l$, haemoglobin concentration 10 g/dl, mean cell volume (MCV) 66 fl and platelet count $53 \times 10^9/l$. The haemoglobin H percentage was 9% and the $\alpha : \beta$ chain synthesis ratio was 0.16. (a) Dimorphic red cells with one of the hypochromic cells containing several Pappenheimer bodies. (b) Dimorphic red cells with normocytic normochromic cells and microcytic target cells. (By courtesy of Dr A. Hendrick.)

turally normal genes was further supported by an experiment in which a human chromosome 16 from a case of acquired haemoglobin H disease was transferred to mouse erythroleukaemia cells with resultant normal expression of human α genes. The great majority of patients with acquired haemoglobin H disease, more than 90%, have been male. The explanation of all of these observations was revealed, when it was demonstrated that the cause of acquired haemoglobin H disease is an acquired somatic mutation of the *ATRX* gene [21,22].

Acquired haemoglobin H disease is associated with variable anaemia and reticulocytosis. Microcytosis is common, but not invariable, whereas in-

herited haemoglobin H disease is invariably associated with microcytosis. The red cells usually show marked anisocytosis, poikilocytosis and hypochromia. The blood film is often dimorphic, a feature that is not seen in the inherited form of the disease. There are three possible explanations for the dimorphism: (i) the frequency of association of acquired haemoglobin H disease with sideroblastic erythropoiesis; (ii) the possibility that there is coexistence of abnormal clonal cells, showing a defect in α chain synthesis, and surviving normal cells with normal haemoglobin synthesis; and (iii) the possibility that the erythroid precursors with a defect in the synthesis of the α chain and haemoglobin represent a

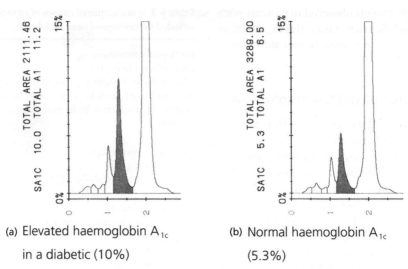

(a) Elevated haemoglobin $A_{1c}$

in a diabetic (10%)

(b) Normal haemoglobin $A_{1c}$

(5.3%)

**Fig. 6.4** High performance liquid chromatography (HPLC) chromatograms showing (a) increased haemoglobin $A_{1c}$ in a diabetic patient and (b) normal haemoglobin $A_{1c}$ in a control sample.

**Table 6.4** Causes of real and apparent increased and decreased percentages of haemoglobin $A_{1c}$.

|  | **Increased percentage** | **Decreased percentage** |
|---|---|---|
| Factitious | Presence of a variant haemoglobin with a retention time overlapping with that of haemoglobin $A_{1c}$ | Presence of various variant haemoglobins, including haemoglobins S, C, Takamatsu, G-Szuhu, Himeyi, O-Padova, Camden, Riyadh, J-Meerut, Sherwood Forrest, Manitoba and G-Coushatta [55] |
| True | Diabetes mellitus Aged population of red cells, e.g. recent onset of pure red cell aplasia Iron deficiency anaemia HIV infection [52] | Shortened red cell life span |

HIV, human immunodeficiency virus.

carbons. Endogenous production of carbon monoxide as a result of catabolism of haemoglobin (specifically haem) and, to a lesser extent, myoglobin is a physiological process, so that a low level of carboxyhaemoglobin is detectable in everyone [36,56]. Healthy non-smokers have around 1% of carboxyhaemoglobin, with higher levels (around 5%) being observed in pregnancy and in the presence of haemolytic anaemia [57] or a haematoma [58]. Fetuses and neonates have higher levels than adults [58]. A much higher level of carboxyhaemoglobin in the blood occurs if there is exposure to exogenous carbon monoxide. Increased levels of carboxyhaemoglobin may result from exposure to:
• car exhaust fumes (deliberate or accidental, including snow-blocked car exhaust pipe [59] — the risk is less when a catalytic converter is fitted);
• coal, gas, peat and charcoal fires, water heaters, central heating boilers, heating appliances, other combustion engines — particularly when ventilation is poor and if a fire intended for outdoor use is used indoors or in a sealed tent;

- inhaled smoke in house fires;
- industrial fumes, including both propane and methane used as fuels and methylene chloride (a common component of paint remover and other solvents, which is metabolized by the liver to carbon monoxide) [56];
- cigarette smoke.

Cigarette smokers often have carboxyhaemoglobin levels of 5–10%, but sometimes up to 20%. Part of the risk to the fetus of cigarette smoking in pregnancy is attributable to carbon monoxide [58]. Much higher levels, which may be fatal, are seen in suicide attempts using car exhaust fumes and with accidental exposure to industrial chemicals or the combustion products of poorly ventilated domestic heaters. Carbon monoxide poisoning is caused by suicide attempts in about one-half of instances, is associated with burns in about one-quarter of cases and results from other unintentional exposure to carbon monoxide in another quarter [60]. A high concentration of carboxyhaemoglobin gives the blood a cherry-red colour. Symptoms include headache, lethargy, nausea and vomiting, followed by drowsiness, convulsions, coma and death.

The affinity of haemoglobin for carbon monoxide is 200–250 times as great as its affinity for oxygen. The process of formation of carboxyhaemoglobin is slowly reversible. The production of carboxyhaemoglobin moves the oxygen dissociation curve to the left and makes it more hyperbolic. This is because, once two carbon monoxide molecules are bound to haem groups, the molecule changes to an oxy conformation, increasing the affinity for oxygen. This means that, in individuals with an increased percentage of carboxyhaemoglobin, the degree of tissue hypoxia is greater than would be expected from the percentage of carboxyhaemoglobin present. The increased oxygen affinity caused by binding to carbon monoxide is more important than the decreased affinity attributable to 2,3-DPG in explaining the varying $P_{50}$ (the $P_{O_2}$ at which haemoglobin is 50% saturated) seen in normal individuals [36]. Carboxyhaemoglobin does not function in oxygen transport and, in addition, oxygen delivery to tissues is impaired, as is shown by the altered shape of the dissociation curve. The effects of tissue hypoxia are further aggravated by the binding of carbon monoxide to myoglobin and to mitochondrial cytochromes [57,61]. The impaired tissue oxygen delivery in individuals with a chronic increase in the percentage of carboxyhaemoglobin means that there is an erythropoietin-driven increase in the rate of haemoglobin synthesis and the haemoglobin concentration is increased. This may mean that increased blood viscosity compounds the effects of reduced delivery of oxygen to tissues.

When the concentration of oxygen in the inspired air is lower, the effects of any influences likely to raise the carboxyhaemoglobin concentration are greater (e.g. poor combustion of a stove in a sealed tent would have a greater effect at altitude). Conversion of carboxyhaemoglobin to oxyhaemoglobin is accelerated by removal from the source of carbon monoxide and by ventilation with oxygen, or by hyperbaric oxygen treatment. The half-life of carboxyhaemoglobin is 240–320 min when breathing air, 80–100 min when breathing 100% oxygen and about 20 min with hyperbaric oxygen [61]. Hyperbaric oxygen therapy has been demonstrated to reduce neurological damage [62]. An increased rate of ventilation, for example as a consequence of vigorous exercise or artificial ventilation, lowers the percentage of carboxyhaemoglobin (assuming that the individual has been removed from the source of carbon monoxide and is breathing inspired air with a low content of carbon monoxide).

If pregnant women are exposed to carbon monoxide, effects in the fetus are even more severe [56]. There is an exaggerated leftwards shift of the oxygen dissociation curve with resultant severe tissue hypoxia. There is a similar increased vulnerability to carbon monoxide poisoning during the first few months of life, when fetal haemoglobin levels remain high, and later in life in individuals with a persistent elevation of fetal haemoglobin [61].

Haemoglobin Zurich is an interesting example of the interaction between inherited and acquired abnormalities of the haemoglobin molecule. It has a greater affinity for carbon monoxide than does haemoglobin A and, paradoxically, this protects cigarette smokers from haemolysis.

Carboxyhaemoglobin is detected and measured by spectroscopy (Fig. 6.5). However, it should be noted that the severity of carbon monoxide poisoning correlates poorly with the carboxyhaemoglobin percentage and this should not be used to judge the necessity for hyperbaric oxygen therapy [63]. Pulse

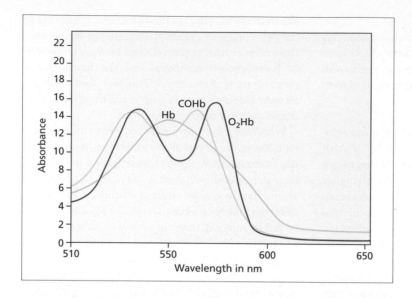

**Fig. 6.5** Spectroscopy showing carboxyhaemoglobin (COHb), oxyhaemoglobin ($O_2$Hb) and deoxyhaemoglobin (Hb).

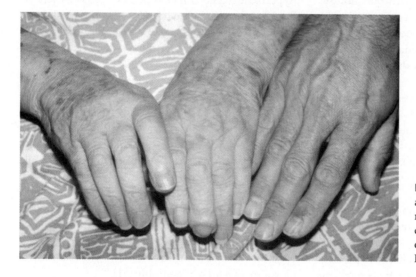

**Fig. 6.6** Hands of a patient with anaemia and mild methaemoglobinaemia caused by dapsone in comparison with the hand of a healthy subject. (By courtesy of Professor L. Hirst.)

oximetry is inaccurate in measuring oxyhaemo-globin when carboxyhaemoglobin is present, as the technique does not distinguish between carboxy-haemoglobin and oxyhaemoglobin [56]. This is be-cause the wavelengths employed by most pulse oximeters are selected to distinguish between oxy-genated and non-oxygenated haemoglobin and not between oxyhaemoglobin and other forms of haemoglobin. A co-oximeter measures the percent-ages of carboxyhaemoglobin, oxyhaemoglobin and deoxyhaemoglobin.

## Methaemoglobinaemia

Methaemoglobin is formed by the oxidation of haem iron, i.e. by conversion from the ferrous ($Fe^{2+}$) to the ferric ($Fe^{3+}$) form. Auto-oxidation of haemoglobin occurs, the α chain being oxidized more rapidly than the β chain in an intact molecule. Auto-oxidation is increased by a rise in temperature, increased 2,3-DPG and reduced pH [58]. The rate of production of methaemoglobin is increased by sepsis. Oxidation of haemoglobin is increased by exposure to exogenous oxidants. Various red cell enzymes convert methaemoglobin back to haemoglobin, so that the level is normally less than 1%.

Methaemoglobin does not function in oxygen transport and, in addition, the presence of methaemoglobin leads to a left shift of the oxygen dissociation curve, which further impairs oxygen delivery to tissues; this is because oxidation of some haems in a partly oxidized tetramer favours the oxy conformation of the tetramer. High levels of methaemoglobin are associated with chocolate-coloured blood, cyanosis (or pseudocyanosis) (Figs 6.6 and 6.7), headache, tachycardia, dyspnoea, tachypnoea and, finally, coma and death. Symptoms are considerably greater when an acute rise in the percentage of methaemoglobin occurs than when there is chronic methaemoglobinaemia. A concentration of 1.5–2 g/dl causes cyanosis (in comparison with the 5 g/dl of deoxyhaemoglobin that is needed to produce cyanosis). Methaemoglobin is detected by spectroscopy (Fig. 6.8) or by co-oximetry, which permits the detection of carboxyhaemoglobin, methaemoglobin and sulphaemoglobin. It should be noted that, as for patients with carboxyhaemoglobinaemia, pulse oximetry and conventional blood gas analysis are misleading in patients with methaemoglobinaemia [64,65]. Pulse oximetry overestimates

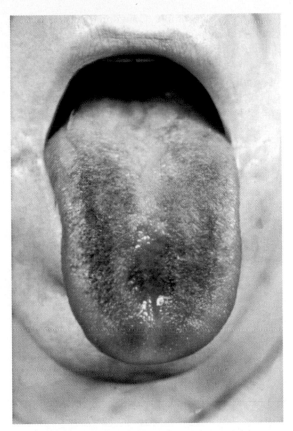

**Fig. 6.7** Tongue of a patient with methaemoglobinaemia.

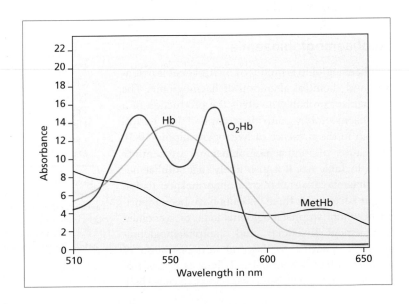

**Fig. 6.8** Spectroscopy showing methaemoglobin (MetHb), oxyhaemoglobin ($O_2Hb$) and deoxyhaemoglobin (Hb).

the oxygen saturation. Congenital and acquired causes of methaemoglobinaemia are shown in Table 6.5. It is also possible that methaemoglobinaemia may be the result of endogenous oxidant production by gut bacteria, as two patients have been reported in whom combined methaemoglobinaemia and sulphaemoglobinaemia responded to the oral administration of antibiotics [80].

The congenital methaemoglobinaemias caused by methaemoglobin reductase (NADH-cytochrome $b_5$ reductase) deficiency usually have 10–20% of methaemoglobin. The reduced oxygen-carrying capacity of the blood leads to secondary polycythaemia. In type I deficiency, methaemoglobinaemia is the only clinical manifestation, whereas, in type II deficiency, in which tissues other than red cells are affected, there is also neurological impairment and growth retardation. Both have an autosomal recessive inheritance.

Infants are more susceptible to methaemoglobinaemia than adults. This is only partly because haemoglobin F is more susceptible to oxidation. It is related more to the reduced level of methaemoglobin reductase at this age.

Individuals with an inherited methaemoglobin reductase deficiency have an increased susceptibility to oxidant drugs and chemicals.

Patients with severe symptoms from methaemoglobinaemia are treated with intravenous methylene blue. In life-threatening situations, exchange transfusion can be employed.

## Sulphaemoglobinaemia

Sulphaemoglobin is produced by irreversible oxidation and chemical alteration of haemoglobin. The mechanism probably involves the production of a ferrohaemoglobin–peroxide complex that is sulphated in the presence of hydrogen sulphide [80]. The causes of sulphaemoglobinaemia are summarized in Table 6.6. It is also likely that sulphaemoglobinaemia can result from an abnormal population of gut bacteria, as three patients have been reported in whom sulphaemoglobinaemia, or combined methaemoglobinaemia and sulphaemoglobinaemia, responded to the oral administration of antibiotics [80]. Abnormal gut flora as a result of constipation has also been suspected as a cause [52].

**Table 6.5** Some causes of an increased concentration of methaemoglobin. (Derived from references [36,58,64,66–79] and other sources.)

**Inherited**
Haemoglobin M
As a feature of an unstable haemoglobin
Deficiency of NADH-cytochrome $b_5$ reductase
    Type I (deficiency of red cells only)
    Type II (generalized tissue deficiency)
Deficiency of cytochrome $b_5$ (single patient) [76]

**Acquired**
Residence at high altitude [77]
Exposure to oxidant drugs and chemicals
    Nitrites such as sodium nitrite*, amyl nitrite‡, butyl nitrite‡, isobutyl nitrite‡ (therapeutic doses of nitrites may produce up to 5% methaemoglobin)
    Nitric oxide (NO) (by inhalation)
    Nitrates (converted to nitrites by hepatic metabolism), e.g. excessive amount of sodium nitrate used as preservative for sausage meat; nitrate-contaminated well water† including when it is used for home dialysis or for reconstituting powdered milk for infants)
    Nitroglycerine (intravenously)
    Nitroprusside
    Nitrate-rich diet (particularly in young babies)
    Phenacetin (now withdrawn from market)
    Paracetamol (acetaminophen)
    Dapsone
    Sulphonamides [75]
    Primaquine
    Flutamide [68]
    Clofazimine
    Local or topical anaesthetics
        Topical benzocaine [75]
        Prilocaine [74]
        Procaine
        Lidocaine
    Riluzole (overdose) [78]
    Copper
    Naphthalene
    Petrol octane booster (contains aniline)
    Henna
    Lysol (50% cresol in linseed oil, potassium hydroxide and water) [79]

*Used for curing meat, as a food preservative, as an insecticide and to inhibit corrosion (may contaminate water in pipes and tanks when it is used as a corrosion-inhibiting solution) [74].
‡Including 'recreational' use.
†The risks from well water relate to the application of nitrogenous fertilizers to surrounding farmland [36].

The drugs that can cause methaemoglobinaemia can also cause sulphaemoglobinaemia. The most common cause is exposure to drugs such as phenacetin and dapsone. Occupational exposure to sulphur-containing compounds can also be responsible. Flutamide, an anti-androgen used for the treatment of carcinoma of the prostate, has been reported to cause sulphaemoglobinaemia and methaemoglobinaemia [68]. A single case of sulphaemoglobinaemia and

**Table 6.6** Causes of an increased concentration of sulphaemoglobin.

| |
| --- |
| **Inherited** |
| Autosomal dominant inherited sulphaemoglobinaemia [36] |
| As a feature of some unstable haemoglobins, e.g. haemoglobin Olmstead [36] |
| |
| **Acquired** |
| Exposure to drugs and chemicals (as for methaemoglobinaemia) |
| Sulphur-containing ointments |
| Occupational exposure to hydrogen sulphide |
| Septicaemia (in a neonate) [81] |

methaemoglobinaemia, apparently caused by intravenous all-*trans*-retinoic acid, has also been reported [72]. Sulphaemoglobin lacks co-operativity [52] and does not function in oxygen transport. However, it leads to reduced oxygen affinity of non-sulphinated monomers, ameliorating the effect on tissue oxygen delivery. It has been postulated that sulphaemoglobinaemia would be much more deleterious in patients with sickle cell disease, because favouring of the deoxy conformation would also favour the maintenance of polymerization [58]. A concentration of 0.5–1.6 g/dl or above can cause cyanosis (or pseudocyanosis). At very high levels, the beneficial effect on oxygen affinity is negated by an extremely right-shifted oxygen dissociation curve. In severe acute sulphaemoglobinaemia, there are neurological effects, pulmonary oedema and death [58].

Sulphaemoglobin can be detected by spectroscopy (Fig. 6.9) and co-oximetry. Pulse oximetry is inaccurate, the oxygen saturation being overestimated [65].

Methylene blue is ineffective in the treatment of sulphaemoglobinaemia but, as most patients are asymptomatic, specific treatment is not indicated.

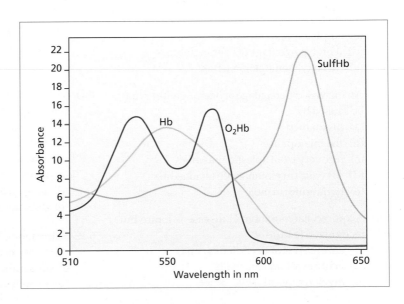

**Fig. 6.9** Spectroscopy showing sulphaemoglobin (sulfHb), oxyhaemoglobin (O₂Hb) and deoxyhaemoglobin (Hb).

## Check your knowledge

One to five answers may be correct. Answers to al-most all questions can be found in this chapter or can be deduced from the information given. The correct answers are given on p. 252.

6.1 Cyanosis may be caused by
(a) methaemoglobinaemia
(b) sulphaemoglobinaemia
(c) carboxyhaemoglobinaemia
(d) increased haemoglobin $A_{1c}$
(e) a low-affinity haemoglobin

6.2 A reduced percentage of haemoglobin $A_2$ can be caused by
(a) haemochromatosis
(b) diabetes mellitus
(c) anaemia of chronic disease
(d) iron deficiency
(e) sideroblastic anaemia

6.3 An increased percentage of haemoglobin F in a neonate may be caused by
(a) intrauterine hypoxia
(b) post-mature baby
(c) maternal diabetes
(d) maternal alcohol intake
(e) maternal cigarette smoking

6.4 Oxygen affinity of whole blood is increased by
(a) a high percentage of haemoglobin F
(b) methaemoglobinaemia
(c) sulphaemoglobinaemia
(d) a high percentage of haemoglobin $A_{1c}$
(e) carboxyhaemoglobinaemia

6.5 An increased percentage of haemoglobin F may be caused by
(a) pregnancy
(b) the menopause
(c) recovery from aplastic anaemia
(d) juvenile myelomonocytic leukaemia
(e) hydatidiform mole

6.6 Acquired haemoglobin H disease is a rare but recognized feature of
(a) chronic lymphocytic leukaemia
(b) acute myeloid leukaemia
(c) myelodysplastic syndromes

(d) non-Hodgkin's lymphoma
(e) congenital sideroblastic anaemia

6.7 Carbon monoxide may be derived from
(a) metabolism of haemoglobin
(b) metabolism of glucose
(c) poorly ventilated domestic heaters
(d) exhaust fumes of motor vehicles
(e) cigarette fumes

6.8 An increased percentage of haemoglobin $A_{1c}$ can result from
(a) haemolytic anaemia
(b) exposure to carbon monoxide
(c) recent onset of pure red cell aplasia
(d) poorly controlled diabetes mellitus
(e) β thalassaemia trait

6.9 Carboxyhaemoglobin
(a) is formed during the transport of carbon dioxide from tissues to the lungs
(b) is produced by the catabolism of myoglobin
(c) is not present in healthy individuals
(d) causes the blood to be chocolate-brown in colour
(e) cannot be reconverted to oxyhaemoglobin

6.10 Methaemoglobinaemia can result from
(a) recreational use of nitrites
(b) domestic heaters in poorly ventilated rooms
(c) occupational exposure to nitrates
(d) cigarette smoking
(e) an inherited abnormality of haemoglobin structure

6.11 The increased percentage of carboxyhaemoglo-bin in cigarette smokers
(a) is greater at increased altitude
(b) can lead to an increased haemoglobin concentration
(c) can reach 50% of total haemoglobin
(d) is reduced by a period of vigorous exercise
(e) does not have any disadvantageous effects

6.12 Sulphaemoglobinaemia
(a) may occur together with methaemo-globinaemia
(b) usually causes severe symptoms

(c) can be corrected by intravenous injection of methylene blue

(d) can be caused by dapsone therapy

(e) alters the absorption spectrum of haemoglobin

## Further reading

Bunn HF and Forget BG. *Hemoglobin: Molecular, Genetic and Clinical Aspects*. W. B. Saunders, Philadelphia, PA, 1986.

Nagel RL and Jaffé ER. CO-, NO-, met-, and sulf-hemoglobinemias: the dyshemoglobinemias. In: Steinberg MH, Forget BG, Higgs DR and Nagel RL, eds. *Disorders of Hemoglobin: Genetics, Pathophysiology, and Clinical Management*. Cambridge University Press, Cambridge, 2001, pp. 1214–1233.

## References

1 Peters RE, May A and Jacobs A (1986) Increased $\alpha$ : non-$\alpha$ globin chain synthesis ratios in myelodysplastic syndromes and myeloid leukaemias. *J Clin Pathol* **39**, 1233–1235.

2 Steensma DP, Viprakasit V, Hendrick A, Goff DK, Leach J, Gibbons RJ and Higgs DR (1995) Deletion of the $\alpha$-globin gene cluster as a cause of acquired $\alpha$-thalassaemia in myelodysplastic syndrome. *Blood* **103**, 1518–1520.

3 Markham RE, Butler F, Goh K and Rowley P (1983) Erythroleukemia manifesting as $\delta\beta$ thalassemia. *Hemoglobin* **7**, 71–78.

4 Aoyagi Y, Akimoto H, Yamaoka K, Koike A, Kanayama M, Miyaji T and Yamamoto K (1989) Refractory anemia with ringed sideroblasts complicated by $\delta\beta$-thalassaemia-like hemoglobinopathy. *Rinsho Ketsueki* **30**, 674–679.

5 Hoyle C, Kaeda J, Leslie J and Luzzatto L (1991) Case report: acquired $\beta$ thalassaemia trait in MDS. *Br J Haematol* **79**, 116–117.

6 Honig GR, Suarez CR, Vida LN, Lu S-J and Liu ET (1998) Juvenile myelomonocytic leukemia (JMML) with the hematologic phenotype of severe $\beta$ thalassemia. *Am J Hematol* **58**, 67–71.

7 White JC, Ellis M, Coleman PN, Beaven GH, Gratzer WB, Shooter EM and Skinner ER (1960) An unstable haemoglobin associated with some cases of leukaemia. *Br J Haematol* **6**, 171–177.

8 Beaven GH, Stevens BL, Dance N and White JC (1963) Occurrence of haemoglobin H in leukaemia. *Nature* **199**, 1297–1298.

9 Rosenweig AI, Heywood JD, Motulsky AG and Finch CA (1968) Hemoglobin H as an acquired defect in alpha-chain synthesis. *Acta Haematol* **8**, 91–101.

10 Hamilton RW, Schwartz E, Atwater J and Erslev AJ (1971) Acquired Hb H disease. *N Engl J Med* **285**, 1217–1221.

11 Boehme WM, Piira TA, Kurnik JE and Bethlenfalvay NC (1978) Acquired hemoglobin H disease in refractory sideroblastic anemia. A preleukemic marker. *Arch Intern Med* **138**, 603–606.

12 Lindsey RJ, Jackson JM and Raven JL (1978) Acquired haemoglobin H disease complicating a myeloproliferative syndrome: a case report. *Pathology* **10**, 329–334.

13 Weatherall DJ, Old J, Longley J, Wood WH, Clegg JB, Pollock A and Lewis MJ (1978) Acquired haemoglobin H disease in leukaemia: pathophysiology and molecular basis. *Br J Haematol* **38**, 305–322.

14 Veer A, Kosciolek BA, Bauman AW and Rowley PT (1979) Acquired hemoglobin H disease in idiopathic myelofibrosis. *Am J Hematol* **6**, 199–206.

15 Dash S and Dash RJ (1980) Idiopathic myelofibrosis without splenomegaly and with an acquired haemoglobin disorder. *Indian J Cancer* **17**, 193–195.

16 Yoo D, Schechter GP, Amigable AN and Nienhuis AW (1980) Myeloproliferative syndrome with sideroblastic anemia and acquired hemoglobin H disease. *Cancer* **45**, 78–83.

17 Kueh YK (1982) Acute lymphoblastic leukemia with brilliant cresyl blue erythrocytic inclusions — acquired hemoglobin H disease? *N Engl J Med* **307**, 193–194.

18 Higgs DR, Wood WG, Barton C and Weatherall DJ (1983) Clinical features and molecular analysis of acquired hemoglobin H disease. *Am J Med* **75**, 181–191.

19 Anognou NP, Ley TJ, Chesbro B, Wright G, Kitchens C, Liebhaber S et al. (1983) Acquired $\alpha$-thalassaemia in preleukemia is due to decreased expression of all four $\alpha$-globin genes *Proc Natl Acad Sci USA* **80**, 6051–6055.

20 Mercieca J, Bain B, Barlow G and Catovsky D (1996) Teaching cases from the Royal Marsden and St Mary's Hospitals, Case 10: microcytic anaemia and thrombocytosis. *Leuk Lymphoma* **18**, 185–186.

21 Gibbons RJ, Pellagatti A, Garrick P, Wood WG, Malik N, Ayyub H et al. (1995) Identification of acquired somatic mutations in the gene encoding chromatin-remodeling factor ATRX in the alpha-thalassaemia myelodysplasia syndrome (ATMDS). *Nat Genet* **34**, 446–449.

22 Steensma DP, Higgs DR, Fisher CA and Gibbons RJ (2004) Acquired somatic *ATRX* mutations in myelodysplastic syndrome associated with α thalassemia (ATMDS) convey a more severe hematologic phenotype than germline *ATRX* mutations. *Blood* **103**, 2019–2026.

23 Helder J and Deisseroth A (1987) SI nuclease analysis of α-globin gene expression in preleukemic patients with acquired hemoglobin H disease after transfer to mouse erythroleukemia cells. *Proc Natl Acad Sci USA* **84**, 2387–2390.

24 Belickova M, Schroeder HW, Guan YL, Brierre J, Berney S, Cooper MD and Prchal JF (1994) Clonal hematopoiesis and acquired thalassaemia in common variable immunodeficiency. *Mol Med* **6**, 56–61.

25 Badens C, Mattei MG, Imbert AM, Lapoumeroulie C, Martini N, Michel G and Lena-Russo D (2002) A novel mechanism for thalassaemia intermedia. *Lancet* **359**, 132–133.

26 Wilson MG, Schroeder WA and Graves DA (1968) Postnatal change of haemoglobin F and A$_2$ in infants with Down's syndrome (G trisomy). *Pediatrics* **42**, 349–353.

27 Weller SDV, Apley J and Raper AB (1966) Malformations associated with precocious synthesis of adult haemoglobin. *Lancet* **i**, 777–779.

28 Nienhuis AW and Benz EJ (1997) Regulation of hemoglobin synthesis during the development of the red cell (third of three parts). *N Engl J Med* **297**, 1430–1436.

29 Fagan DG, Lancashire RJ, Walker A and Sorohan T (1995) Determinants of fetal haemoglobin in newborn infants. *Arch Dis Child* **72**, F111–F114.

30 Cochran DL, Conrad ME and Matney J (1997) Hemoglobin F and risk factors for sudden infant death syndrome. *Lab Med* **28**, 53–57.

31 Giulian GG, Gilbert EF and Moss RL (1987) Elevated fetal hemoglobin levels in sudden infant death syndrome. *N Engl J Med* **316**, 1122–1126.

32 Cheron G, Bachoux I, Maier M, Massonneau M, Peltier JY and Girot R (1989) Fetal hemoglobin in sudden infant death syndrome. *N Engl J Med* **320**, 1011–1012.

33 Zielke HR, Meny RG, O'Brien MJ, Smialek JE, Kutlar F, Huisman THJ and Dover GJ (1989) Normal fetal hemoglobin levels in the sudden infant death syndrome. *N Engl J Med* **321**, 1359–1364.

34 Papayannopoulou T, Vichinsky E and Stamatoyannopoulos G (1980) Fetal Hb production during acute erythroid expansion I. Observation in patients with transient erythroblastopenia and postphlebotomy. *Br J Haematol* **44**, 535–546.

35 Weatherall D and Clegg JB. *The Thalassaemia Syndromes*. Blackwell Science, Oxford, 1981.

36 Bunn HF and Forget BG. *Hemoglobin: Molecular, Genetic and Clinical Aspects*. W. B. Saunders, Philadelphia, PA, 1986.

37 Perrine SP, Greene MF and Faller DV (1985) Delay in fetal globin switch in infants of diabetic mothers. *N Engl J Med* **312**, 334–338.

38 Peters F, Rohloff D, Kohlmann T, Renner F, Jantschek G, Kerner W and Fehm HL (1998) Fetal hemoglobin in starvation ketosis in young women. *Blood* **91**, 691–694.

39 Kellen JA, Bush RS and Malkin A (1980) Alkali-resistant hemoglobin (Hb F) in cancer patients. *Cancer* **45**, 1448–1450.

40 Kendall AG and Bastomsky CH (1981) Haemoglobin A$_2$ in hyperthyroidism. *Hemoglobin* **5**, 571–577.

41 Little JA, Dempsey NJ, Tuchman M and Ginder GD (1995) Metabolic persistence of fetal hemoglobin. *Blood* **85**, 1712–1718.

42 Luna-Fineman S, Shannon KM, Atwater SK, Davis J, Masterson M, Ortega J et al. (1999) Myelodysplastic and myeloproliferative disorders of childhood: a study of 167 patients. *Blood* **93**, 459–466.

43 Poli-Neto A, Nonoyama K, Oshiro M, Ebner-Filho W, Miguita K, Watanabe CI and Barretto OC de O (1998) Increased fetal hemoglobin levels in H.I.V. patients. *Br J Haematol* **102**, 96.

44 Aksoy M and Erdem S (1978) Followup study of the mortality and the development of leukemia in 444 pancytopenic patients with chronic exposure to benzene. *Blood* **52**, 285–292.

45 Alperin JB, Dow PA and Petteway MB (1977) Haemoglobin A$_2$ levels in health and various hematologic disorders. *Am J Clin Pathol* **67**, 219–226.

46 Steinberg MH and Adams JG (1991) Hemoglobin A$_2$: origin, evolution, and aftermath. *Blood* **78**, 2165–2177.

47 Routy JP, Monte M, Beaulieu R, Toma E, St-Pierre L and Dumont M (1993) Increase of hemoglobin A2 in human immunodeficiency virus-I-infected patients treated with zidovudine. *Am J Hematol* **43**, 86–90.

48 Howard J, Henthorn JS, Murphy S and Davies SC (2005) Implications of increased haemoglobin A2 levels in HIV-positive women in the antenatal clinic. *J Clin Pathol* **58**, 556–558.

49 Bain BJ, Benzie A, Wilkinson M and Phelan L (2005) Haemoglobin A$_2$ in HIV-positive patients, receiving or not receiving anti-retroviral chemotherapy. In preparation.

50 Ali MAM and Schwertner E (1974) Hemoglobin A2 level: a proposed test for confirming the diagnosis of iron deficiency. *Am J Clin Pathol* **63**, 549–553.

51 Cech P, Testa U, Dubart A, Schneider P, Bachmann F and Guerrasio A (1982) Lasting Hb F reactivation and Hb A2 reduction induced by the treatment of Hodgkin's disease in a woman heterozygous for beta-thalassemia and the Swiss type of the heterocellular hereditary persistence of fetal haemoglobin. *Acta Haematol* **67**, 275–284.

52 Nagel RL and Steinberg MH. Hemoglobins of the embryo and fetus and minor hemoglobins of adults. In: Steinberg MH, Forget BG, Higgs DR and Nagel RL, eds. *Disorders of Hemoglobin: Genetics, Pathophysiology, and Clinical Management*. Cambridge University Press, Cambridge, 2001, pp. 197–230.

53 Karsten J, Anker AP and Odink RJ (1996) Glycosylated haemoglobin and transient erythroblastopenia of childhood. *Lancet* **347**, 273.

54 Coban E, Özdogan M and Timuragaoglu A (2004) Effect of iron deficiency anemia on levels of hemoglobin A1c in nondiabetic patients. *Acta Haematol* **112**, 126–128.

55 Moriwaki Y, Yamamoto T, Shibutani Y, Harano T, Takahashi S and Hada T (2000) Abnormal haemoglobins, Hb Takamatsu and Hb G-Szuhu, detected during the analysis of glycated haemoglobin (HbA1C) by high performance liquid chromatography. *J Clin Pathol* **53**, 854–857.

56 Ernst A and Zibiak JD (1998) Carbon monoxide poisoning. *N Engl J Med* **339**, 1603–1608.

57 Blumenthal I (2001) Carbon monoxide poisoning. *J R Soc Med* **94**, 270–272.

58 Nagel RL and Jaffé ER. CO-, NO-, met-, and sulf-hemoglobinemias: the dyshemoglobinemias. In: Steinberg MH, Forget BG, Higgs DR and Nagel RL, eds. *Disorders of Hemoglobin: Genetics, Pathophysiology, and Clinical Management*. Cambridge University Press, Cambridge, 2001, pp. 1214–1233.

59 Choo V (1996) Snow-blocked car exhaust causes CO poisoning. *Lancet* **347**, 384.

60 Pullinger R (1996) Something in the air: survival after dramatic, unsuspected case of accidental carbon monoxide poisoning. *Lancet* **312**, 897–898.

61 Leach RM, Rees PJ and Wilmshurst P (1998) Hyperbaric oxygen therapy. *Br Med J* **317**, 1140–1143.

62 Weaver LK, Hopkins RO, Chan KJ, Churchill S, Elliot CG, Clemmer TP *et al.* (2002) Hyperbaric oxygen for acute carbon monoxide poisoning. *N Engl J Med* **347**, 1057–1067.

63 Pitkin AD, Broome JR and Salmon J (1999) Hyperbaric oxygen therapy in intensive care. Part II: carbon monoxide poisoning. *Br J Intensive Care* **9**, 189–195.

64 Sin DD and Shafran SD (1996) Dapsone- and primaquine-induced methemoglobinemia in HIV-infected individuals. *J Acquir Immune Defic Syndr Hum Retrovirol* **12**, 477–481.

65 Hohl RJ, Sherburne AR, Feely JE, Huisman THJ and Burns CP (1998) Low pulse oximeter-measured hemoglobin oxygen saturations with hemoglobin Cheverly. *Am J Hematol* **59**, 181–184.

66 Cummings MH, Day S, Norton S, Cook G and Alexander WD (1994) Petrol octane booster and methemoglobinemia. *J Intern Med* **235**, 279–280.

67 Zinkham WH and Oski FA (1996) Henna: a potential cause of oxidative hemolysis and neonatal hyperbilirubinemia. *Pediatrics* **97**, 707–709.

68 Kouides PA, Abboud CN and Fairbanks VF (1996) Flutamide-induced cyanosis refractory to methylene blue therapy. *Br J Haematol* **94**, 73–75.

69 Nakajima W, Ishida A, Arai H and Takada G (1997) Methaemoglobinaemia after inhalation of nitric oxide in infant with pulmonary hypertension. *Lancet* **350**, 1002–1003.

70 Sanders P and Faunt J (1997) An unusual cause of cyanosis (isosorbide dinitrate induced methaemoglobinaemia). *Aust NZ J Med* **27**, 596.

71 Bacon R (1997) Nitrate preserved sausage meat causes an unusual food poisoning incident. *Comm Dis Rep* **77**, R45–R47.

72 Hogan CJ, Wiley JS and Billington T (1997) Intravascular haemolysis complicating treatment of acute promyelocytic leukaemia. *Aust NZ J Med* **27**, 450–451.

73 Moreira V de A, de Medeiros BC, Bonfim CMS, Pasquini R and de Medeiros CR (1998) Methemoglobinemia secondary to clofazimine treatment with chronic graft-versus-host disease. *Blood* **92**, 4872–4873.

74 Finan A, Keenan P, O'Donovan FO, Mayne P and Murphy J (1998) Methaemoglobinaemia associated with sodium nitrite in three siblings. *Br Med J* **317**, 1138–1139.

75 Donnelly GB and Randlett D (2000) Methemoglobinemia. *N Engl J Med* **343**, 337.

76 Hurford WE and Kratz A (2003) Case 23-2004: a 50-year-old woman with low oxygen saturation. *N Engl J Med* **351**, 380–387.

77 Gourdin D, Vergnes H and Gutierez N (1975) Methaemoglobin in a man living at high altitude. *Br J Haematol* **29**, 243–246.

78 Viallon A, Page Y and Bertrand JC (2000) Methemoglobinemia due to riluzole. *N Engl J Med* **343**, 665–666.

79 Chan TK, Mak LW and Ng RP (1971) Methemoglo-binemia, Heinz bodies and acute massive intravascular hemolysis in Lysol poisoning. *Blood* **38**, 739–744.

80 Levine D, Brunton AT, Kruger A and Hersant M (2000) Recurrent sulphaemoglobinaemia treated with neomycin. *J R Soc Med* **93**, 428.

81 Tangerman A, Bongaerts G, Agbeko R, Semmekrot B and Severijnen R (2002) The origin of hydrogen sulfide in a newborn with sulfhaemoglobin induced cyanosis. *J Clin Pathol* **55**, 631–633.

## Answers to questions

| 6.1 | | | 6.3 | | | 6.5 | | | 6.7 | | | 6.9 | | | 6.11 | | |
|-----|---|---|-----|---|---|-----|---|---|-----|---|---|-----|---|---|------|---|---|
| | (a) | T | | (a) | T | | (a) | T | | (a) | T | | (a) | F | | (a) | T |
| | (b) | T | | (b) | F | | (b) | F | | (b) | F | | (b) | T | | (b) | T |
| | (c) | F | | (c) | T | | (c) | T | | (c) | T | | (c) | F | | (c) | F |
| | (d) | F | | (d) | F | | (d) | T | | (d) | T | | (d) | F | | (d) | T |
| | (e) | T | | (e) | T | | (e) | T | | (e) | T | | (e) | F | | (e) | F |

| 6.2 | | | 6.4 | | | 6.6 | | | 6.8 | | | 6.10 | | | 6.12 | | |
|-----|---|---|-----|---|---|-----|---|---|-----|---|---|------|---|---|------|---|---|
| | (a) | F | | (a) | T | | (a) | F | | (a) | F | | (a) | T | | (a) | T |
| | (b) | F | | (b) | T | | (b) | T | | (b) | F | | (b) | F | | (b) | F |
| | (c) | T | | (c) | F | | (c) | T | | (c) | T | | (c) | T | | (c) | F |
| | (d) | T | | (d) | T | | (d) | F | | (d) | T | | (d) | F | | (d) | T |
| | (e) | T | | (e) | T | | (e) | F | | (e) | F | | (e) | T | | (e) | T |

# 7 Organization of a haemoglobinopathy diagnostic service

The organization of a haemoglobinopathy diagnostic service depends on the ethnic mix of the population served and also on whether the service is hospital based or a regional scheme, whether antenatal and neonatal screening are required and whether children are included in those tested. It is essential that laboratories have clearly defined written protocols that are followed. These will differ depending on the patient population, the nature of the service that is required and the technology employed. Protocols will differ according to the primary laboratory technique employed, whether this be haemoglobin electrophoresis, high performance liquid chromatography (HPLC) or isoelectric focusing (IEF). It is important to remember that, in a diagnostic laboratory, the identification of a variant haemoglobin is often presumptive rather than definitive and that it may not be possible, or indeed clinically relevant, to identify every variant haemoglobin detected. The protocols that are followed should ensure that the great majority of clinically relevant disorders of haemoglobin synthesis are detected. It is not realistic to hope that *all* relevant abnormalities will be detected. For example, in antenatal screening, silent β thalassaemia will generally be missed. Laboratory tests for haemoglobinopathies should not be performed in a knowledge vacuum. It is essential to know the age of the patient, the ethnic origin, the red cell indices and the clinical features, if any. It is essential to know if the patient has been transfused in the recent past. Only with this information will the testing be clinically relevant and appropriately interpreted. This chapter discusses mainly the provision of a hospital-based service in a multi-ethnic community in which the population to be tested includes neonates and children and also pregnant women and their partners. In laboratories serving populations of a single ethnic origin, the laboratory procedures will be adapted to local requirements.

All abnormal results of haemoglobinopathy testing should be conveyed to the patient or, in the case of a child, to the patient's parents in written form together with an appropriate explanation. To avoid unnecessary repeat testing, it may also be useful to give the patient written confirmation of significant negative results, for example that haemoglobin S is not present. Haemoglobinopathy cards are a useful way to give the patient documentation of the results. These should give the patient's name, the date of testing, the test results and, if necessary, an interpretation. It is also useful to include the haemoglobin concentration and the mean cell haemoglobin (MCH) (or mean cell volume (MCV)). In the case of normal results in microcytic patients from ethnic groups in which α thalassaemia trait occurs, it is useful to add a statement: 'This test does not exclude α thalassaemia trait'.

## Antenatal haemoglobinopathy/ thalassaemia screening and fetal diagnosis

The aim of antenatal screening is to detect inherited abnormalities in the parents that might lead to such severe disease in the fetus that termination of pregnancy would be justified and might be requested by the parents. In some instances, specifically when haemoglobin Bart's hydrops fetalis is predicted in the fetus, continuing the pregnancy may also put the mother's own health and even life at risk.

In some countries with a high prevalence of disorders of globin chain synthesis, screening is usually performed before pregnancy is undertaken. In countries with adequate resources, this can be achieved by population screening, as is carried out, for example, in Cyprus. In countries with fewer economic resources, it may be possible to make testing cost-effective by targeting individuals most in need of

**Table 7.1** Haemoglobinopathies of such severity that the likelihood of their occurrence in a fetus should be predicted.

Haemoglobin Bart's hydrops fetalis

β thalassaemia major and intermedia including that resulting from β thalassaemia/haemoglobin E compound heterozygosity

Sickle cell disease
  Sickle cell anaemia
  Sickle cell/haemoglobin C disease
  Sickle cell/β thalassaemia
  Sickle cell/δβ thalassaemia
  Sickle cell/haemoglobin Lepore
  Sickle cell/ haemoglobin D-Punjab
  Sickle cell/ haemoglobin O-Arab

**Table 7.2** Disorders of globin chain synthesis that should be detected in prospective parents in order to predict the occurrence of severe disease in their offspring.

$\alpha^0$ thalassaemia trait and haemoglobin H disease
β thalassaemia trait
δβ thalassaemia trait
Haemoglobin Lepore
Haemoglobin E
Haemoglobin S
Haemoglobin C
Haemoglobin D-Punjab
Haemoglobin O-Arab
Unstable haemoglobins

**Table 7.3** Less severe haemoglobinopathies for which the prediction of the condition in a fetus is not usually considered to be essential.

Haemoglobin H disease
Mild sickling conditions
  Sickle cell/haemoglobin E compound heterozygosity
  Sickle cell/deletional hereditary persistence of fetal
  haemoglobin compound heterozygosity
Haemoglobin E homozygosity
Haemoglobin C homozygosity

testing. For example, in countries, such as Pakistan, in which consanguineous marriages are common and specific disorders of globin chain synthesis, e.g. β thalassaemia, tend to segregate in families, screening can be targeted on extended families with an index case [1]. However, in many countries, screening is commonly undertaken only when the potential mother is already pregnant. Tests must therefore be performed rapidly in order to permit testing of the partner and to offer fetal diagnosis and termination of pregnancy, when appropriate, whilst the pregnancy is still in its early stages. Fetal diagnosis carries a small risk of inducing miscarriage of a fetus, possibly a normal fetus. For this reason, fetal diagnosis should generally only be undertaken when the potential parents wish to consider termination of pregnancy. Counselling of parents should be based on the provision of very full information on the likely outcome of pregnancy and the likely severity of any fetal disease. It may be useful for potential parents to be referred to relevant patient support groups. Counselling should be non-directive.

The conditions that should be predicted in a fetus are shown in Table 7.1 and the abnormalities that should therefore be detected in the mother are given in Table 7.2. It follows that, when one of these abnormalities is detected in the mother, appropriate testing of the potential father will follow. Table 7.3 shows conditions that are generally mild and for which prediction is not generally considered to be necessary.

Tables 7.1 and 7.3 represent the consensus view in the UK [2–4], but there are some areas of controversy. Severe haemoglobin H disease is one such area. In countries or ethnic groups in which there is a high prevalence of both $\alpha^0$ and $\alpha^T\alpha$ or $\alpha^+$ thalassaemia heterozygosity, prediction of haemoglobin H disease can be attempted. However, it should be noted that mild haemoglobin H disease would not generally be considered a sufficiently severe disease to justify termination of pregnancy. The prediction of thalassaemia intermedia is also a difficult area, as this condition varies greatly in severity and the severity of the phenotype associated with a specific genotype is not always predictable. This uncertainty must be conveyed to prospective parents. Tables 7.1 and 7.3 are not exhaustive, but cover the great majority of likely clinical situations. Parents with rare abnormalities, for example an unstable haemoglobin, need to be assessed individually. In any antenatal screening programme, it should be remembered that genetic testing causes anxiety, particularly if a woman is already pregnant. In addition, the cost of genetic testing may be considerable and no health service has unlimited resources. This must always be borne in mind when drawing up protocols. It may not be justifiable to test a large number of couples for rare disorders in order to attempt to identify a very small proportion of patients with a significant abnormality. Screening for $\alpha^0$ thalassaemia provides an example of where zeal should be tempered by consideration of what is reasonable. This condition occurs in native British, Afro-Caribbeans and Indians, but is very uncommon in all of these ethnic groups. Both Afro-Caribbeans and Indians have a high percentage of $\alpha^+$ thalassaemia, and screening the large number of individuals with microcytosis that is likely to be attributable to heterozygosity or homozygosity for $\alpha^+$ thalassaemia in the hope of identifying rare individuals with $\alpha^0$ thalassaemia trait is not usually considered to be justifiable [4]. Individual circumstances may dictate that certain couples are tested, e.g. if there is consanguinity, if native British originate in Lancashire or Cheshire or if a person of Caribbean origin may have Chinese ancestry.

Uptake of antenatal diagnosis is dependent on cultural factors and on the severity of the condition that is predicted. In an audit of prenatal diagnosis for haemoglobinopathies in the UK, the uptake was 90% amongst Cypriots, 41–65% amongst Indians, 26% amongst Pakistanis and 9% amongst Bangladeshis [5]. Uptake is also higher in high prevalence areas of the UK, possibly because of the availability of well-informed doctors and counsellors. In general, uptake is higher when $\beta$ thalassaemia major is predicted than when sickle cell disease is predicted. Uptake is almost universal when haemoglobin Bart's hydrops fetalis is predicted, although it should be noted that occasional parents choose diagnosis followed by intrauterine transfusion rather than termination of pregnancy.

A protocol based on cellulose acetate electrophoresis for the identification of variant haemoglobins and $\beta$ thalassaemia trait, applicable in both antenatal screening and other circumstances, is shown in Fig. 7.1, and a similar protocol applicable when HPLC is the primary diagnostic tool is given in Fig. 7.2. Protocols including possible policies for the diagnosis of $\alpha^0$ thalassaemia trait are shown diagrammatically in Figs 7.3 and 7.4. The cut-off point adopted in the UK for $\alpha^0$ thalassaemia screening is an MCH of less than 25 pg. A study in Hong Kong indicated that about 1.8% of individuals with $-\!-^{SEA}/(2/110)$ would be missed by this strategy [6]; a cut-off point of 27 pg for the MCH or 80 fl for the MCV is therefore preferred in Hong Kong.

When testing of a pregnant woman reveals a potentially significant condition, it is useful to issue, with the test result, a proforma that can be followed by antenatal clinic staff during the further management of the patient. A typical form in use at St Mary's Hospital NHS Trust is shown in Fig. 7.5. Such proformas help to ensure correct patient management and can also be used for audit purposes.

In countries that have regulations governing DNA analysis, these should be followed if testing is DNA based. It is particularly important that very full information about the implications of testing is given when family studies are to be undertaken, as these sometimes reveal non-paternity. This is necessary for protein-based testing as well as for DNA-based testing.

## Neonatal screening

The purpose of neonatal screening is principally the detection of sickle cell disease, as early diagnosis has been shown to reduce mortality during infancy and early childhood. Neonatal screening can be performed on a cord blood sample (taken by syringe and needle or evacuated container and needle from an umbilical cord vessel after carefully wiping any maternal blood from the surface of the cord), an anticoagulated capillary blood sample, a dried spot of capillary blood (e.g. on a Guthrie card) or, in sick hospitalized babies, a venous sample (Table 7.4). Cord blood should not be squeezed from the end of the cut cord because of the risk of contamination with maternal blood. A capillary sample obtained by heel prick, blotted on to filter paper and permitted to dry, is usually most convenient. Often one blood spot on a Guthrie card (used for the diagnosis of congenital metabolic diseases) is used for this purpose. When such a dried blood spot is used, a circle of blood-impregnated filter paper is punched out and the haemoglobin is eluted.

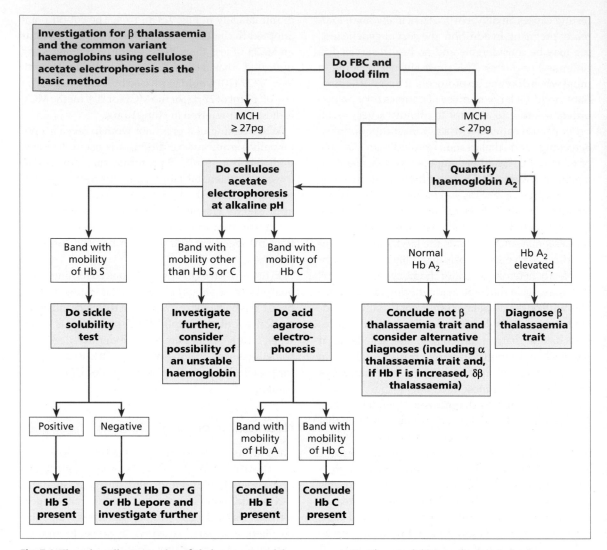

**Fig. 7.1** Flow chart illustrating how β thalassaemia and the common variant haemoglobins can be detected using haemoglobin electrophoresis on cellulose acetate at alkaline pH as the basic method. FBC, full blood count; Hb, haemoglobin; MCH, mean cell haemoglobin.

Universal neonatal screening has been recommended when more than 15% of neonates are born to ethnic minority mothers [7] and, in the UK, nationwide universal screening is now being introduced [8]. In other circumstances, considerations of cost may dictate selective screening. Screening can be performed before the baby leaves hospital in a hospital-based scheme or together with screening for inherited metabolic defects in a community-based scheme. The most suitable techniques are those that are sensitive and can be performed with small blood samples, e.g. HPLC and IEF [9–11]. A suitable protocol is shown in Fig. 7.6. Cellulose acetate electrophoresis can also be used, but the eluate of a dried blood spot may be too dilute for this technique and, in addition, it is less sensitive than HPLC and IEF for the detection of the low percentages of haemoglobin A that may be present in premature

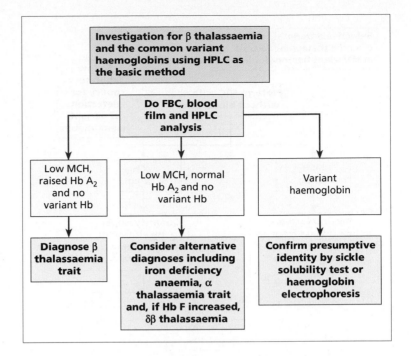

**Fig. 7.2** Flow chart illustrating how β thalassaemia and the common variant haemoglobins can be detected using high performance liquid chromatography (HPLC) as the basic method. FBC, full blood count; Hb, haemoglobin; MCH, mean cell haemoglobin.

neonates. It is also less sensitive for the detection of small amounts of variant haemoglobins, levels down to 4% being detected in one study, whereas HPLC and IEF detected haemoglobin variants down to levels of less than 2% [10]. Haemoglobin Bart's is unstable on storage and may therefore be missed, regardless of technique, if there is a delay in testing [8]. In selecting a method for neonatal screening, consideration must be given to the workload and to whether it is convenient to use the same technique for both neonatal screening and other screening. A consideration of both the requirement for sensitivity and the need to use the same instrumentation for other purposes means that HPLC is often the technique chosen. The use of sensitive techniques is particularly important in screening premature babies in whom the percentage of haemoglobin A or of any variant haemoglobin is likely to be low. Screening of these babies should be performed soon after birth to avoid the possibility of a sample being taken after a blood transfusion. The presence of more haemoglobin A than F or a prominent haemoglobin $A_2$ band in a neonatal sample should raise the possibility that there has been contamination with maternal blood or

that a post-transfusion sample has been sent to the laboratory.

All haemoglobin variants detected by the initial screening method should be further investigated by a supplementary alternative method to make their presumptive identification more reliable. It should be noted that a sickle solubility test should not be used in neonates because of the high probability of false negative results. Potentially significant haemoglobinopathies should be confirmed by a second sample, conveniently around the age of 6–8 weeks. Repeat testing should also be performed on all babies whose initial sample shows no haemoglobin A. In addition, it is prudent to repeat tests if the predominant haemoglobin present is haemoglobin F with very small amounts of haemoglobins A and S, as it can be difficult to distinguish sickle cell trait from sickle cell/$\beta^+$ thalassaemia in this circumstance. The initial report on such a sample should be circumspect. The detection of only haemoglobins S and F in a neonate is most often attributable to sickle cell anaemia. However, compound heterozygosity for haemoglobin S and either $\beta^0$ thalassaemia or deletional hereditary persistence of fetal haemoglobin

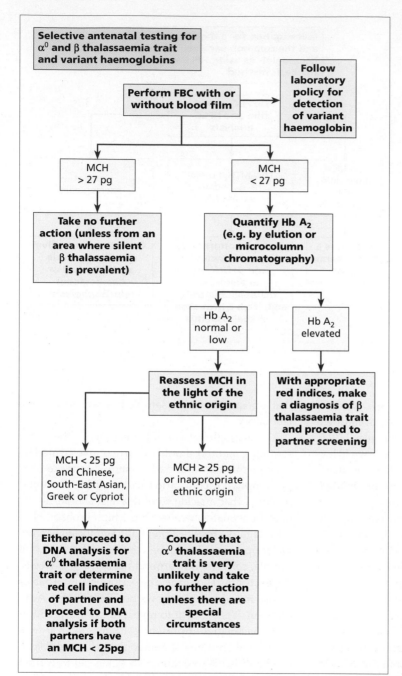

**Fig. 7.3** Flow chart illustrating selective antenatal testing for $\alpha^0$ and $\beta$ thalassaemia trait; haemoglobin $A_2$ is quantified and specific tests for $\alpha^0$ thalassaemia trait are performed only when the mean cell haemoglobin (MCH) is appropriately reduced. FBC, full blood count; Hb, haemoglobin.

also produces this pattern. In addition, it has been noted that some babies with sickle cell/$\beta^+$ thalassaemia compound heterozygosity also have only haemoglobins S and F detectable at birth, particularly if cellulose acetate electrophoresis is the detection method employed [12].

An essential part of any neonatal screening programme is a well-organized system of follow-up and appropriate management of babies found to have a significant abnormality. Information and an appropriate explanation must also be given to the parents of babies found to have sickle cell trait or other

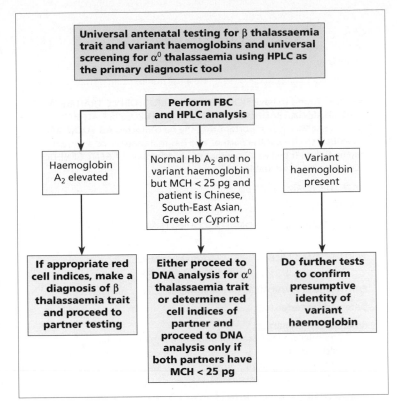

**Fig. 7.4** Flow chart illustrating universal antenatal testing for β thalassaemia trait and universal antenatal screening for $\alpha^0$ thalassaemia trait; haemoglobin A$_2$ is quantified on all samples, but specific investigations for $\alpha^0$ thalassaemia are carried out only when the mean cell haemoglobin (MCH) is appropriately reduced. FBC, full blood count; Hb, haemoglobin; HPLC, high performance liquid chromatography.

heterozygous conditions. It is important for all those involved in neonatal screening schemes to remember that β thalassaemia trait will not be detected by testing in neonates or young infants. If it is known that one or both parents have β thalassaemia trait, this should be borne in mind when issuing a report.

## Pre-anaesthetic testing

It is important to detect all patients with sickle cell disease before anaesthesia in order to ensure that the necessity for pre-operative blood transfusion is considered and that the patient is kept warm, well hydrated and well oxygenated both during surgery and in the post-operative period. Although patients with sickle cell anaemia and other severe sickling disorders will usually already have been diagnosed prior to presenting with a condition requiring immediate surgery and anaesthesia, this is not necessarily so in

patients with sickle cell/haemoglobin C disease and sickle cell/β⁺ thalassaemia. Such patients may have a normal haemoglobin concentration, so that diagnosis, in an emergency situation, cannot rest on a sickle solubility test and full blood count (FBC) alone. Supplementing these tests with a blood film makes provisional identification of these compound heterozygous states more accurate.

It is also conventional to test any patient at risk of having sickle cell trait prior to anaesthesia, in order to ensure that hypoxia does not occur during surgery. It could, however, be argued that *no* patient should be permitted to become hypoxic and that sickle screening is therefore unnecessary if sickle cell disease can be excluded.

In testing for haemoglobin S, it is necessary to bear in mind the very wide range of ethnic groups in which this variant haemoglobin may occur (see Chapter 4). If routine surgery is being planned, all patients of an appropriate ethnic group should have

**St Mary's Hospital NHS Trust**

Dear Sister,                          Date.......................................................

Patient................................   Hospital number..............................

Has been found to have SICKLE TRAIT/HAEMOGLOBIN C TRAIT/BETA THALASSAEMIA TRAIT/HAEMOGLOBIN E TRAIT/POSSIBLE ALPHA⁰ THALASSAEMIA. It is important that she be contacted **AS SOON AS POSSIBLE** to check if the partner also has thalassaemia or a variant haemoglobin. If he has a haemoglobinopathy then URGENT GENETIC COUNSELLING is advisable.

DATE THIS FORM RECEIVED...................

PARTNER'S ANCESTRY............................

DATE WOMAN REATTENDED FOR COUNSELLING....................

                                                              Tick
PARTNER AVAILABLE             Agrees to test........
                             Does not agree to test........

PARTNER NOT AVAILABLE, give reason....................................

Date partner tested...............................

Result of test on partner
       no relevant thalassaemia or abnormal haemoglobin
       sickle trait
       β thalassaemia trait
       other abnormality (specify)...........

IF ABNORMAL, WHO COUNSELLED THE COUPLE REGARDING ANTENATAL DIAGNOSIS ?...........................

ANTENATAL DIAGNOSIS HAS BEEN ARRANGED             **YES/NO**

IF NOT, WAS IT BECAUSE THE COUPLE DID NOT WANT IT ?   **YES/NO**

**PLEASE FILE THIS IN THE PATIENT'S NOTES AND USE IT FOR REFERENCE**

**Fig. 7.5** An example of the type of form that is useful for documenting antenatal haemoglobinopathy testing in a patient's hospital records.

an FBC, sickle solubility test and haemoglobin electrophoresis. If emergency anaesthesia is required, the patient should be assessed for clinical features suggestive of an undiagnosed sickling disorder. If there are no such features, an FBC and sickle solubility test should be performed; if the haemoglobin concentration is reduced, a blood film should be examined. If the patient has clinical features compatible with a sickling disorder, an FBC, blood film and sickle solubility test should be performed. The purpose of the blood film in these circumstances is to facilitate the diagnosis of patients with sickle cell disease with a normal haemoglobin concentration who might otherwise be assumed to have sickle cell trait. When resources permit, a definitive diagnosis of sickle cell disease should be made prior to surgery. This is more likely to be feasible in laboratories using HPLC rather than haemoglobin electrophoresis as the primary diagnostic method. If a definitive diagnosis cannot be made rapidly, but sickle cell disease is suspected, surgery should proceed on the assumption that the patient does have sickle cell disease and

**Table 7.4** Methods applicable to neonatal haemoglobinopathy diagnosis.

|  | Advantages and disadvantages |
| --- | --- |
| *Method of obtaining blood* | |
| By needle and syringe from cord vessel | Contamination with maternal blood can occur if technique is not meticulous; inadvertently obtaining a sample after a baby has been transfused is generally avoided; there may be more certainty of testing every neonate if a cord blood sample is used |
| Heel prick sample into a heparinized capillary tube | Transport and labelling of the sample are more difficult, but the sample does not suffer the dilution that occurs when a dried blood spot is eluted; contamination by maternal blood is avoided, but it is important to avoid inadvertently taking a sample after a blood transfusion has been given |
| Heel prick sample blotted on to filter paper and dried | Transport and labelling are easy, but dried samples are more likely to be denatured giving blurred bands; contamination by maternal blood is avoided, but it is important to avoid inadvertently taking a sample after a blood transfusion has been given; the blood sample can be obtained at the same time as sampling for metabolic testing, e.g. for phenylketonuria |
| *Method of detecting variant haemoglobins* | |
| High performance liquid chromatography | Very sensitive technique; variant haemoglobins are quantified |
| Isoelectric focusing | Very sensitive technique |
| Cellulose acetate electrophoresis | An eluate from a Guthrie spot may be too dilute for this technique; less sensitive to low concentrations of a normal or variant haemoglobin |

appropriate attention should be paid to oxygenation and hydration. When full testing is not possible in an emergency situation, it is important to ensure that an adequate pre-transfusion sample is available for full testing on the next working day. A laboratory protocol for pre-anaesthetic testing is shown in Fig. 7.7. These procedures will mean that the provisional diagnosis is correct in the majority of patients. Some patients with sickle cell disease with a high percentage of haemoglobin F or sickle cell/β⁺ thalassaemia with a high percentage of haemoglobin A may be missed, but they are the patients most likely to have mild disease and least likely to suffer complications in relation to surgery and anaesthesia. It should also be noted that false negative results with a sickle solubility test can be seen in young infants. However, a false negative test is only expected with quite a low haemoglobin S percentage when anaesthetic complications would be unlikely. Definitive testing by haemoglobin electrophoresis or HPLC is required, but emergency surgery can proceed.

## Other haemoglobinopathy investigations

### Investigation of haemolytic anaemia

Haemolytic anaemia can be consequent on the presence of an unstable haemoglobin. When this is suspected, the following tests should be performed:

- FBC, blood film and reticulocyte count;
- haemoglobin electrophoresis or HPLC;
- isopropanol and heat instability tests;
- haemoglobin $A_2$ estimation;
- a test for Heinz bodies, repeated after incubation for 24 h at 37°C, if initially negative;
- family studies;
- tests to exclude other causes of a haemolytic anaemia.

### Investigation of unexplained cyanosis

Unexplained cyanosis can be caused by a low-

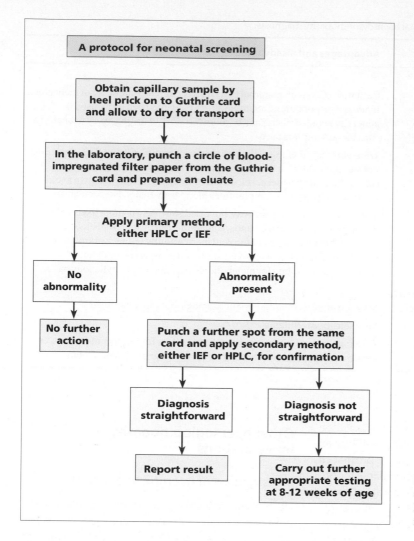

**Fig. 7.6** A protocol for neonatal screening. HPLC, high performance liquid chromatography; IEF, isoelectric focusing.

oxygen-affinity haemoglobin, methaemoglobinaemia or sulphaemoglobinaemia. Some inherited methaemoglobins are also unstable. Relevant investigations include:

• FBC, blood film and reticulocyte count;
• haemoglobin electrophoresis or HPLC;
• haemoglobin electrophoresis after conversion of all haemoglobin to methaemoglobin;
• isopropanol and heat instability tests;
• spectrophotometry for the detection and quantification of sulphaemoglobin and methaemoglobin;

• oxygen dissociation curve and estimation of $P_{50}$ (the $Po_2$ at which haemoglobin is 50% saturated);
• partial pressure of oxygen in arterial blood to exclude hypoxia as a cause of cyanosis;
• family studies.

## Investigation of unexplained polycythaemia

Polycythaemia can be consequent on a high-affinity haemoglobin or, rarely, on homozygosity for hereditary persistence of fetal haemoglobin. Some high-

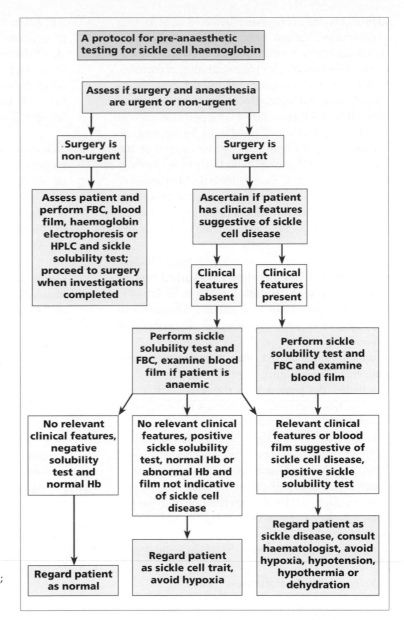

**Fig. 7.7** A protocol for pre-anaesthetic testing for patients with sickle cell trait or sickle cell disease prior to routine or emergency surgery. FBC, full blood count; Hb, haemoglobin concentration; HPLC, high performance liquid chromatography.

oxygen-affinity haemoglobins are also unstable. Relevant investigations include:
- FBC, blood film and reticulocyte count;
- haemoglobin electrophoresis or HPLC;
- isopropanol and heat instability tests;
- oxygen dissociation curve and estimation of $P_{50}$;
- family studies;

- investigation to exclude other causes of polycythaemia.

## Identification of an unknown variant haemoglobin

Uncommon haemoglobins that are not readily

identifiable are occasionally detected in screening programmes. Variant haemoglobins may also be detected because of an aberrant result when measuring haemoglobin $A_{1c}$ for the monitoring of diabetes. It is not always necessary, or indeed possible, to identify a variant haemoglobin, but it is necessary to determine whether or not it is of potential clinical significance. Routine tests should be applied, as shown in Figs 7.1 and 7.2, in order to identify the common variant haemoglobins likely to be clinically important, including haemoglobin S, C, D-Punjab, E, O-Arab, Lepore and Constant Spring. If the variant haemoglobin remains unidentified after following one of these protocols, the following factors should be considered:

• whether there is any personal or family history suggestive of a clinically significant variant haemoglobin (e.g. anaemia, jaundice, polycythaemia);
• whether there is an elevated reticulocyte count or any blood film abnormality suggestive of haemolysis;
• whether there are red cell indices suggestive of a thalassaemic condition;
• whether the patient is in the reproductive age range or has close relatives who may be considering pregnancy.

Further tests that might be indicated include a sickle solubility test (as not all sickling haemoglobins have the mobility of haemoglobin S) and a test for an unstable haemoglobin. Other tests that might be selectively applied if the variant haemoglobin has not been identified by electrophoresis and HPLC include:

• oxygen dissociation curve and determination of $P_{50}$;
• haemoglobin absorption spectrum;
• electron spray mass spectrometry;
• DNA sequencing;
• globin chain electrophoresis;
• tryptic digestion and peptide fingerprinting;
• study of rate of synthesis of globin chains.

## Check your knowledge

One to five answers may be correct. Answers to almost all questions can be found in this chapter or can be deduced from the information given. The correct answers are given on p. 266.

7.1 An antenatal haemoglobinopathy screening programme should detect
(a) $\alpha^0$ thalassaemia
(b) $\alpha^+$ thalassaemia
(c) $\beta^0$ thalassaemia
(d) $\beta^+$ thalassaemia
(e) $\delta\beta$ thalassaemia

7.2 Sickle cell disease, which could complicate surgery and anaesthesia, may be observed in
(a) Arabs
(b) Greeks
(c) Cypriots
(d) North Africans
(e) Afro-Caribbeans

7.3 Haemoglobin electrophoresis plus high performance liquid chromatography at 6 weeks of age could provide a definitive diagnosis of
(a) $\beta$ thalassaemia trait
(b) sickle cell/hereditary persistence of fetal haemoglobin
(c) sickle cell/$\beta^0$ thalassaemia
(d) sickle cell/haemoglobin C disease
(e) sickle cell trait

7.4 It is important that an antenatal haemoglobinopathy screening programme detects
(a) haemoglobin C trait
(b) haemoglobin D-Punjab trait
(c) haemoglobin E trait
(d) haemoglobin G-Philadelphia trait
(e) haemoglobin Lepore trait

7.5 In an antenatal haemoglobinopathy screening programme, investigation for $\alpha^0$ thalassaemia trait should be carried out in
(a) Chinese
(b) Laotians
(c) Cambodians
(d) Japanese
(e) Vietnamese

7.6 A patient with a high-oxygen-affinity haemoglobin could have normal results for
(a) cellulose acetate electrophoresis at alkaline pH
(b) oxygen dissociation curve

(c) agarose gel electrophoresis at acid pH

(d) measurement of $P_{50}$

(e) isopropanol test

7.7 A neonatal haemoglobinopathy screening programme should aim to detect cases of

(a) α thalassaemia trait

(b) β thalassaemia trait

(c) sickle cell anaemia

(d) sickle cell/$β^0$ thalassaemia compound heterozygosity

(e) hereditary persistence of fetal haemoglobin

7.8 In an antenatal haemoglobinopathy screening programme, investigation for $α^0$ thalassaemia trait should be carried out in

(a) Greeks

(b) Cypriots

(c) Spaniards

(d) Portuguese

(e) Austrians

7.9 Suitable primary methods for neonatal haemoglobinopathy screening include

(a) cellulose acetate electrophoresis at alkaline pH

(b) citrate agar or agarose gel electrophoresis at acid pH

(c) isoelectric focusing

(d) high performance liquid chromatography

(e) sickle solubility test

7.10 Emergency pre-anaesthetic screening should detect patients with

(a) sickle cell trait

(b) β thalassaemia trait

(c) sickle cell disease

(d) sickle cell/haemoglobin C disease

(e) haemoglobin C disease

# References

1 Ahmed S, Saleem M, Modell B and Petrou M (2002) Screening extended families for genetic hemoglobin disorders in Pakistan. *N Engl J Med* **347**, 1162–1168.

2 Globin Gene Disorder Working Party of the BCSH General Haematology Task Force (1994) Guidelines for the fetal diagnosis of globin gene disorders. *J Clin Pathol* **47**, 199–204.

3 The Thalassaemia Working Party of the BCSH General Haematology Task Force (1994) Guidelines for the investigation of the α and β thalassaemia traits. *J Clin Pathol* **47**, 289–295.

4 Working Party of the General Haematology Task Force of the British Committee for Standards in Haematology (1998) The laboratory diagnosis of haemoglobinopathies. *Br J Haematol* **101**, 783–792.

5 Modell B, Petrou M, Layton M, Varnavides L, Moisely C, Ward RHT *et al.* (1998) Audit of prenatal diagnosis for haemoglobin disorders in the United Kingdom: the first twenty years. *Ann NY Acad Sci* **850**, 420–422.

6 Ma ESK, Chan AYY, Ha SY, Lau YL and Chan LC (2001) Thalassemia screening based on red cell indices in the Chinese. *Haematologica* **86**, 1310–1311.

7 *Report of a Working Party of the Standing Medical Advisory Committee on Sickle Cell, Thalassaemia and other Haemoglobinopathies.* HMSO, London, 1993.

8 Henthorn JS, Almeida AM and Davies SC (2004) Neonatal screening for sickle cell disorders. *Br J Haematol* **124**, 259–263.

9 International Committee for Standardization in Haematology (1988) Recommendations for neonatal screening for haemoglobinopathies. *Clin Lab Haematol* **10**, 335–345.

10 Chapman C and Chambers K (1997) Neonatal haemoglobinopathy screening methods. *MDA Evaluation Report MDA/97/64*, Medical Devices Agency, London.

11 Campbell M, Henthorn JS and Davies SC (1999) Evaluation of cation-exchange HPLC compared with isoelectric focusing for neonatal hemoglobinopathy screening. *Clin Chem* **45**, 9251–9275.

12 US Department of Health and Human Services (1993) Guideline: laboratory screening for sickle cell disease. *Lab Med* **24**, 515–522.

## Answers to questions

| 7.1 | | | 7.3 | | | 7.5 | | | 7.7 | | | 7.9 | |
|-----|-----|-----|-----|-----|-----|-----|-----|-----|-----|-----|-----|-----|-----|
| | (a) | T | | (a) | F | | (a) | T | | (a) | F | | (a) | T |
| | (b) | F | | (b) | F | | (b) | T | | (b) | F | | (b) | F |
| | (c) | T | | (c) | F | | (c) | T | | (c) | T | | (c) | T |
| | (d) | T | | (d) | T | | (d) | F | | (d) | T | | (d) | T |
| | (e) | T | | (e) | T | | (e) | T | | (e) | F | | (e) | F |

| 7.2 | | | 7.4 | | | 7.6 | | | 7.8 | | | 7.10 | |
|-----|-----|-----|-----|-----|-----|-----|-----|-----|-----|-----|-----|-----|-----|
| | (a) | T | | (a) | T | | (a) | T | | (a) | T | | (a) | T |
| | (b) | T | | (b) | T | | (b) | F | | (b) | T | | (b) | F |
| | (c) | T | | (c) | T | | (c) | T | | (c) | F | | (c) | T |
| | (d) | T | | (d) | F | | (d) | F | | (d) | F | | (d) | T |
| | (e) | T | | (e) | T | | (e) | T | | (e) | F | | (e) | F |

# 8 Self-assessment: test cases

## Questions

All the case studies relate to real patients presenting real diagnostic problems. The reader is advised that not all are straightforward. Careful thought and, if necessary, reference back to earlier chapters is advised before looking at the answers given in the second half of this chapter.

## Exercise 8.1

You are provided with a diagrammatic representation of the results of haemoglobin electrophoresis on cellulose acetate at alkaline pH, haemoglobin electrophoresis on agarose gel at acid pH and sickle solubility tests on a control sample and samples from patients 1–11.

Give the most likely explanation or explanations for each case. No patient had been transfused and all were adults. (For patient 3, note the quantity of the variant haemoglobin.)

Patient 1............................................................
Patient 2............................................................
Patient 3............................................................
Patient 4............................................................
Patient 5............................................................
Patient 6............................................................
Patient 7............................................................
Patient 8............................................................
Patient 9............................................................
Patient 10...........................................................
Patient 11...........................................................

| | Cellulose acetate electrophoresis – alkaline | | | | Agarose gel electrophoresis – acid | | | | |
| --- | --- | --- | --- | --- | --- | --- | --- | --- | --- |
| | A | F | S | C | F | A | S | C | Sickle solubility test |
| Control | | | | | | | | | |
| 1 | | | | | | | | | Positive |
| 2 | | | | | | | | | Negative |
| 3 | | | | | | | | | Negative |
| 4 | | | | | | | | | Positive |
| 5 | | | | | | | | | Positive |
| 6 | | | | | | | | | Positive |
| 7 | | | | | | | | | Negative |
| 8 | | | | | | | | | Negative |
| 9 | | | | | | | | | Negative |
| 10 | | | | | | | | | Positive |
| 11 | | | | | | | | | Negative |

## Exercise 8.2

You are provided with haemoglobin electrophoresis at alkaline pH, a sickle solubility test and a high performance liquid chromatography (HPLC) trace from two Afro-Caribbean patients, patient 1 and patient 2.

Give the most likely diagnosis in each.

Patient 1.....................................................

Patient 2.....................................................

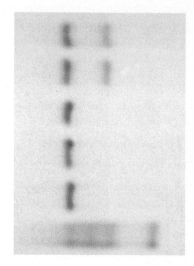

Patient 1

Patient 2

Patient 3

Patient 4

Patient 5

AFSC control

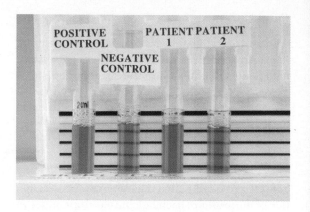

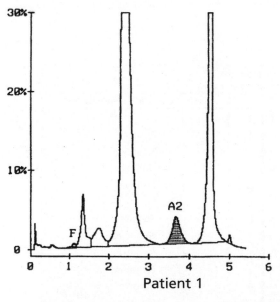

Patient 1

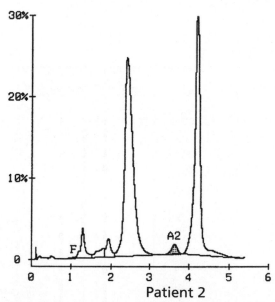

Patient 2

Retention time (minutes)

## Exercise 8.3

You are provided with a blood film and the results of electrophoresis at alkaline pH (lane d) on a 33-year-old pregnant Bangladeshi woman with the following red cell indices: red blood cell count (RBC) 4.39 × 10$^{12}$/l, haemoglobin concentration (Hb) 11 g/dl, haematocrit (Hct) 0.32, mean cell volume (MCV) 74 fl, mean cell haemoglobin (MCH) 25.1 pg and mean cell haemoglobin concentration (MCHC) 33.2 g/dl.

What is the most likely diagnosis? What test would you perform to confirm the diagnosis? What abnormality in the partner would be most likely to lead to serious disease in the fetus?

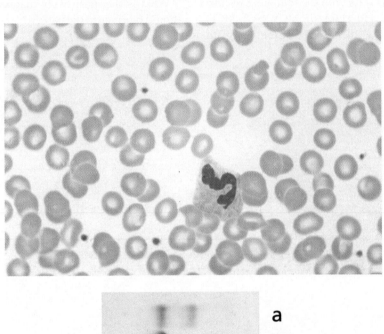

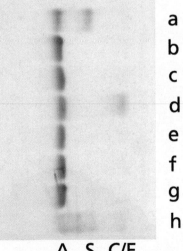

## Exercise 8.4

A young woman was referred to a haematologist because of borderline anaemia (Hb 10–11.5 g/dl) and microcytosis that had not responded to oral iron. The patient stated that, as far as she knew, her ancestry was totally English, although her father had once been told that he had 'Spanish blood'. The haematologist stopped the iron therapy and a week later performed various tests with the following results: RBC $5.37 \times 10^{12}$/l, Hb 11.6 g/dl, MCV 69 fl, MCH 21.7 pg, MCHC 31.2 g/dl, red cell distribution width (RDW) 19.2% (normal range 11.1–14.9%) and serum ferritin 28 μmol/l (normal range 10–300 μmol/l). You are provided with the blood film and the electrophoretic pattern on cellulose acetate at alkaline pH (lane b). The haemoglobin $A_2$ was estimated at 1.8% and 2.5% on two occasions (normal range 2.3–3.5%). Haemoglobin F was 11.4% by alkali denaturation with a heterogeneous distribution on a Kleihauer test.

What is the most likely diagnosis? What advice should be given to the patient?

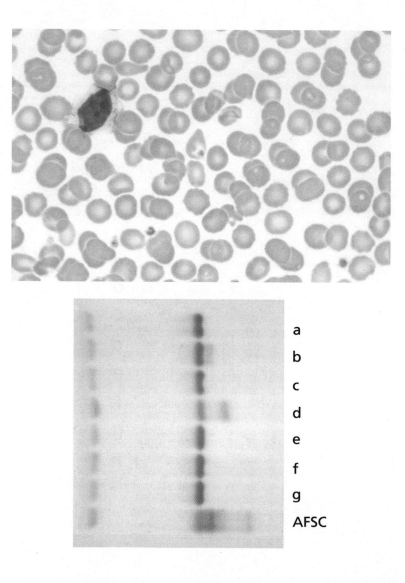

## Exercise 8.5

You are provided with the blood film, the electrophoretic pattern at alkaline pH (lane d) and the HPLC trace of a 34-year-old woman from Gibraltar with the following red cell indices: RBC $4.83 \times 10^{12}$/l, Hb 10.5 g/dl, Hct 0.35, MCV 72 fl, MCH 21.7 pg and MCHC 30.1 g/dl. Electrophoresis at acid pH was normal.

What is the most likely diagnosis? What is the clinical significance of this result?

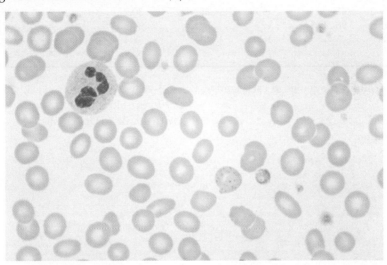

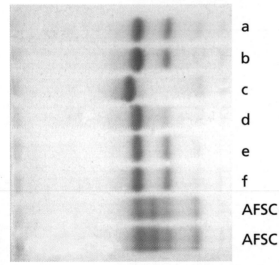

a

b

c

d

e

f

AFSC

AFSC

```
**** Beta Thal Short 70259-B4 ****
DATE:18/12/98        TIME:19:25:29

TECH ID#        0
VIAL#           7
SAMPLE ID# 00083527089000000000

ANALYTE ID      %       TIME        AREA

F               5.0     1.09        80175
P2              5.9     1.30        96045
P3              4.4     1.80        70937
Ao             71.2     2.52      1159967
A2             14.3     3.56       201297

            TOTAL AREA            1608421

F           5.0%    A2           14.3%
```

## Exercise 8.6

You are provided with blood films, red cell indices and the results of haemoglobin electrophoresis on a middle-aged man, who was complaining of fatigue, and three of his children.

| Family member | RBC ($10^{-12}$/l) | Hb (g/dl) | MCV (fl) | MCHC (g/dl) | Haemoglobin electrophoresis |
|---|---|---|---|---|---|
| Father (a) | 5.47 | 10.7 | 65 | 30.2 | A + A$_2$ (A$_2$ 5.2%) |
| Daughter (age 17) (b) | 3.96 | 11.7 | 87 | 34.3 | A + A$_2$ (A$_2$ 2.5%) |
| Daughter (age 15) (c) | 5.43 | 10.9 | 64 | 31.4 | A + A$_2$ (A$_2$ 5.1%) |
| Son (age 10) (d) | 4.61 | 12.9 | 88 | 33.9 | A + A$_2$ (A$_2$ 2.3%) |

What is the most likely diagnosis in each family member?

Father.........................................................

17-year-old daughter......................................

15-year-old daughter......................................

10-year-old son.............................................

(With thanks to Dr F. Toolis.)

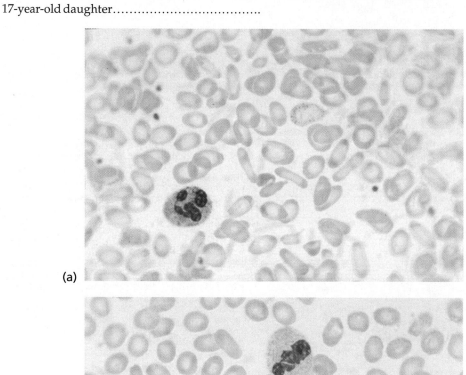

(a)

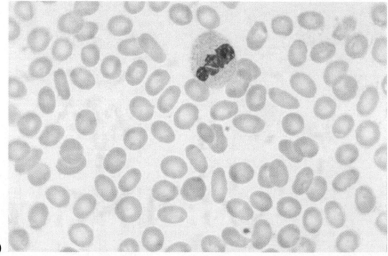

(b)

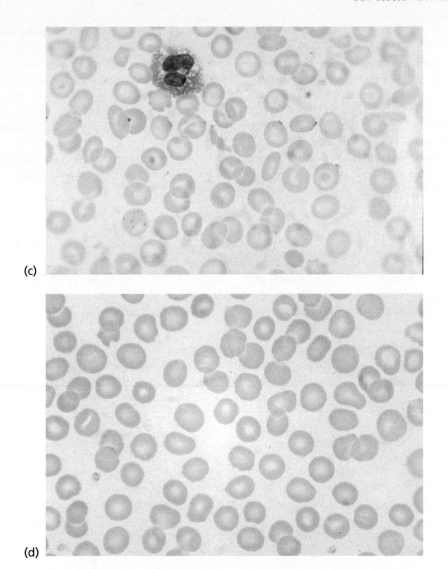

(c)

(d)

## Exercise 8.7

A 74-year-old white American was hospitalized because of back pain caused by osteoporosis. A blood film showed hypochromia and a full blood count (FBC) showed RBC $2.9 \times 10^{12}$/l, Hb 6.9 g/dl, Hct 0.21, MCV 74 fl, MCH 23 pg and RDW 18.4% (normal range 11.1–14.9%). She was transfused with 2 units of red cells and was discharged. Several weeks later she was readmitted with a haemoglobin of 5.9 g/dl and was found to have a bleeding gastric ulcer. She was transfused with 5 units of blood over 3 days. Subsequently, haemoglobin electrophoresis showed a band with the mobility of haemoglobin S and a sickle cell solubility test was positive. Haemoglobins were quantified by HPLC as follows: haemoglobin A 89.7%, haemoglobin $A_2$ 2.9%, haemoglobin F 0.4% and haemoglobin S 7.0%.

What explanations of these results would you consider and what further investigations would you perform?

## Exercise 8.8

You are provided with a blood film, haemoglobin electrophoresis on cellulose acetate at alkaline pH (lane b), haemoglobin electrophoresis on agarose gel at acid pH (lane b) and the results of globin chain synthesis studies (by courtesy of Professor L. Luzzatto) from an Afro-Caribbean patient with the following red cell indices: RBC $5.43 \times 10^{12}$/l, Hb 10.7 g/dl, Hct 0.34, MCV 63 fl, MCH 19.7 pg and MCHC 31.2 g/dl.

What is the diagnosis?

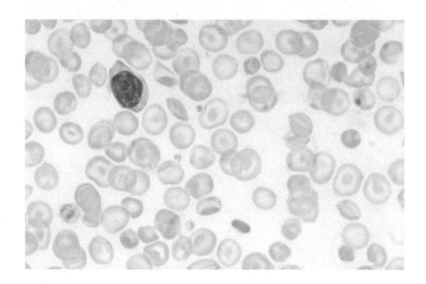

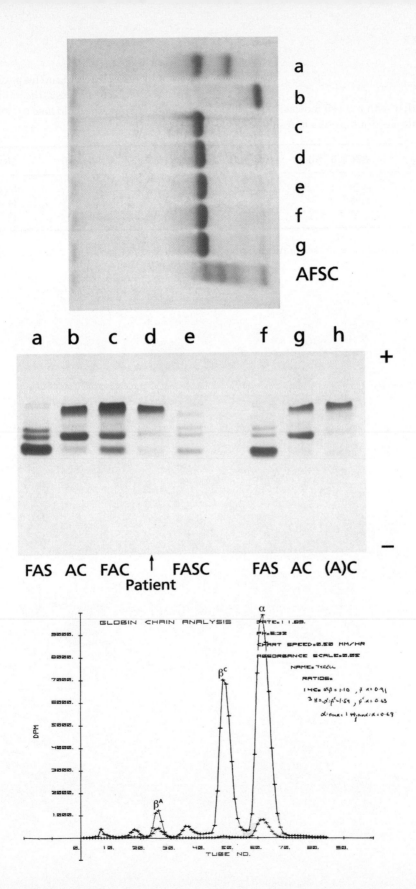

## Exercise 8.9

You are provided with red cell indices, blood films, cellulose acetate electrophoresis and results of sickle solubility tests on a child and his parents. In the cellulose acetate electrophoresis, the mother is lane a, the father lane b and the child lane f.

| Family member | RBC (10⁻¹²/l) | Hb (g/dl) | MCV (fl) | MCH (pg) | Sickle solubility test |
|---|---|---|---|---|---|
| Mother (a) | 4.39 | 11.7 | 80 | 26.6 | Negative |
| Father (b) | 4.96 | 14.6 | 88 | 29.4 | Positive |
| Child (c) | 2.05 | 7.2 | 98 | 35.2 | Positive |

What is the likely diagnosis in each family member?

Mother.................................................................

Father.................................................................

Child.................................................................

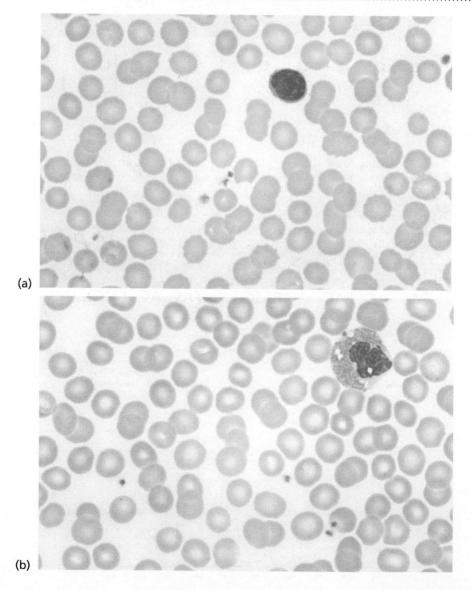

(a)

(b)

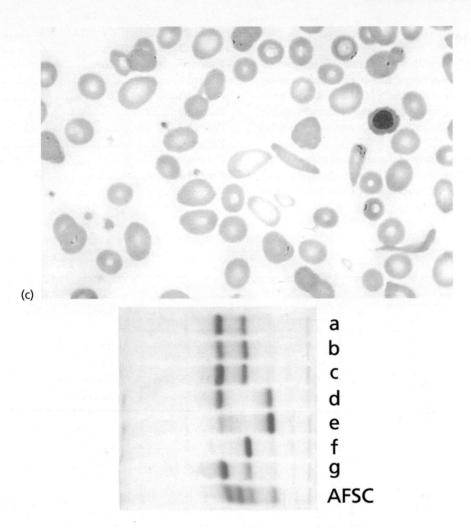

(c)

## Exercise 8.10

You are provided with a diagrammatic representation of the results of haemoglobin electrophoresis on cellulose acetate at alkaline pH, haemoglobin electrophoresis on agarose gel at acid pH and a sickle solubility test on a control sample and samples from patients 1–11.

Give the most likely explanation or explanations for each case. No patient had been transfused and all were adults. For the purposes of this exercise, ignore the thickness of the bands.

Patient 1.....................................................
Patient 2.....................................................
Patient 3.....................................................
Patient 4.....................................................
Patient 5.....................................................
Patient 6.....................................................
Patient 7.....................................................
Patient 8.....................................................
Patient 9.....................................................
Patient 10....................................................
Patient 11....................................................

| | Cellulose acetate electrophoresis – alkaline | | | | Agarose gel electrophoresis – acid | | | | Sickle solubility test |
|---|---|---|---|---|---|---|---|---|---|
| | A | F | S | C | F | A | S | C | |
| Control | ● | ● | ● | ● | ● | ● | ● | ● | |
| 1 | | ● | ● | ● | | ● | ● | ● | Positive |
| 2 | | | ● | ● | | ● | ● | | Positive |
| 3 | | | ● | ● | | ● | ● | | Positive |
| 4 | | | ● | ● | | | ● | | Positive |
| 5 | | | ● | | ● | | | ● | Negative |
| 6 | ● | | ● | ● | | ● | | ● | Negative |
| 7 | | | ● | ● | | ● | | ● | Positive |
| 8 | | | ● | | | | | ● | Negative |
| 9 | | | ● | | | ● | | | Negative |
| 10 | | | ● | | | | ● | | Negative |
| 11 | | | ● | | | | ● | ● | Positive |

## Exercise 8.11

A young man had a routine blood count performed. This was noted to show abnormal red cell indices, leading to haemoglobin electrophoresis being performed. Three of the patient's grandparents were of Indian ethnic origin. The other was half-Indian and half-Chinese. There was no history of consanguinity. The red cell indices were as follows:

RBC $5.56 \times 10^{12}$/l, Hb 11.0 g/dl, Hct 0.36, MCV 65 fl, MCH 19.8 pg and MCHC 30.7 g/dl. The haemoglobin $A_2$ was 5.5%. You are provided with the patient's blood film and haemoglobin electrophoresis on cellulose acetate at alkaline pH (lane c).

Suggest two possible explanations of the abnormality observed. What is the likely clinical significance?

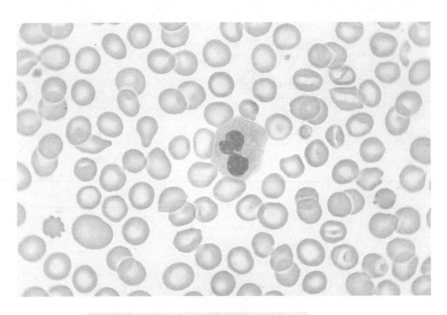

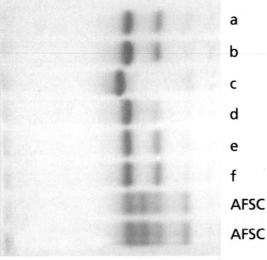

a

b

c

d

e

f

AFSC

AFSC

## Exercise 8.12

A 23-year-old Afro-Caribbean woman had a positive sickle solubility test and the following red cell indices: RBC $4.42 \times 10^{12}/l$, Hb 11.5 g/dl, Hct 0.35, MCV 78 fl, MCH 26 pg and MCHC 31.8 g/dl. You are provided with the blood film and an electrophoretic strip at alkaline pH (lane e).

What is the most likely explanation of the abnormal red cell indices and electrophoretic abnormality?

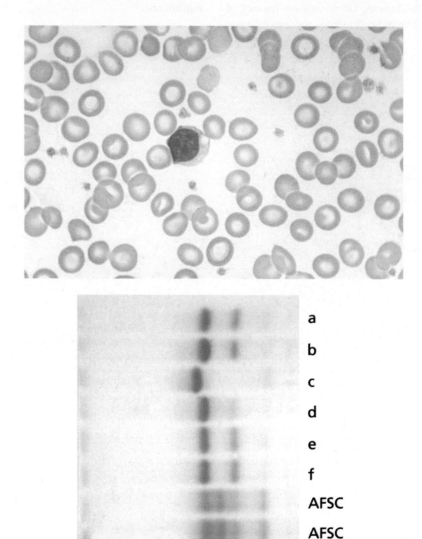

## Exercise 8.13

A 67-year-old man of Northern European Caucasian origin presented with a history of breathlessness and ankle oedema. On physical examination, he was pale but no other abnormality was detected. His FBC was as follows: white blood cell count (WBC) $5.7 \times 10^9/l$, RBC $5.3 \times 10^{12}/l$, Hb 9.4 g/dl, Hct 0.36, MCV 68.6 fl, MCH 17.7 pg, MCHC 26.1 g/dl and platelet count $651 \times 10^9/l$. You are provided with his peripheral blood film and bone marrow aspirate. The bone marrow was hypercellular with an increased number of megakaryocytes, some of which were hypolobated. The bone marrow differential count showed 90% erythroid cells; 4% of the remaining cells were blasts. Erythroblasts showed increased siderotic granulation, including a low percentage of ring sideroblasts. Haemoglobin electrophoresis showed 15% haemoglobin H and a haemoglobin H preparation showed typical inclusions. The $\alpha : \beta$ chain synthesis ratio was 0.49.

What abnormalities are shown by the blood and bone marrow films? Explain the nature of the patient's condition. (By courtesy of Dr J. Mercieca.)

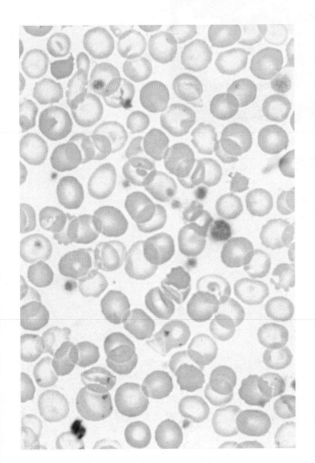

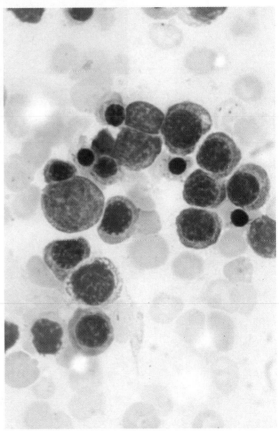

## Exercise 8.14

You are provided with a blood film and a computed tomography (CT) scan of the abdomen, performed without any contrast medium, from a young African man with sickle cell anaemia.

Explain the blood film and CT scan features in relation to each other.

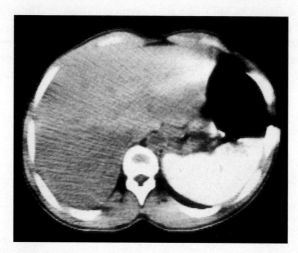

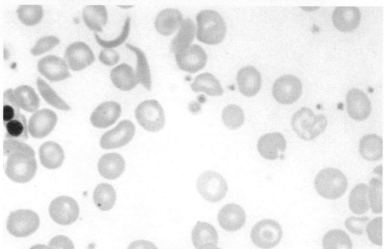

## Exercise 8.15

You are provided with a blood film, haemoglobin electrophoresis on cellulose acetate at alkaline pH (lane e) and haemoglobin electrophoresis on agarose gel at acid pH (lanes 6 and 8) from a young Afro-Caribbean woman with anaemia and recurrent limb pains.

What is the most likely diagnosis?

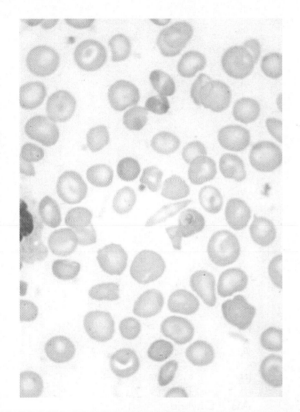

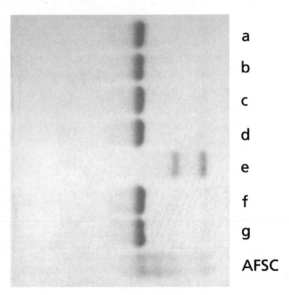

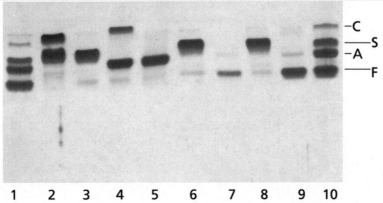

## Exercise 8.16

You are provided with a blood film and haemoglobin electrophoresis on cellulose acetate at alkaline pH (Patient, sixth lane) from an African woman who had been hospitalized with a breast abscess. The red cell indices were as follows: RBC $4.23 \times 10^{12}$/l, Hb 10.7 g/dl, MCV 75 fl, MCH 25.3 pg, MCHC 33.5 g/dl and RDW 15.3%. A sickle solubility test was positive. Haemoglobin electrophoresis on agarose gel at acid pH showed *two* major bands with the mobilities of haemoglobins A and S.

What is the most likely diagnosis? What is the significance of this diagnosis? What are the possible explanations of the microcytosis?

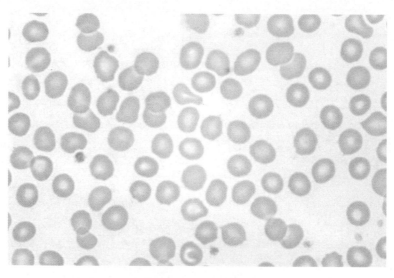

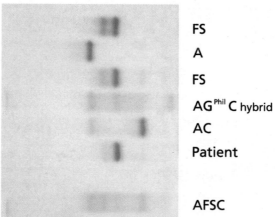

FS

A

FS

AG^Phil C hybrid

AC

Patient

AFSC

## Exercise 8.17

You are provided with the blood film and haemoglobin electrophoresis at alkaline pH (Patient, fifth lane from left) of an Afro-Caribbean woman in the first trimester of pregnancy. On agarose gel at acid pH, there were two bands with the mobilities of haemoglobins A and S. The sickle solubility test was positive.

What is the most likely diagnosis? What is the significance to the patient?

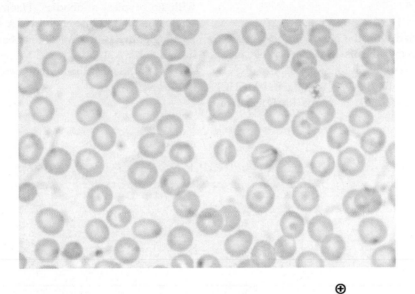

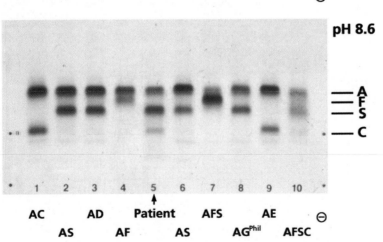

## Exercise 8.18

A 32-year-old pregnant Chinese woman had normal haemoglobin electrophoresis (haemoglobin $A_2$ 2.1%) and the following red cell indices: RBC $5.71 \times 10^{12}$/l, Hb 11.5 g/dl, Hct 0.38, MCV 66 fl, MCH 20.1 pg and MCHC 30.4 g/dl.

What diagnoses are likely? What tests should be performed in her partner and why?

## Exercise 8.19

You are provided with the blood film of an Afro-Caribbean woman in the first trimester of pregnancy. Her red cell indices were as follows: RBC $4.2 \times 10^{12}$/l, Hb 12 g/dl, MCV 88 fl, MCH 28.6 pg and MCHC 32.4 g/dl. She was found to be rhesus (Rh) D negative with no atypical antibodies. Haemoglobinopathy screening showed haemoglobins A, F and $A_2$, with haemoglobin F being 23% of total haemoglobin and haemoglobin $A_2$ 1.6%.

What is the most likely diagnosis? What are the implications?

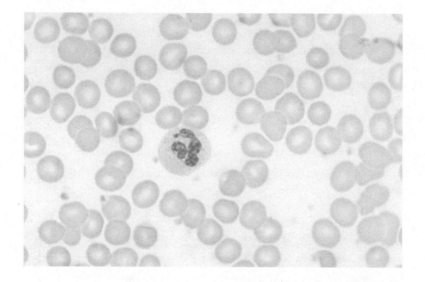

## Exercise 8.20

You are provided with the blood film of a 2-year-old Northern European Caucasian boy noted by his parents to be miserable and fretful. On examination, he had hepatosplenomegaly, moderate enlargement of the lymph nodes and an eczematous rash. There was a family history of neurofibromatosis and the child himself was noted to have occasional *café-au-lait* spots. The results of FBC were: WBC $28.3 \times 10^9/l$, Hb $8.4$ g/dl, MCV 78 fl and platelet count $96 \times 10^9/l$. Monocytes and neutrophils were both increased. Haemoglobin electrophoresis showed 12% haemoglobin F and 1.0% haemoglobin $A_2$. The carbonic anhydrase band on the stained electrophoretic strip appeared to be reduced.

What is the likely diagnosis?

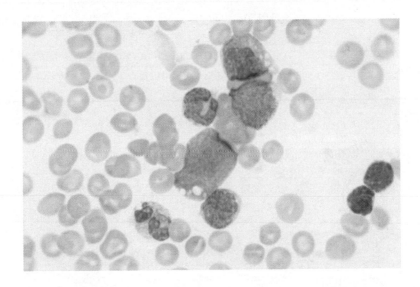

## Exercise 8.21

You are provided with the blood film of a 17-year-old girl with an English mother and a Pakistani father. She had been found to be anaemic when she required extraction of wisdom teeth. There was no hepato-megaly or splenomegaly. The red cell indices and results of haemoglobin $A_2$ quantification in the girl and her parents are tabulated.

Suggest reasons that might explain why the girl is more anaemic than her father. (With thanks to Dr M. Makris.)

| | Daughter | Father | Mother |
|---|---|---|---|
| RBC $(10^{-12}/l)$ | 4.04 | 5.99 | 4.22 |
| Hb (g/dl) | 8.5 | 12.0 | 13.6 |
| MCV (fl) | 68.8 | 62.9 | 93.1 |
| MCH (pg) | 21.0 | 20.2 | 32.2 |
| Haemoglobin $A_2$ (%) | 4.7 | 4.4 | 2.3 |
| Haemoglobin F (%) | 3.2 | <1.0 | <1.0 |

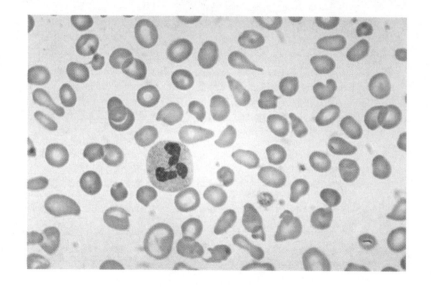

## Exercise 8.22

You are provided with an HPLC trace of a patient with the following red cell indices: RBC $4.56 \times 10^{12}/l$, Hb 11.3 g/dl, Hct 0.34, MCV 75 fl, MCH 24.7 pg and MCHC 33.2 g/dl. Haemoglobin F was 18.3% and haemoglobin $A_2$ was 2.6% by HPLC and 1.8% by microcolumn chromatography.

What is the likely diagnosis?

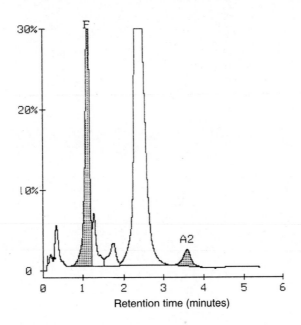

## Exercise 8.23

You are provided with blood films from a girl aged 18 years (a) and her mother (b). The girl's father had a normal blood film. Other details are tabulated.

What is the most likely diagnosis in the mother? What is the most likely diagnosis in the daughter?

|  | Daughter | Mother | Father |
|---|---|---|---|
| Ethnic origin | Italian-African | Italian | West African |
| RBC ($10^{-12}$/l) | 3.65 | 5.78 | 5.1 |
| Hb (g/dl) | 7.0 | 10.5 | 15.3 |
| MCV (fl) | 60 | 56 | 90 |
| MCH (pg) | 19.2 | 18.2 | 30 |
| MCHC (g/dl) | 31.9 | 32.3 | 32.6 |
| Ferritin (µmol/l) | 430 | 33 | 50 |

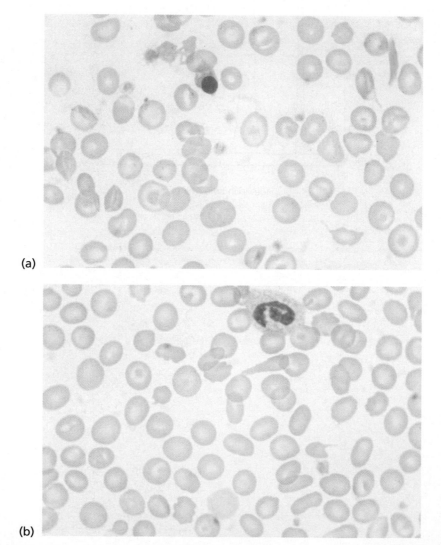

(a)

(b)

## Exercise 8.24

You are provided with the blood film of a patient with the following red cell indices: RBC $5.39 \times 10^{12}$/l, Hb 12.6 g/dl, Hct 0.37, MCV 69 fl, MCH 23.4 pg and MCHC 34 g/dl. Haemoglobin electrophoresis showed haemoglobin A 23%, haemoglobin S 73% and haemoglobin $A_2$ 4%.

What is the most likely diagnosis?

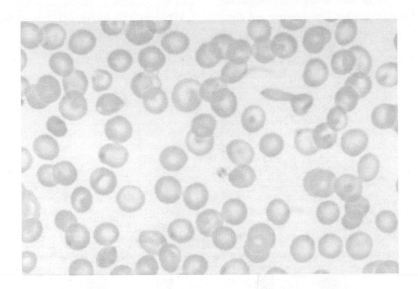

## Exercise 8.25

A 3-year-old English boy was brought to the paediatric accident and emergency department by his father who had found him playing in the garden shed several hours previously. The child had complained of abdominal pain and had vomited. Thereafter, he appeared restless and lethargic. On examination in the emergency department, he was noted to have central cyanosis, tachycardia, tachypnoea and hypotension. He was afebrile. Heart sounds were normal and there was no abnormality on auscultation of the lungs. Arterial blood gas analysis showed a normal partial pressure of oxygen and reduced partial pressure of carbon dioxide. An FBC showed the following: WBC $14.3 \times 10^9$/l, Hb 11.0 g/dl, MCV 85 fl, MCH 27 pg and platelet count $360 \times 10^9$/l. The laboratory scientist performing the blood count and blood gas analysis noted that the blood was chocolate-brown in colour.

What is the most likely diagnosis? What test should be done? What treatment should be given?

## Exercise 8.26

You are provided with the results of cellulose acetate electrophoresis at alkaline pH, agarose gel electrophoresis at acid pH and an HPLC trace of an Irish woman known to have had a high haemoglobin concentration for some time. On agarose gel electrophoresis, the patient's blood sample is second from the right between an AC sample (left) and an FASC control sample (right). Her WBC and platelet count were normal. The red cell indices were as follows: RBC $4.71 \times 10^{12}/l$, Hb 16.1 g/dl, Hct 0.46, MCV 96.8 fl, MCH 34.1 pg, MCHC 35.2 g/dl and RDW 12.2%.

What is the likely diagnosis? (With thanks to Mairead O'Reilly, Cork.)

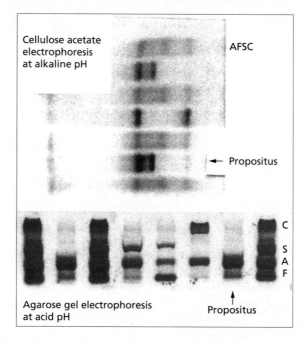

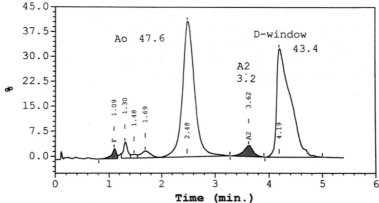

## Exercise 8.27

You are provided with an HPLC trace of an anaemic pregnant African woman (haemoglobin 9.8 g/dl, MCV 79 fl). The 'P2 fraction' on Bio-Rad Variant II HPLC analysis was 41.4% with the abnormal peak having a retention time of 1.35 min. On cellulose acetate electrophoresis at alkaline pH, the A band was broadened by a slightly faster component. Agarose gel electrophoresis at acid pH was normal.

Is this likely to indicate pregnancy-related diabetes or is there an alternative explanation?

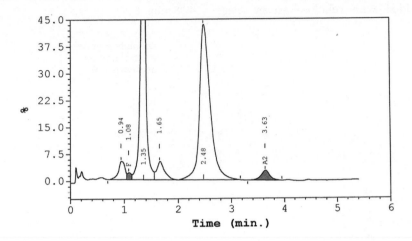

## Exercise 8.28

Three previously healthy children whose father was a butcher became profoundly cyanosed, with a deteriorating level of consciousness, within a short time of each other. Rapid recovery occurred following intravenous injection of methylene blue.

What is the likely cause of the cyanosis? What is the probable underlying cause?

## Exercise 8.29

The blood of a 34-year-old pregnant Caucasian woman was sent for antenatal thalassaemia and haemoglobinopathy screening in a hospital with a policy of universal screening. Her red cell indices were as follows: RBC $4.23 \times 10^{12}/l$, Hb 13.4 g/dl, Hct 0.39, MCV 92 fl, MCH 31.6 pg and MCHC 34.6 g/dl. You are provided with cellulose acetate elec-trophoresis at alkaline pH and agarose gel elec-trophoresis at acid pH.

Make a provisional diagnosis.

After reaching a provisional diagnosis, examine the HPLC trace provided and assess whether the provisional diagnosis is confirmed. State the significance of your findings. The variant haemo-globin was 41.9% and had a retention time of 4.38 min.

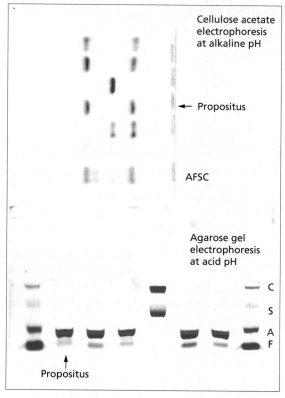

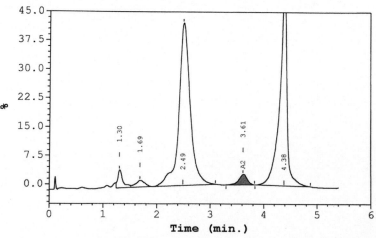

## Exercise 8.30

Haemoglobinopathy investigation was requested on a 15-year-old boy hospitalized with vomiting and diarrhoea. His ethnic origin was not totally clear; he was stated to be 'black' and had a name that suggested he might be of Arab ancestry or from a Moslem country. The red cell indices were as follows: RBC $5.18 \times 10^{12}$/l, Hb 8.6 g/dl, Hct 0.286, MCV 55 fl, MCH 16.6 pg, MCHC 30 g/dl and RDW 24%. His blood film showed hypochromia, microcytosis,

numerous target cells, basophilic stippling and some irregularly contracted cells. You are provided with haemoglobin electrophoresis on cellulose acetate at alkaline pH and an HPLC trace (performed on washed cells). The smaller peak on the right-hand side of the chromatogram was in the S window and was 20%; a sickle solubility test was positive. Haemoglobin F was 3% and haemoglobin $A_2$ was quantified as 4%.

Explain your findings and give a provisional diagnosis.

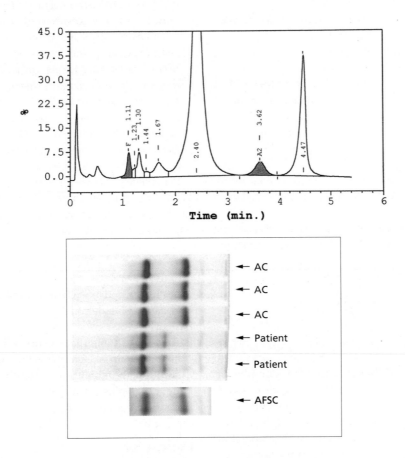

## Exercise 8.31

Pre-operative haemoglobinopathy screening was requested in a 26-year-old woman. She was found to have a haemoglobin $A_2$ of 5.3% and haemoglobin F of 2.5%. Her red cell indices were as follows: RBC $4.64 \times 10^{12}/l$, Hb 12.9 g/dl, Hct 0.41, MCV 89 fl, MCH 27.7 pg and MCHC 31.2 pg/dl.

Does she have β thalassaemia trait? How would you proceed?

## Exercise 8.32

The following is an extract from the *Manchester Guardian* of 30 September 1902.

### TRAGIC DEATH OF E. ZOLA
ACCIDENTALLY ASPHYXIATED
MADAME ZOLA NEARLY SHARES HIS FATE

*We regret to announce the death, under circumstances of a most tragic character, of the renowned French novelist, M. Emile Zola. The following telegram explains how M. Zola died:*

**Paris**

*M. Emile Zola was this morning found dead in his house from accidental asphyxiation. Madame Zola is seriously ill.*

*2.00 p.m. The death of M. Zola appears to have been caused by poisonous gases emitted from a stove, the pipe of which is stated to have fitted badly. It is believed that doctors will be able to save the life of Madame Zola, who was also affected by the noxious vapour.*

*From such details as have hitherto been obtained it seems that M. and Madame Zola returned yesterday from the country where they had been staying for about three months. Their house in Rue de Bruxelles was very cold, not having been inhabited for so long, and as there was a considerable fall in the temperature, M. Zola ordered the fire to be lighted in the grate of the bedroom, which is a vast apartment. The footman set about lighting the fire, but it did not draw at all well. After dinner, which M. and Madame Zola ate with good appetite they retired to rest. That was about 10 o'clock.*

*This morning at 9.30 a.m. some workmen went to the house to execute certain repairs which had been ordered to be carried out in M. Zola's room. The servants, who were already a little alarmed at having heard no sound in the bedroom, knocked loudly at the door, which, as they received no response, they broke in . . . M. Zola was found lying half out of bed . . . He was quite dead. . . . Madame Zola was found lying in bed showing no signs of life . . . The frightened servants instantly threw open the windows and gave the alarm.*

What is the 'noxious vapour' to which death is attributed? Explain the mechanism of death. Did the servants take the right action?

## Answers

### Exercise 8.1

Patient 1: AS.

Patient 2: AD or AG (heterozygosity for a number of haemoglobins designated D or G, both α and β chain variants, for example D-Punjab, D-Iran, D-Copenhagen, D-Norfolk or G-Philadelphia). Note that the quantities of the variant and haemoglobin A are similar, and so a β chain variant is favoured.

Patient 3: A plus Lepore.

Patient 4: SS or $S\beta^0$ thalassaemia.

Patient 5: SD (e.g. S plus D-Punjab as the proportions are equal and a β chain variant is favoured).

Patient 6: AS plus G-Philadelphia.

Patient 7: AD plus G-Philadelphia (i.e. heterozygosity for a β chain variant designated D or G, e.g. D-Punjab, and an α chain variant designated D or G, e.g. G-Philadelphia).

Patient 8: AC.

Patient 9: AE (note that the quantity of the variant haemoglobin is usually less than in C trait and, in addition, the mobility at acid pH is different).

Patient 10: A plus C-Harlem.

Patient 11: A plus O-Arab.

### Exercise 8.2

Patient 1: AS (sickle cell trait).

Patient 2: A plus D-Punjab (the HPLC trace is typical of D-Punjab heterozygosity).

### Exercise 8.3

Haemoglobin E trait is most likely because of the

ethnic origin, the thalassaemic indices, the mobility of the variant haemoglobin at alkaline pH and the relatively low percentage of the variant haemoglobin (it appears to be around 30%). Haemoglobin C and haemoglobin O-Arab are much less likely. The provisional diagnosis could be confirmed by haemoglobin electrophoresis at acid pH or HPLC.

The condition of most potential significance in the partner would be β thalassaemia trait, as the compound heterozygous state for haemoglobin E and β thalassaemia often leads to the clinical picture of thalassaemia intermedia or even thalassaemia major.

## Exercise 8.4

The findings are indicative of heterozygosity for δβ thalassaemia as there are thalassaemic indices with elevation of haemoglobin F but not haemoglobin $A_2$. It would be sensible to test the patient's father and, if he were normal, the patient's mother to help confirm the diagnosis.

The patient's father was tested and was found to have the same haematological abnormality as the patient. The clinical significance is very similar to that of β thalassaemia heterozygosity. The patient should not take iron unless she is demonstrated to be iron deficient and should be warned of the possibility of thalassaemia intermedia or major in the fetus if her partner should happen to be heterozygous for β (or δβ) thalassaemia. If she were to become pregnant, it should be noted that her high fetal haemoglobin percentage would be likely to result in a positive Kleihauer test. If she were Rh D negative, she would need an alternative test for detection of feto-maternal haemorrhage.

## Exercise 8.5

There is a band with the mobility of S at alkaline pH, which we can deduce has the same mobility as A at acid pH. On the HPLC trace, it is seen that the variant haemoglobin is eluting in the haemoglobin $A_2$ window and is 14.3% of total haemoglobin. Clearly, it is not haemoglobin $A_2$ on the grounds of the proportion of the variant and its electrophoretic mobility. These findings are indicative of haemoglobin Lepore trait.

The significance is similar to that of β thalassaemia trait.

For a bonus point, you might have noted that the 'P2 fraction' eluting after haemoglobin F, representing glycosylated haemoglobin, is also quite high.

## Exercise 8.6

Father: β thalassaemia trait plus hereditary elliptocytosis.
Daughter aged 17: hereditary elliptocytosis.
Daughter aged 15: β thalassaemia trait.
Son aged 10: normal.

The father's blood film shows anisocytosis, poikilocytosis including elliptocytes and ovalocytes, microcytosis and hypochromia. There is a teardrop poikilocyte showing basophilic stippling. His haemoglobin $A_2$ is elevated. The film is more strikingly elliptocytic than is usual in β thalassaemia trait and consideration of the conditions he has transmitted to two of his children indicates that he is likely to have both β thalassaemia trait and hereditary elliptocytosis.

## Exercise 8.7

The clinical history and initial laboratory findings suggest a diagnosis of iron deficiency anaemia. The subsequent demonstration of a variant haemoglobin, identified as haemoglobin S, is likely to be correct as it is based on electrophoresis, HPLC and a sickle solubility test. An explanation needs to be found for haemoglobin S being present in such a low concentration. There are two possible explanations:
• she has been transfused with blood from a donor with sickle cell trait;
• she herself has sickle cell trait and the percentage of the variant haemoglobin has been lowered by the recent transfusion.

It is unlikely that the patient has sickle cell disease as there is nothing in the history to suggest this. The fact that she is identified as 'white' does not exclude her from having haemoglobin S. However, haemoglobin electrophoresis on a residual blood sample from each of the donor bags confirmed that the patient had been transfused with blood from a donor with sickle cell trait.

It is not rare for clinical staff to request investigation for a haemoglobinopathy when there is no clear clinical indication for the test, nor is it rare for a test to be requested, inappropriately, on a blood sample taken *after* transfusion. The laboratory should be alert for this explanation of anomalous results.

Ahmad E and Sykes E (1999) Clinical pathology rounds: low level of hemoglobin S in a white woman. *Lab Med* **30**, 572–575.

## Exercise 8.8

The blood film shows target cells, irregularly contracted cells and a haemoglobin C crystal. Electrophoresis on cellulose acetate at alkaline pH shows only haemoglobin C, but on agarose gel faint bands with the mobilities of F and A are also present, in addition to the major C band. A laboratory error might be suspected as the explanation of this discrepancy, but in fact agarose gel electrophoresis is more sensitive than cellulose acetate electrophoresis for the detection of a low concentration of normal and variant haemoglobins. Globin chain synthesis studies confirmed that the patient was a compound heterozygote for $\beta^C$ and $\beta^+$ thalassaemia with greatly reduced synthesis of $\beta^A$ globin chain.

## Exercise 8.9

The mother has D or G trait. The father has sickle cell trait. The child obviously has a sickling disorder and must have inherited D from the mother and S from the father. The blood film of the child indicates that there has been interaction between haemoglobin S and the other variant haemoglobin, producing a clinically significant disorder. This is likely to be haemoglobin S/haemoglobin D-Punjab compound heterozygosity. Other haemoglobins designated D and G do not interact adversely with haemoglobin S. Haemoglobin D-Punjab was confirmed on further testing.

This case shows the importance of performing electrophoresis at acid pH in patients who, on cellulose acetate electrophoresis, have a single band with the mobility of haemoglobin S. Misdiagnosis of compound heterozygous states as sickle cell anaemia may lead to paternity being questioned in cases in which the father does not have haemoglobin S, with serious social and possibly legal consequences.

## Exercise 8.10

Patient 1: SC.
Patient 2: SE.
Patient 3: S plus C-Harlem or SS plus G-Philadelphia (or other D/G α chain variant).
Patient 4: S plus O-Arab.
Patient 5: CC plus G-Philadelphia.
Patient 6: AC plus G-Philadelphia.
Patient 7: SC plus G-Philadelphia.
Patient 8: CC or $C\beta^0$ thalassaemia.
Patient 9: EE or $E\beta^0$ thalassaemia.
Patient 10: O-Arab homozygote or O-Arab/$\beta^0$ thalassaemia.
Patient 11: C plus C-Harlem.

## Exercise 8.11

The electrophoretic strip shows only haemoglobin $A_2$ and a variant haemoglobin that is slightly faster than haemoglobin A. There is no common variant haemoglobin with this mobility. The two possible explanations are:
• compound heterozygosity for $\beta^0$ thalassaemia and an uncommon variant haemoglobin;
• homozygosity for an uncommon haemoglobin.

In the absence of consanguinity, it is unlikely that the patient would be homozygous for an uncommon variant haemoglobin. DNA analysis confirmed that he was heterozygous for $\beta^0$ thalassaemia and electron spray mass spectrometry (by courtesy of Dr Barbara Wild) identified the variant haemoglobin as haemoglobin Tacoma.

As these investigations are said to have resulted from a 'routine blood count', it appears that the patient is asymptomatic (this was confirmed) and the variant haemoglobin is therefore not likely to be of any clinical significance. The β thalassaemia trait, however, could have genetic significance.

## Exercise 8.12

The patient has sickle cell trait as she has a positive sickle solubility test and a variant haemoglobin with the mobility of haemoglobin S. However, the haemoglobin S percentage is unusually low. This, together with the thalassaemic indices, suggests that as well as having sickle cell trait she is homozygous for $\alpha^+$ thalassaemia. The genotype $-\alpha/-\alpha$ is found in 1–2% of Afro-Caribbeans. The genotype $--/\alpha\alpha$ is very rare in this ethnic group and so is a much less likely explanation. The S band is so faint that, except for the positive sickle solubility test, haemoglobin Lepore might have been suspected.

## Exercise 8.13

The blood film is dimorphic and shows target cells, Pappenheimer bodies and giant platelets. The bone marrow shows marked erythroid hyperplasia. Inherited haemoglobin H disease is unlikely in view of the ethnic origin and the presence of haematological abnormalities indicative of a haematological neoplasm. Because blasts are a high percentage of non-erythroid cells, the disease was classified, according to the French–American–British (FAB) classification, as M6 acute myeloid leukaemia rather than as myelodysplastic syndrome. It is of interest that the patient has both myelodysplastic features (anaemia and ring sideroblasts) and myeloproliferative features (thrombocytosis with giant platelets). This represents an 'overlap syndrome', i.e. a condition with overlapping myelodysplastic/myeloproliferative features evolving into acute myeloid leukaemia. This patient illustrates the particular association of acquired haemoglobin H disease and erythroleukaemia.

Bain BJ (1999) The relationship between the myeloproliferative syndromes and the myeloproliferative disorders. *Leuk Lymphoma* **34**, 443–449.

Mercieca J, Bain B, Barbour G and Catovsky D (1996) Teaching cases from the Royal Marsden and St Mary's Hospitals. Case 10: Microcytic anaemia and thrombocytosis. *Leuk Lymphoma* **21**, 185–186.

## Exercise 8.14

The blood film shows that the patient has the features expected in sickle cell anaemia, including hyposplenic features (a target cell and a Howell–Jolly body). The CT scan shows that, rather than having splenic atrophy, the patient's spleen is of normal size and abnormally dense. This unusual appearance suggests that there is deposition of calcium in the spleen, an unusual result of recurrent splenic infarction. Despite the normal-sized spleen, the patient has functional hyposplenism.

## Exercise 8.15

It is clear from the history and the blood film that the patient has some type of sickle cell disease. Haemoglobin electrophoresis at alkaline pH suggests possible compound heterozygosity for haemoglobins S and C. However, at acid pH, it is clear that there is no haemoglobin C present. Compound heterozygosity for haemoglobin S and C-Harlem should be suspected (and was the answer given in the first edition of this book). However, further investigation, including family studies, citrate agar electrophoresis and mass spectrometry, led to a diagnosis of compound heterozygosity for haemoglobin S and haemoglobin O-Arab. The variable mobility of haemoglobin O-Arab on electrophoresis at acid pH can cause problems in the diagnosis of compound heterozygous states. These problems do not arise in the simple heterozygous state as haemoglobin C-Harlem has a positive sickle solubility test and haemoglobin O-Arab does not.

## Exercise 8.16

The patient is a compound heterozygote for haemoglobin S and a β chain variant, haemoglobin D or G. As she is asymptomatic and the blood film does not show any features of sickle cell disease, the second haemoglobin is likely to be a variant that does not interact with haemoglobin S, rather than haemoglobin D-Punjab, which does interact. Although the precise variant was not identified in this case, it was shown by HPLC not to be haemoglobin D-Punjab.

Only the haemoglobin S heterozygosity is likely to be clinically significant. If she requires a general anaesthetic for drainage of the breast abscess, the anaesthetist will wish to know that she has sickle cell trait. This would also be of potential genetic significance.

The anaemia and microcytosis could be caused by the effects of the infection, if it has been going on for some time, leading to anaemia of chronic disease. Alternatively, the patient could have a coincidental iron deficiency anaemia. α Thalassaemia trait is also quite likely in this ethnic group.

## Exercise 8.17

The patient is heterozygous for both $\beta^S$ and $\alpha^{G\text{-Philadelphia}}$, hence the three bands on electrophoresis at alkaline pH. The haemoglobin G-Philadelphia is very unlikely to be of any clinical significance. However, if the patient's partner also has sickle cell trait, there is a one in four risk of the fetus having sickle cell anaemia. There would also be significant genetic implications if the patient's partner has β thalassaemia trait, haemoglobin C, haemoglobin D-Punjab or haemoglobin O-Arab. The couple concerned might wish to consider termination of pregnancy if significant fetal disease were predicted.

Red cell indices and haemoglobin electrophoresis should be performed followed, if indicated, by consideration of antenatal diagnosis of any significant abnormality in the fetus.

## Exercise 8.18

As the patient has marked microcytosis, but a normal haemoglobin concentration, she is unlikely to have iron deficiency. The red cell indices are suggestive of thalassaemia and, as she has a normal haemoglobin $A_2$ concentration, it is likely that she has α thalassaemia. As she is Chinese, she could be heterozygous for $\alpha^0$ thalassaemia ($--/\alpha\alpha$) or homozygous for $\alpha^+$ thalassaemia ($-\alpha/-\alpha$). The microcytosis is too marked for heterozygosity for $\alpha^+$ thalassaemia to be a likely diagnosis. The implications are shown in the table below.

| Abnormality present in mother | Findings in partner | Possible abnormality in fetus |
|---|---|---|
| $-\alpha/-\alpha$ | $\alpha\alpha/\alpha\alpha$ | $-\alpha/\alpha\alpha$ (α thalassaemia trait) |
| | $-\alpha/\alpha\alpha$ | $-\alpha/\alpha\alpha$ or $-\alpha/-\alpha$ (α thalassaemia trait) |
| | $-\alpha/-\alpha$ | $-\alpha/-\alpha$ (α thalassaemia trait) |
| | $--/\alpha\alpha$ | $-\alpha/\alpha\alpha$ (α thalassaemia trait) or $-\alpha/--$ (haemoglobin H disease) |
| $--/\alpha\alpha$ | $\alpha\alpha/\alpha\alpha$ | $\alpha\alpha/\alpha\alpha$ (normal) or $--/\alpha\alpha$ (α thalassaemia trait) |
| | $-\alpha/\alpha\alpha$ | $\alpha\alpha/\alpha\alpha$ (normal), $-\alpha/\alpha\alpha$ (α thalassaemia trait), $--/\alpha\alpha$ (α thalassaemia trait) or $--/-\alpha$ (haemoglobin H disease) |
| | $-\alpha/-\alpha$ | $-\alpha/\alpha\alpha$ (α thalassaemia trait) or $--/-\alpha$ (haemoglobin H disease) |
| | $--/\alpha\alpha$ | $\alpha\alpha/\alpha\alpha$ (normal), $--/\alpha\alpha$ (α thalassaemia trait) or $--/--$ (haemoglobin Bart's hydrops fetalis) |
| | β thalassaemia trait | *Beware*: a diagnosis of β thalassaemia trait in the partner does not exclude his also having α thalassaemia trait; molecular analysis to exclude $--/\alpha\alpha$ is indicated |

## Exercise 8.19

The high haemoglobin F with normal red cell indices is likely to be caused by deletional hereditary persistence of fetal haemoglobin. This has no clinical significance except that the Kleihauer test will be positive. The patient is Rh D negative and an alternative technique will have to be used after delivery to detect and quantify fetal cells in the maternal circulation.

## Exercise 8.20

The findings are those of juvenile myelomonocytic leukaemia (previously known as juvenile chronic myeloid leukaemia). An increased haemoglobin F percentage for age is one of the criteria that can be used to make this diagnosis.

## Exercise 8.21

It appears that both the daughter and the father are heterozygous for β thalassaemia trait as they both have microcytosis and an increased haemoglobin $A_2$ percentage. This was confirmed on molecular analysis, both having the IVS1 5 G→C mutation. Possible explanations of the more severe phenotype in the daughter include:

• coinheritance of a 'silent' β thalassaemia allele from the mother;
• coinheritance of homozygosity or heterozygosity for triple α.

The latter explanation was found to be correct; the mother and the daughter were heterozygous for triple α. This condition was harmless in the mother but, in the daughter, aggravated the chain imbalance attributable to the β thalassaemia trait and led to a more severe phenotype.

Bain BJ, Swirsky D, Bhavnani N, Layton M, Parker N, Makris M *et al.* (2001) British Society for Haematology Slide Session, Annual Scientific Meeting, Bournemouth, 2000. *Clin Lab Haematol* **23**, 265–269.

## Exercise 8.22

The findings are those of heterozygosity for δβ thalassaemia. Hereditary persistence of fetal haemoglobin is excluded by the 'thalassaemic' red cell indices.

## Exercise 8.23

The most likely diagnosis in the mother is β thalassaemia trait and in the daughter is compound heterozygosity for haemoglobin S and β thalassaemia. In fact, she has $S/\beta^0$ thalassaemia.

## Exercise 8.24

Haemoglobin $S/\beta^+$ thalassaemia compound heterozygosity.

## Exercise 8.25

The most likely diagnosis is methaemoglobinaemia caused by exposure to a toxic substance found in the garden shed.

Methaemoglobin should be tested for by spectrometry or co-oximetry. A co-oximeter is an instrument that passes monochromatic light at four wavelengths through the test sample and is thus able to quantify carboxyhaemoglobin, methaemoglobin, oxyhaemoglobin and reduced haemoglobin.

The correct treatment is intravenous methylene blue.

Wentworth P, Roy M, Wilson B, Padusenko J, Smeaton A and Burchell N (1999) Clinical pathology rounds: toxic methemoglobinemia in a 2-year-old child. *Lab Med* **30**, 311–315.

## Exercise 8.26

A variant haemoglobin is present, suggesting that the polycythaemia is the result of a high-affinity haemoglobin. This was haemoglobin Kempsey and, although the variant haemoglobin appears in the 'D window' of the HPLC trace, its curious shape is characteristic of haemoglobin Kempsey.

## Exercise 8.27

The grossly increased 'P2 fraction' has nothing to do with diabetes, although it would give a factitious result on haemoglobin $A_{1c}$ quantification. It should be recognized as a variant haemoglobin. It was identified by mass spectrometry as haemoglobin Hope. (With thanks to Dr Barbara Wild.)

## Exercise 8.28

The recovery with methylene blue suggests methaemoglobinaemia.

Given the father's occupation, the likely underlying cause is accidental exposure to sodium nitrite, used for curing meat.

In the family described, the sodium nitrite had been introduced into the domestic environment for use as an insecticide and had been emptied into a sugar bowl by one of the children.

Finan A, Keenan P, O'Donovan FO, Mayne P and Murphy J (1998) Methaemoglobinaemia associated with so-dium nitrite in three siblings. *Br Med J* **317**, 1138–1139.

## Exercise 8.29

The variant haemoglobin has electrophoretic characteristics suggestive of haemoglobin E, but it is odd that the patient is Caucasian. In addition, the proportions of haemoglobin A and the variant haemoglobin appear to be similar, a very unlikely finding if this were haemoglobin E. The results of HPLC analysis exclude the possibility of haemoglobin E as there is a variant haemoglobin in the 'S window'. These are the features of haemoglobin E-Saskatoon, which does not have the genetic implications of haemoglobin E. This case shows that, even with two independent methods, a provisional identification may be incorrect.

## Exercise 8.30

The HPLC trace and haemoglobin electrophoresis show the presence of haemoglobin S at an unusually low level of 20%. Haemoglobin $A_2$ appears slightly elevated, but its quantification can be inaccurate in the presence of haemoglobin S. There is a slight increase in haemoglobin F. There is an abnormal fraction eluting early, which has the form expected of haemoglobin Bart's (although no haemoglobin Bart's was visible on haemoglobin electrophoresis). A haemoglobin H preparation was negative. These findings are the consequence of sickle cell trait plus the genotype of haemoglobin H disease. The reported levels of haemoglobin S in this condition vary between 10% and 25%. Haemoglobin H is present in only very trivial amounts.

## Exercise 8.31

The possibility of elevation of haemoglobin $A_2$ for another reason (e.g. treatment of retroviral infection) should be considered. Alternatively, could the indices be atypical because of coexisting liver disease, megaloblastic anaemia (unlikely as the haemoglobin concentration is normal) or hydroxycarbamide therapy (not very likely in a young pre-operative patient)?

The explanation was found, on DNA analysis, to be coexisting $\alpha$ and $\beta$ thalassaemia trait, known to normalize the red cell indices but not the elevated haemoglobin $A_2$ that would be expected in $\beta$ thalassaemia trait. Specifically, she had $-\alpha/\alpha\alpha$ and the $\beta^+$ mutation, $-29A \rightarrow G$.

## Exercise 8.32

The noxious vapour was carbon monoxide.

Carbon monoxide poisoning causes death by asphyxiation. Carboxyhaemoglobin has no oxygen-combining activity and, in addition, increases the oxygen affinity of the remaining haemoglobin, further impairing oxygen delivery to tissues.

The servants' instinctive action in throwing open the windows has a sound physiological basis as carboxyhaemoglobin is slowly converted to oxyhaemoglobin on breathing room air. Removing Madame Zola to another room may have been even more effective.

# Index